BEAUTIFUL, POWERFUL YOU

A NURSE'S GUIDE TO RECLAIM YOUR POWER & TRANSFORM YOUR HEALTH

TRICIA QUICK

BALBOA.PRESS

A DIVISION OF HAY HOUSE

Balboa Press books may be ordered through booksellers or by contacting:

Balboa Press
A Division of Hay House
1663 Liberty Drive
Bloomington, IN 47403
www.balboapress.com
844-682-1282

Print information available on the last page.

ISBN: 979-8-7652-4619-1 (sc)
ISBN: 979-8-7652-4618-4 (hc)
ISBN: 979-8-7652-4620-7 (e)

Library of Congress Control Number: 2023919463

Balboa Press rev. date: 12/20/2023

"You never change things by fighting the existing reality. To change something, build a new model that makes the existing model obsolete."
— Richard Buckminster Fuller

This book is dedicated to all of the beautiful souls who have touched my heart and changed my life over the last 25 years. I am forever grateful for all that you've taught me and for your immense love, even when you were suffering in the hardest of times. You helped me want to be a better person in the world.

CONTENTS

Afterword

REFERENCE LOVE

iNTRODUCTiON

While I was writing this book, I went through just about every emotion imaginable. At times, it felt as though I was grieving something. The more I wrote, the more my heart spoke and the biggest thing that it told me was that I was no longer in the best place for *me*. What I wanted to do to help people wasn't in the realm of the industry I was working in. I was surrounded by sick people who all needed help and all I could think about was what was missing and being kept from them.

As any nurse might tell you, our job is a rollercoaster ride like no other, physically, mentally, and emotionally. The things we witness, what we go through with our patients, and the magnitude of emotion that we feel affect us on a pretty deep level. Especially, if we're the kind of nurse that is empathic and transparent.

We're the ones who are by your side when you're sick, after you receive your diagnosis, holding your hand in the most difficult of times, comforting you, and ensuring that you have the most peaceful and healing outcome possible.

Unfortunately, I was one of those nurses that knew there was so much more information out there that people deserved to know about. There was more to health and healing than just pills and procedures. I waited patiently to see if things might change through the years, but not much did.

I felt that people should be given the chance to be able to heal themselves on every level, as a lot of the time, illness is much deeper than it looks on the surface. People deserved to know what was happening to their body and what they could do to get through and out of the mess they found themselves in. There was a lot that could help them find their way back to their health and wholeness, and most of all, to themselves.

It began early on for me when I first started my career and realized that the food people were eating, their emotional and mental state, and the way that they lived their life was strongly affecting where they were at in health and mind.

There was always a part of me, where I knew in my heart that so much helpful information was being held back from people. There were simple, beautiful things that could've helped so many of them get back on their feet and truly help themselves to heal.

I stuck it out and kept on going because what else was I going to do besides nursing? The amazing and beautiful people that I cared for made it all worth it in the end. I met some truly amazing people through the years, so many of them touched my heart and soul in a way that I would've never experienced without this work.

From the deepest part of my soul, I just wanted these beautiful people to get better and come out on the other side of their illness. I wanted them to be able to see the absolute beautiful soul that they were and that they had more power in them than they had believed. There was healing potential just waiting to be accessed if only they were given the chance to see it.

I wanted people to see beyond the limitations that were placed upon them and to know that there was *so much more* to their health and healing process than what's been revealed. I knew how important it was for them to feel supported and cared for through their healing process, and I wanted to be there to help them through all of it.

However, I hit some walls within my scope of practice and found that I couldn't hold these values up as much as I wanted to.

I spent a lot of time throughout my career studying and reading about ancient healing practices, alternative and holistic science and medicine, and the beautiful theories and methods that had been left out of the equation. I knew that what I was taught in my profession was *not all there was*. I saw the powerful connections to our health around food, plant medicine, oxygen and sunlight, and how everything we think, feel, and experience affect our state of health and our wellbeing. Once I saw all of this, there was no turning back.

As the years went by, I continued to witness the downfall of good people who didn't deserve to fall apart in the way that they were.

Watching people's health slowly fail, as they came in and out of the hospital for the same problem, became so painful to witness.

For years I knew there was more. More to how people could get themselves better, more that would strengthen their organs and systems, and more that could help them heal the broken parts of themselves. It wasn't just about a symptom or diagnosis. I wanted to offer people a deeper, broader perspective around how they looked at and cared for their health.

I wanted people to know how to connect into themselves more. How to look deeper into whatever it was that was going on with them. I wanted them to know of the powerful and wonderful things that they themselves, could do and change, to get to a better place than where they were.

Unfortunately, or fortunately, I saw way early on in my career that there was so much missing in the health care profession. If I'm honest, it really began to disappoint me. Twenty-five years went by and nothing more was added or discovered that would help people get out of being in the sick, awful place they were in. Just new drugs and procedures, but that was it.

I grew more frustrated and jaded as time went on, but I didn't let it affect how I was with my patients. Even though my joy, satisfaction, and love for the profession grew weaker, I made sure that I cared for my patients in the best way that I could.

I think we've finally reached a breaking point; people are sick of being sick and tired and just taking a handful of pills. More patients that came through my hands were seeking more information and were curious about different therapies and methods that might be able to help them. It brought a lot of joy to my world, however, the process of obtaining care outside of the conventional world was sometimes difficult to find. Not to mention, it was all out of pocket which made it hard on people who were already struggling.

I witnessed too many people go through the most painful of times. I saw lives lost that didn't deserve to be. I couldn't help but feel heartbroken around all of the sadness that was happening. Of course, this is the game in the world of health care. There are tragedies occurring on a constant basis, but there are also lots of wonderful, healing moments that I personally experienced, that brought some joy to the profession. However, I truly couldn't help but focus on the injustices and things that were going wrong because there were times that absolutely shook me to the core.

I felt that there were too many good people needlessly losing their lives. So many things that were going on with these people were being overlooked and sadly missed. I felt like a lot of people weren't getting the help in the ways that they truly needed it because the guys in charge weren't noticing.

My love and concern for my patients ran pretty deep. You can ask any of them to this day… I was a dedicated and heartfelt nurse like many of us are. I did whatever it was within my power to help people, sometimes even going out of my way to extend love and assistance. There was even a time where I visited with some of my patients when I wasn't working, back when I worked home health and hospice. I loved doing things that would bring them joy and make them feel loved such as in bringing them food or running errands for them. I would even buy different items that I knew would bring them relief and comfort.

I loved getting to know my patients on a deeper, emotional, and personal level. It was such a gift to me. I wanted to know things so I could find ways to help them in whatever ways presented themselves. I knew so much of the things that would help them heal would be revealed in our open and heartfelt conversations.

I wanted to understand how they got to the place that they were in; what led up to it, the things that were going wrong, their emotional and mental situations, what their diet was like, how they felt about themselves… basically overall assess where they were at mentally, physically, emotionally, *and* even spiritually.

You can honestly learn so much about a person if you just give them the chance to be seen and heard. There truly is so much information in a person's story as to why they're suffering and as to how they got there. Their story also carries many of the *solutions* and *answers* that we need to recognize, to help them work on healing themselves.

You see, when you get to know several angles of what's going on in a person's life, you can more easily figure out what it is that needs to get done. You can look at areas that need to be worked on, emotional situations that need to be worked through, all kinds of things that need shifting and changing, and what could really use some extra attention.

When we look at people in this way and treat them as a whole, we deal with the root cause and transform and heal things on a deeper level.

So, that's really the mindset that I come from.

I feel that so much of what people go through in their life is connected to where their health is at and how their life is going in the present moment. People's entire life experiences and all that took place for them over the years, have an enormous impact on the state of their health and wellbeing.

Of course, I always saw the obvious like the food, lifestyle, and genetic weaknesses. It's very important to look at how people eat and what they eat, what they did or didn't do to their body, and what health issues they had from early on. One of the biggest factors in people's health comes from their upbringing and younger years. We don't realize that our health is being set up for us when we're children, so everything that happens to us and our bodies affects our health as adults.

Clearly, there are so many more levels and layers to the health of people than is being taken into account.

My patients were like family to me. It wasn't always just about what I had to do for them as a nurse, it was about being present with another beautiful human who was struggling and scared. Some of them needed all of the love and concern they could get, and personally, all I wanted to do was comfort them and make everything better for them somehow. Even at times, I did my best to get them to laugh, as I knew that laughter is such a healing medicine.

Needless to say, as time went on in my career, I became more frustrated with the limitations in the thinking, solutions, and interventions that were given to people. It was too easy to notice the lack of connection *to* the people, as well as a lack of concern for what was really going on with them beyond their physical manifestations.

It got to a point where practically every day felt like a struggle for me, and it only got worse over the years. I continued to stick it out, because how else was I going to make decent money and help take care of people?

Well, the fact of the matter is that illness isn't always cut and dry or black and white, and as we know, things can't always be fixed with the medications or the interventions offered in the conventional medical world. Surely, people deserve to know about the natural, holistic methods and practices that are out there and how powerfully helpful they can be. People should know how food and diet alone, can move mountains. There are so many beautiful things that can be done to help people get through their illnesses, and come out a new man or woman on the other side.

These past few years have been such a roller coaster ride for everyone. Fear became the norm, people have been in constant overload and stress, and things are seemingly always being thrown at us on one level or another. It's not a wonder why people are really struggling so much right now. If it's not one thing to be scared of, it's another. People can't seem to get a break and it's weakening everyone on so many levels.

Because of this, I feel this is the time where we need to decide to do a few things for ourselves. Stand up for ourselves and do better than we've been doing to take care of ourselves.

We don't have to stay stuck in fear, illness, or struggle, we can choose to take a different path. We just need to learn how to focus our energy on more of what's important to us and work on things that will help us step back into our power, so we can get ahead of things instead of lagging behind.

We can even use the fear as a catalyst.

We should be spending our time and energy on getting to know ourselves better and in learning things that will help us get our health and our lives back on track.

The truth is, we already have the power inside of us to be able to do that, all we have to do is access it. We have the power to heal the many parts of ourselves that need it, and that's literal and true science.

When we learn to access our potential, (and I promise it isn't as difficult as you might think), we can do some pretty amazing things. We can finally learn how to *truly* love and take care of ourselves, connect deeper into our gifts, and to realize the enormous strength that we all have inside of us.

There's no one truth or answer out there for everyone, but we can always find a way to create a better life for ourselves. We can establish new goals that will help us redesign our life at any moment in time. Because, in the end, it's up to us. We get to make our own choices and decide what is best for us and what isn't. All we need to do is work on learning to listen to ourselves, and we'll find that the answers we need come to us much easier.

I hope this book can highlight just how powerful and amazing we are. That we can do more in our power to change our lives and our health than we ever thought we could.

We're not meant to play small, nor stay sick or fearful. We're meant to be powerful and (re)learn how to heal ourselves, because we deserve nothing less. It's time that we see ourselves for the true, magnificent, and amazing beings that we are.

The world wouldn't be the same without you. So, get out there and step into the next chapter of your life with confidence, strength, and grace. You got this!

Just a few more things …

This book is not here to advise, nor be a medical guide of any kind. It's meant to expand our awareness in how we see and care for our health. We have unlimited, untapped potential and power just waiting to be discovered.

I'm definitely not everyone's cup of tea. I don't speak within the mainstream mindset, nor come from the usual medical thought processes like you might expect from a nurse who's worked full on in the industry the last twenty-five years. I have much of the conventional knowledge, however I see through several different lenses and perspectives. I've learned more than I can even speak to over the last twenty-five years.

We ultimately get to choose what's best for us, what's true for us, and what isn't.

We all deserve to have a peaceful, healthy, and abundant existence.

We are all worthy of love.

We live on the most beautiful and bountiful planet. It nourishes our bodies, soothes our souls, and gives us all that we need to live, thrive, and heal abundantly and freely.

Our mind can either create something beautiful, or it can ruin and destroy something.

Every experience is meant to teach us a lesson, expand our awareness, or inspire us into action.

Lessons are gifts, no matter how difficult they may be.

You are your own boss. You get to decide what you will and won't allow into your life. You are the one in charge of how your life looks.

It's important that you put in the energy and effort that you need to help keep yourself healthy, happy, and being able to do what you love in life.

You know yourself better than anyone else.

It's always okay to seek the help that we need.

We all have the ability to take care of ourselves and completely love ourselves.

It's never too late to learn. We can learn things at any age.

Seek information, ponder upon different perspectives, and see what vibes with you.

There are some truly amazing things coming to light, on *every* level. Don't forget to hold onto your hats.

It's really a good idea to focus on the good that is happening over the bad.

What we put our energy and focus onto, will find its way into our reality.

Give thanks for everything you have, in all ways, on all days.

One of the greatest gifts we can gift to ourselves, is forgiveness. It's true.

Not everything we hear is the truth. It's important to learn to discern information with our intuition.

Always trust your gut first and foremost. It gets stronger the more you use it.

The truth will always prevail in the end.

There's more to life, than what we see in front of us.

Know that you can always shift your outlook.

Change is the only constant. It's only ever good to be comfortable with change.

You have the power to *create* change. Decide what kind of changes you want to see in yourself and in the world around you.

Decide what you want in your life. Create and build a plan for it.

You can create anything if you put your heart, mind, and soul into it.

You have more power than you know.

You're as old as you think you are. Age is not a number, it's how you carry yourself, treat life, live healthfully, and thrive regardless of the number of years you've been alive. *We are not our age, we are our energy.*

When you want or intend for something, acknowledge it like you've already got it.

Sometimes, we are our own biggest roadblock. It's time to get out of the way.

You are not your name, profession, or any other label that's attached to you.

We're not a body with a soul, we're a soul with a body.

We are made up of stardust!

No one is better than or more special than you! Realize the gold that you are.

You never need permission from another to feel worthy of being loved, being healed, or having the best in life.

Regardless of what you've done or failed to do in your life, you are worthy of all the good that's out there.

OUR INCREDIBLE BODY

"Embrace and love your body. It's the most amazing thing you'll ever own."
—Anonymous

TO KNOW, LOVE, & APPRECIATE OUR BODY

The human body—what an absolute powerhouse it is! It's a unique and complex organism guided by a divine, innate intelligence with miraculous self-healing capabilities. It's our best friend, there for us day in and day out, with every breath and every step we take. It helps us navigate through life, through all of its ups and downs, and no matter where we land or fall, it's there.

Whatever we give to it or put it through, it survives. Our body is always working to be at the top of its game and be at its absolute best for us. It's working every second of the day, with no breaks, doing all that it has to do while working hard to repair itself, especially while we're asleep.

Our body is always in the midst of a thousand different jobs to maintain its balance and function. It does everything in its power to ensure that we have as smooth and as easy of a ride, as possible. It only ever wants us to be healthy and to be able to live our best life.

Connecting back to seeing our bodies in this light, is essential. Many of us have been so out of touch with ourselves and our bodies for far too long, barely seeing them for the beautiful miracle that they are. Our body deserves to be acknowledged, loved, and cherished, for it's the only one we have. Without it, we wouldn't be here.

Everything we do affects and influences how it thrives and what happens to it. Physically, mentally, and emotionally, everything we consume has an impact on it. Even what we speak and think about affects our body. Our body is influenced by so much in ways we hadn't even thought of.

It's a great time to realize that everything we do affects it. We can look more clearly at just how much or how little we're doing for it. Are we contributing to our body's wellbeing? Are the things we're eating or doing, beneficial to our bodies? Or, are we causing them more stress, harm, or difficulty?

It's easy to see that our bodies take care of everything for us. We barely even have to think about it. It's on auto-pilot being amazing and keeping us in the game, that is, until things get too overwhelming for it.

After years of being neglected or abused in one form or another, our body just isn't able to do its jobs the same way as it once did. It becomes overloaded, stressed out, and sometimes even ends up having major difficulties. We so often get caught up in the stresses and occurrences of our everyday lives, that we forget to actually pay much attention to it. We practically ignore it, other than the basics of eating, drinking, and sleeping, and some people can barely even take care of those parts. It's as though we've forgotten what we're supposed to do for it, sometimes even so busy and distracted that we forget to breathe.

So, what happens to our body when we're too busy to pay attention to it?

Well, it still does its day-to-day jobs, at least it tries to, and continues maintaining everything to the best of its ability. However, after a while, things may begin to come undone. The burden of our ignorance and all the stress we place on it, begin to overload it. Now it needs our help in an even bigger way. We end up with more on our plate, more stress is added to our life, and we finally realize that without our health in a good position, we can't go on living life the way we've become so used to.

So, why wait until it gets to that point? Our body deserves our love, attention, and acknowledgment from the start. However, most of us didn't learn much about this along the way to be able to recognize and act upon this. So, becoming aware of our body and its amazing capabilities is a perfect place for us to start. When we acknowledge it more than we have in the past, it instantly adds a new level of love, appreciation, and concern to the equation that wasn't there before. In doing this, we create a new level of consciousness where we can put forth more energy, thoughtfulness, and compassion, showing it the kindness that it so deserves.

Of course, you might already be on top of taking care of and listening to your body, and how beautiful is that. Maybe you always have, or maybe some of us have more recently stepped into this place. It does seem that a lot of us are finding ourselves called to take notice of and take better care of our bodies. We're suddenly finding ways to do more to help them, and to get to know them better.

It's true that we're at a point in time where taking the best care of our physical body needs to be on the top of the list. Without our body in a strong, healthy physical state, we really can't go on living the life we want to, or at least, happily. We have to step in for it more, support it, and take better care of things. We need to treat our body with more respect and kindness. Afterall, it lives for us, serving us on so many levels, working day in and out, and so powerfully so. Our body deserves our unconditional love, time, and attention… I cannot stress that enough.

We're at a very powerful time in history. Right now, it really feels like we're all feeling compelled to move towards a more powerful level of awareness and understanding around our bodies and their needs. It's as though it's happening almost automatically for us and without much thought. We have more of a connection to our bodies, emotions, and minds than we've had in the past. Actually, I believe we're reaching back into the wisdom of the past, the wisdom that our ancestors had, and the wisdom that we have deeply embedded in our DNA and consciousness. It may sound a little out there, but things are changing on so many levels at this time. We're coming to realize just how intricate our body is, as it contains more than just our organs and cells.

We've unfortunately spent eons so disconnected from our bodies. We might feed them and get some sleep in, maybe even exercise, but is that really enough? It's time to acknowledge and realize that we need a deeper connection to our body and to increase our awareness around it. When we connect to it on a deeper level, we start recognizing its absolute beauty and potential, and as a result, we find more ways to support it and shower it with love.

Acknowledging the fact that we had a disconnection to our body immediately opens up our connection to it. In doing this, we are better able to tune in and listen more intently to its messages and signals, hearing more clearly what our body is trying to tell us. We're able to connect in more deeply, even more quickly to what it is that our body

3

needs from us. We'll even find ourselves knowing more specifically what we need to do for it. Our desire for this connection with our body will grow and expand, and good things begin to happen.

When our body finally captures our attention and senses that we will listen to it more during challenging times, the answers seem to reveal themselves. This deeper connection empowers us to take more proactive steps in caring for our body and addressing its needs. When we were extremely disconnected from it, even the most obvious signs and signals were missed and ignored. However, with a renewed connection, we find ourselves feeling more capable than we had previously considered ourselves to be.

It's so easy to get caught up in the distractions of the world, especially at this very moment in time. It's hard to ignore the heaviness and stresses that are constantly circulating around us. Sometimes, days can pass by before we realize that we haven't done much to check in with ourselves or our bodies. We've absolutely all been there, considering all of the expectations and demands that we encounter on a daily basis. But, as we become more aware of things, the time it takes for us to connect back in, is less. Eventually, with practice, it becomes a habit to check in every day, even several times a day.

Even the smallest of moments that we give to our body, creates a huge impact on it. It strengthens our connection to it. The more connected we are to it, the more we take notice of the things we're doing to it and for it. We also see what it is that we're *not* doing to it or for it, and perhaps what it is that we've been ignoring. Rekindling the connection we have with our body, helps us feel more confident in ourselves. Our compassion for our body grows, and we ultimately become more understanding and concerned for it, which only helps our happiness increase and our entire life to shift, for the better.

What a beautiful thing it is, when we begin our journey towards having a deeper connection with our bodies. It increases our clarity into seeing a lot of the things that we need to change, what we need to stop doing, and what would be good to *start* doing. Deep down, we know *way* more about our bodies and what they need than we give ourselves credit for. When we acknowledge our body and its messages, it allows for things to come up to the surface that we weren't seeing before. The things that need to be seen, heard, and acknowledged. Our bodies finally feel like they have us in their corner.

We are truly these magical, amazing, epic, and divine beings who happen to be one of the most advanced species on the planet. Our body's incredible potential honestly deserves our respect, hands down. Our cuts heal themselves, our colds resolve, even our broken bones grow back together. Our body can regenerate, what a concept! It's always working to grow into a better version of itself.

Sadly, this knowledge has been left out of the equation for the most part, dangling by a thread instead of being the front and center, like it should be. This *is* the most profound and miraculous part of our body and what it can do. This is the magic, my friends. Regeneration, one of our body's most powerful forces.

Our body is way more sophisticated and intelligent than what we've been led to believe. However, on a daily basis, this information is coming into light, and more and more beautiful people in and around us, are sharing this information. We're reconnecting to this wisdom. Even in my medical and nurse training, this wasn't highlighted much, if at all.

Not only are we stepping into recognizing our body's awe-inspiring and amazing potential, we're also beginning to open the doors to accessing some seriously powerful tools and therapies. Ones that have the potential to help us heal and support our bodies on so many levels. The art of caring for our bodies has even become more popular over the past few years, understandably so considering how the past few years have gone for us.

The usual fix-it drugs and methods are as always, recognized for their usefulness, but the truth is, most people are wanting more than that. The people who've been taking medications for years and are still feeling terrible, are now looking for more answers. People are starting to recognize that most of the fix-it solutions offered should more so be used as a *bridge* to get over the other side, not as a life-long solution that never fully resolves the problem. The time to accept less than we deserve when it comes to our health and healing our body, is over. We are coming to realize that we need to work on fixing the problems that are causing our body these issues instead of ignoring them and covering them up.

People are becoming more motivated to want to do something about their problems (as we all should be). We're working on becoming more intentional about what we're doing, eating, thinking, expressing, and putting out into the world, because it's true that all of it affects this beautiful, physical body of ours.

We recognize that we can assist our bodies by altering our habits and making different choices. Additionally, seeking more information becomes a valuable tool. Books, videos, blogs, attending health talks, and participating in events are perfect ways to immerse ourselves in gaining more power through new information. This process helps us comprehend our bodies better and strengthens our connection to them. As we learn about our bodies, what we can do for them, and how to listen and connect more, we gain empowerment.

Contrary to what we've been told, weakness or breakdown in the body is not normal, and it doesn't always need to feel hopeless. At any point, we can decide to work on cleaning out, rebuilding, and regenerating our body, because that's the divinity of it all. We can do this at any point in time and with our help, we can help our body work its way out of being in a not-so-great place. The answers on how we can support our body further along seem to come more naturally, especially when we learn to quiet ourselves enough to listen.

When we disengage from all of the external influences and chatter, we will really become pros at this. Our bodies will *always* talk to us. When we can sit with ourselves for a moment, perhaps meditating on our body, our body's intelligence, gifts, and beautiful messages come through more clearly.

In these quieter times, our body will not by shy about telling us what we need to do for it. Often times these prompts come in a way where thoughts and ideas just pop into our minds. Or, we might read something and think, yes, that's exactly what I need to do. Our body will even guide us to realizing when we need to seek help from other people. We might feel pulled to go see our doctor or are drawn to a certain practitioner. We might feel prompted to search for a certain kind of therapy or clinic. Things just seem to come to mind. We might even run into a friend along the way who happens to mention some kind of help that he or she is getting, that sounds a lot like something that we need.

Our body will always try its best to help us get back on track when we've fallen off, especially before things get too out of control. It's always trying to prevent worse things from happening. It tells us when it disagrees with our actions, the food we're eating, or when we need to do something for it. Our body uses our nervous system to speak to us and send us messages.

So many of us have ignored our body's messages largely in the past. We've either conditioned ourselves to ignore it, or we have the habit to go see our doctor with every cough and sneeze we have. To be honest, we were never really taught much about our body and what it's saying. There's no real class on this throughout school, so the truth is, we've truly known no better. We may have learned a little about what the body does, along with some of its parts, but overall, establishing and keeping a connection to it? Not so much. If we were lucky, maybe our parents taught us, but that too, is very rare. For the most part, we were taught to see someone else when it comes to anything regarding our body.

Our parents likely weren't taught any of this either, so how could they teach it to us? It seems to have been going on this way for generations. The disconnection growing farther apart, and most of us have just become grossly unaware and numb to it.

We've gotten so used to believing that our bodies will just take whatever we throw at them, but the time has come that we're now realizing that this isn't exactly true. We're beginning to notice the end result of a highly toxic diet and no exercise, and it isn't actually a very good one, as we're suddenly riddled with heart disease and can't get around like we used to. People like to blame it on getting older, but that's not really what's going on. And there will always be people who come up with a hundred reasons why their health and body are suffering, never taking accountability, but thankfully, that's not all of us.

A lot of us have been avoiding doing many of the good things our bodies need from us. However, I think we're entering a time where that can't be the way it works anymore. We're beginning to realize that a significant portion of our illness and discomfort actually stems from our own actions and acknowledging this helps us take responsibility for what's going on. It pushes us into a place where we're finally step up and so something about it, and I guarantee, our body couldn't be more grateful for this. It's always better late than never.

Disease and illness are indeed, pretty scary on so many levels, as most don't have a cure. So, what we do for ourselves and our bodies after we find ourselves in a difficult health situation, is truly what matters. Where we turn our focus and the changes we decide to make, are going to make us or break us.

Fear definitely loves to find its way to creep on in, and understandably so. Even if we know we're partly responsible and are willing to do some things about it, our feelings of fear, guilt, and disappointment arise. Now we have some extra burdens to spend our time on, and it becomes quite easy to get lost in all that's happening, on top of our everyday life and its responsibilities.

Of course, it's natural to have these feelings come up. There's overwhelm regarding how we're going to make changes, give up things we love, and find all the time to spend on getting things into a better place. Our feelings do indeed serve us, just as long as we don't stay stuck in them.

We can use the fear as motivation so, it's important that we do our best to release ourselves from the guilt and regret that we have. We can't change the past so we need to put in some work on forgiving ourselves. There's truly no use in beating ourselves up after the fact. We need to use our energy wisely and put it towards getting ourselves better.

If we focus on our issues and our fears surrounding them, unfortunately, we're just adding more stress to our body. Stress as we all know, creates a less productive healing environment, which makes it more difficult for our bodies to work their healing processes. Stress sets off our fight and flight response, which when activated, creates more work for our body on top of all that's already going on. Stress on stress never serves the body, nor strengthens it. It actually weakens it further, and that's never what we want when we're facing health issues.

I do want to lend room to this fact, however. Health and body issues are never a joke, nor is it easy to turn off our stress levels at the blink of an eye. It's good to be patient with ourselves and learn ways in which we can calm our nervous systems down, relax our fight and flight response, and take a hold of the situation. With practice, we can indeed figure this out, as well as get stronger at doing this.

If we allow the fear to take over and do nothing to release some of it, we waste the precious time and energy that we need. We forget that we actually have the strength and power within us (whether we believe it or not) to do something on our own account. We certainly don't need more of a disconnection that we've already been dealing with, and let's face it, if we give into the fear, we render ourselves useless, weakened, and one issue becomes ten.

Fear is suppressive. Worry and fear actually weaken our body even further, especially our immune system, endocrine system, nervous system, as well as our mental and emotional states. Fear takes us off the path that we actually need to be on. The path towards a stronger state of health, physically, emotionally, and mentally. Stress and fear create vulnerability, weakness, and further disconnection.

So, why not instead, flip the script and use our fear to work *for* us instead of against us. We can use our fear as a catalyst, motivating us to get stronger and create new neural pathways that work for our benefit. Using fear as a motivator toward our betterment takes practice and patience, but when we realize how much of a tool fear can be and how it can help us take the best possible care of our bodies, we can utilize the power behind it.

The first time we do something better for ourself, not out of fear but *because* of fear, we gain both strength and confidence. We're finally showing our bodies, and ourselves, that we have more love within us, than fear. The reward of facing our fear and using it for our benefit, is huge.

How we speak to our body while it's undergoing stress and illness, is another important level to things. Of course, how we speak to ourselves and our bodies matters *all* of the time, but what we say when we're sick is especially so much more important, as it is so much more potent. We can either support our body with what we speak or we can knock it down even further. It's easy to be in the negative if we're already so used to it, now even more so when we're feeling more scared and stressed out over things.

Throughout my entire career, I've encountered expressions of absolute disgust and anger directed towards the body when it's not at its best. Personally, I've engaged in such behavior in the past, and I've observed people close to me and tens of thousands of my patients doing the same. It's as if our ego learns to contribute to beating ourselves up when we're going through challenging times.

We literally find ourselves saying things like *"my heart is so weak"*, *"my stupid knee"*, or *"my back is always such a problem"*. In saying these things, we're really doing our bodies a huge disservice. Not only are we working against these parts, we're not supporting our body, which takes away more of our power as well as the energy that we need to help things heal and get better.

When we realize the significance and impact that our words have on us, mainly our body, it changes things. Our perspective shifts and we realize that we need to change how we speak to ourselves. We need to make sure that we take notice of, and do our best to cancel out the old, negative language and bring in a new version. A dialogue that consists of kind, loving, and supportive words that our body needs to hear and that it can actually use towards its benefit.

The more conscious we become of it, the less negative we are to our body. When we decide to get serious about this, it's almost as though the angry, harsh words disappear from our vocabulary. I believe it's in the act of continuously taking notice of them, that does this. I realized that the more I canceled out the negative stuff, speaking the positive became that much easier to do. We even find that we catch ourselves before the words even leave our mouths, and, it only gets better with time. So finally, when our body is having new problems or issues, our compassion kicks in, understanding that our bodies hear the words that we speak to them and that it matters.

In this, we're creating more room to help support our bodies by giving them more of the love and concern that they deserve. The emotional and mental language that we express, affects our body and how it goes forward.

One of the ways we can be proactive in doing this, is to work on it even before health issues arise. We can at any moment in time, express and speak love to our body intentionally. We can do this any time, all of the time, or at least as often as we can think to do it. We can work to add more positive, supportive, and loving statements to our days. Ones that will wholeheartedly help our body feel our gratitude for it and our support, on every level.

If we've never done this sort of thing before, it can certainly seem strange at first. Telling our body how strong and powerful it is will help to open us up to appreciating our body that much more. Our health is supported, our energy levels increase, we feel happier, and our body has a greater rate of success at making it through whatever it's going through. All of this just from speaking loving, supportive words and statements to it.

Our body's intelligence and nervous system respond immensely to this. The environment that we create from bringing in more kind, loving words is a calmer, more balanced, and safer place for our body to be in. Even saying something as simple as *"I love you"*, and feeling those words directed in towards our body, is enough as we don't have to over-complicate things. This one simple statement can change everything. It's so enormously powerful, especially when we're struggling. There is truly nothing better that we can do initially when we're unhappy, hurting, or not feeling well, as these words are so comforting and way more impactful than we might ever realize.

Our body always needs our love.

Afterall, it is a living being that needs us. It needs our care, concern, kind words, loving actions, and attention, just like a child. Our body responds to whatever we send its way, be it negative or positive. Our words, thoughts, and actions create an impact on so many levels.

Even the things we heard and received throughout our lives from other people, have had a strong impact on our bodies. We don't realize that our family's words, thoughts, and emotions around their own bodies, had an impact on us. We may have watched how they took care of their body (or didn't), what they said about it, as well as what they said about other people's bodies, including ours.

A lot of us came from critical families that were focused on the external appearance of our body, over the actual health of it, which gave us the room to believe that the external was the most important aspect. This was all learned of course, and not because they were just downright negative people (or maybe they were). The values of society shoved their way into our families lives, and our lives, creating misdirection and disconnection for many.

Regardless of why it happened or what was said, all of that stuff translated into our subconscious mind and often left us holding onto the same thought patterns and ideas. This is likely how many of us continue to repeat the same unhealthy family patterns in relation to body image and health, even taking on the same illnesses.

However, we are strong, capable adults who can change all of that. We don't have to allow the limitations and judgement of others create our present or our future. The words that were said might have stuck around for a minute, but we can work on releasing them and finally putting some of that negativity to rest. We're learning to function on a new level of acknowledgement. One that supports our body and where we want to go.

It's not hard to see why changing our dialogue is almost essential at this point in time. We have to be the ones who speak those kind, loving, healing words to our bodies. We want our self-talk and the thoughts we have about ourselves to support our healing and empower our bodies.

To understand a bit more about the power that our words and thoughts have on our bodies, I'd love to introduce a well-known man by the name of Dr. Masaru Emoto. Some of you may have already heard of him. Dr. Emoto's work and research clearly shows how human words, emotions, and intentions can greatly impact the molecular structure of water. You may be asking how this applies to us.

In his book, *The Hidden Messages of Water,* Dr. Emoto explains how the tone, emotion, and energy behind our words impacts our body on a powerful level because we are, in essence, largely made up of water, approximately 70%. His research shows how the molecules of the water literally change their structure and formation depending on the words that are spoken and the emotions that are behind them. The frequencies that are created through the words and emotions are what influence the structure.

When positive and supportive statements or words of gratitude were spoken, the structure of the water molecules formed into harmonious, symmetrical, and beautiful patterns. When something negative was spoken, such as harsh or angry words, the water molecule structures became chaotic, malformed, and disorganized, thus showing how powerful our words and emotions can be to our bodies and our cells.

Dr. Joe Dispenza, a well-known author and educator, also gives credit to the profound effect that words, thoughts, and emotions have on us and our body. What we speak about, think about, and ultimately believe to be true, all affect what's going on within our body, as well as in all areas of our life. We have the power to either create something we want, or something we don't, and this greatly pertains to the health and condition of our body.

The body and brain go hand in hand. Our body holds a certain degree of memory and programming through our DNA and of course, from what we've received in our environment growing up. If we came from a place where we received a lot of negative messages and poor emotional support, the language and emotions held in our body will keep us in a suppressed, weakened state, which can subject us to health problems down the line. This is unfortunately, a common place that many of us come from and live in presently. We've likely been stuck with this for decades, if not, our entire life. Even more likely, it's been carried through our family line for generations.

Most of us haven't been aware of the impact that our emotions have on our physical body and what's going on with it. Not to mention, most of us have never heard of this, at least I hadn't heard about it until later in life while doing my own research. It's certainly not mentioned in the medical industry much if at all, though it would serve greatly to be a bigger part of it and could change many people's lives.

It can prove to be difficult to realign our thoughts and emotions at first, especially because so much of this is so deeply embedded, and many of us are so used to negativity and repression being a main part of how we think and feel. However, the reward for transforming this is enormous. Our bodies will thank us and feel the shift instantly. Even if we don't feel it, our bodies will. Creating new thoughts and feelings will help to support our bodies and health on new levels. It's honestly just as important, if not more important than the food we eat.

It's been proven that we can only receive that which is in alignment with our *emotional state,* so in order to incorporate these new, positive thoughts and emotions, we need to retrain our body's emotional state. Retraining our body emotionally requires us to start doing a bit of *pretending* so to speak. To connect into what it would *feel like* to be in a perfectly healthy, blissful, and happy state. What it would feel like to have a healthy body and feel good physically.

We can do this by going through the emotions as though all of the goodness is already happening. While it might appear as though you're pretending, in reality, you're actively fostering well-being for yourself by engaging in this behavior. Your mind and body don't actually know the difference, as they work with the thoughts and emotions that we are presently in or putting forth.

As we do this, we begin moving ourselves out of the negativity and unhealthy emotions, little by little. As we continue practicing this, we suddenly realize that our whole persona shifts. We start realizing that it's not pretend, it's just reprogramming the negative stuff that didn't serve us. Doing this sets us up for success around our health *and our life,* as we rewrite our internal language and dialogue. We don't have to stay stuck in old emotions, thought patterns, and negative thinking about our body or health, no matter how hard it's been. The truth is, it's always been in our hands to be able to do this. We always had the power, and we *have* the power now to remove those old emotions of lack, fear, and sickness and make it a thing of the past.

Most of us want to be in a state of thriving, so it's important that we keep ourselves in as positive of a state as possible, hard as that may sound or seem. Because, if we're always in a poor emotional state thinking negative thoughts, our body is essentially going to feel it, show it, and end up being more stressed out and weaker than it needs to be, putting us in a more vulnerable position.

This is why it's so important that we know how to get ourselves out of a negative, fearful place and improve our self-talk and emotional state. So we can transform our body's entire state of being, and actually help our bodies to get in some healing.

I believe the best time and place to start working on expanding our positive self-talk and emotional awareness is in the mornings, before getting ready and heading out into our day. It sets us up for a more positive outcome bringing in with it, a healthier, happier state of being that will resonate out and through our day. It can help us shift how we experience and receive the day ahead of us.

It's fairly easy; we just need to sit with ourselves for a quiet moment or two and practice *feeling* what it would *feel* like to be happy and in a perfectly state health. Even more importantly, we need to visualize ourselves in these states. What does a perfectly healthy state look like? Well, we can see our bodies free from illness and health issues, see ourselves moving around freely, painlessly, and doing the things that we love in a happy, peaceful state. As we see this, it's important to feel immense gratitude for it, as though it's our true state of being in that very moment.

With time, our visualizations will become clearer and emotions will grow more deeply into a positive state, as we envision this for ourselves. We might even get to a place where we well up with tears in our eyes, because of how peaceful and happy we feel while doing this. Our desire for change in our mental and emotional state, will hit hard. When we stir up the deep emotions of gratitude, we become more aligned with where we want to be.

I know this can be a challenge, because how can we feel this way when we're literally not feeling well, nor in good health. It's understandable to fall into a place of resistance, maybe even because it sounds silly, or just because of all the years of conditioning that we have. Trust me, I've been there. Our mind and body respond this way initially, often times creating distractions or negative thoughts to move us away from doing it. It's because this process is foreign to us and our bodies, so it doesn't resonate to what we've thought, and who we've been all this time. However, the more persistent we are about it and the more we work on it, the easier it gets.

It doesn't hurt to have a guided meditation to help us do this, and Dr. Joe has many available, as well as that there are many others out there who teach this. I like his morning meditation that starts the day off by guiding you into a place of unlimited and positive potential which can be used towards our health, or anything else that we are wanting to build up in our lives. It only takes 20-25 minutes and I cannot express enough, just how powerful it is. Some days it even moves me to tears.

For many of us, a lot of our old programming does dwell in the negative. Besides our probable upbringing that created this, we're bombarded by a daily influx of negative and confusing messages that society puts out around our bodies and our health, including the common health scares, viruses, and so on. So, another beautiful tool we can use in order to move through and passed all of that, to strengthen our bodies and help them to heal, is through practicing gratitude.

Gratitude is so powerful. It can help us retrain our brain, body, emotions, and in turn, our outcomes. We will talk more about gratitude later on, but this is important while we are talking about our bodies. Since we can only accept and believe thoughts that resonate with our emotional state, practicing gratitude and sitting with the emotions of being grateful for our bodies, will without a doubt, strongly affect how our health and body respond.

Just saying thank you to our body and telling it that we love it, is powerful. We can do this at any time of the day and as often as we might think to. The more often, the better. If we know we'll be super busy during the day, doing this in the morning and again at night is amazingly powerful.

I like to practice gratitude when I'm laying down in bed, snuggled up under the covers, both before falling asleep and upon waking, before I actually get out of bed. This helps to create positive feelings throughout my entire being, no matter what lies ahead in my day, and there are *always* things to be grateful for.

Speaking of the end of our day, the last five minutes of our day has a huge impact on our subconscious mind, which does a lot of work while we're asleep. It uses whatever it is that we're thinking about those last few minutes before falling asleep. Our subconscious mind is what programs our feelings, thoughts, and body. So, in knowing this, it makes sense to spend those last few minutes of our day thinking about what we *do* want, as well as what we're grateful for, which includes our body and our health. The same goes for our first few thoughts when we're waking up.

Both times happen to be powerfully influential in what we receive and experience. So why wouldn't we want to develop a new, super easy habit that will add more positivity to our life? One that can actually give us the power to consciously create more good to come our way and into our life. It's so easy to do and we will absolutely begin to notice the difference in our attitude, thinking, and the experiences that we have.

It's easy to understand how our mindset and our emotions can affect our body, how it functions, and how it responds for us. Gratitude creates an emotional imprint that helps to move the mind and body out of the negative emotions that it's been in, into a place of greater appreciation and reward, creating a new space for healing that is needed.

When doing this, we will find ourselves more motivated and drawn to do the things that will help strengthen and support our body. Ultimately, we end up making better decisions for ourselves, such as eating healthier and getting in more exercise.

The thoughts, words, and even the experiences we have in life, affect our cells. Science has proven this. Our body and our cells *feel* the effects of our words and thoughts quite meaningfully. It's vital that we are patient and gentle with ourselves as we develop this new muscle and way of being, as it may take some time to rewire our thinking and our emotions.

Having the desire to do it makes the whole process easier and much more powerful. I believe that most of us would rather be more loving and compassionate towards ourselves and our bodies than we have been in the past. Afterall, this is our natural state of being.

Now that we know the connection that our emotions and thoughts have on our body, we can get to the more obvious stuff, which is the physical. All that we breathe in, eat, put onto our skin, and even allow into our environment energetically, affects our physical state.

Obviously, our body is affected by what we feed it, that's an easy one to understand. However, at this point in time, there are so many levels and complexities to the food we eat. It's not just cut and dry, grown out of the ground like it's original status once was. Once upon a time, it *was* literally farm to table and all food grown was considered organic.

However, in this day and age, we are challenged by of all of the non-foods and processed foods, as well as all of the chemicals that are slathered all over, and infused into our food. This has changed the body and health game completely. It's no longer simple plant biology and chemistry, working with our human biology and chemistry. Not anymore. It *was* once that simple and wonderful, and for the most part, the human body worked harmoniously with all of it. Even if illness did exist, it wasn't anything like what we face today.

As a society, we've fallen into the most sick and diseased states of health than we've ever had before. Our bodies are heavily stressed out, taking in so many chemicals and toxins that it's a wonder some of us are even still alive. Needless to say, our bodies are miraculous in what they can put up with, but why do we have to deal with all of these terrible insults and harm that's put upon us?

Most everyone has a health issue in some form or another. We seem to believe that as we get older, our bodies begin to weaken and become a target for illness and disease. You gotta love hearing someone say, "It's fun getting old." when they're talking about how poorly their health is doing. Sadly, we've been taught not to recognize the fact that our bodies are literally falling apart because of what we've been given to eat, ingest, apply, and drink, not because of our years on the planet.

So, because of all the chemicals and external burdens, health crises show up. In these health crises, we have several systems and organs that are struggling to do their best or failing to do their jobs, and we are desperate to find something to *fix it*. We turn to the doctors and they tell us what's happening if they can figure it out, and away we go. Medications and maybe surgeries or procedures, hoping things will get better, maybe even cured. And maybe it does. Yet, nothing is said about what we need to stop doing, avoid, or actually do to help ourselves get out of this terrible situation or keep us from entering into it again.

It's good to let the doctor look after our disease, but it's what we learn from the health issue or crisis that's important. We need to learn that we weren't listening, that we weren't being good to our body, and that we likely need to stop some of the things we were doing. The doctor can hopefully help us on some level or another, but the overall lesson is in what we learned about ourselves through it.

The truth is, we need to learn what we need to do from this point forward and how we can help ourselves. Just being on the path to realizing this, gaining a little knowledge and having the desire for change, will ultimately bring us power. The power to get ourselves out of being in a bad place, as well as to keep ourselves away from any unnecessary strife or sickness down the line. Because, if we do nothing to change the way we've been treating our bodies, things are guaranteed to show up again, and maybe next time, things will be much worse.

Learning a thing or two about our body is always a good thing. It gives us strength and a good batch of confidence. However, most people shy away from learning about their body because of how it's been portrayed by modern day medicine and science, as complicated. With big, hard to pronounce words, endless different processes and diagnosis names, thousands of medications, and the complex schooling doctors have to go through, what everyday person wouldn't feel overwhelmed and doubtful? I totally get it.

However, we really don't need to understand *all of that* to be able to understand a few vital things about our bodies and ourselves. We can get to know the basics and most important aspects about our body, as well as what we can do to help it. The sheer fact that our body has the capacity to heal itself, is already a huge plus in our favor. Knowing how to support it in doing that, is everything. We can all know some of the ins and outs of the body and what it needs from us, and undoubtedly learn what we can do for it at home. Afterall, the doctor isn't there every moment of every day, taking care of the things that need to get done. That's our job.

A lot of what we're being fed, given to use, and exposed to on a daily basis, is not easy for our bodies to deal with, hence the health issues and breakdown that begins to occur in our systems and organs.

As we get older, we start to notice that our body is having a harder time with things. We feel weaker, we might have pain in several areas, and we can't seem to do the things we used to in the same way. However, we can understand that the copious amounts of chemicals and toxins in our environment and food are huge contributing factors in this. We'll even notice that our emotional and mental health are affected by these toxins that we're ingesting and utilizing.

Still, even when we're older, our body has the intelligence and capability to bounce back after just about anything. We've seen this either having gone through something difficult ourselves, or through witnessing someone who has. Some people can be in a really bad position and somehow their bodies bounce back almost miraculously. Personally, I've seen people on their death beds come back to life. It is possible, we just have to realize how much our hand plays in this.

For one, we can do our best to take in less toxins and bad-for-you stuff that's made available to us. Again, we have a choice in what we give to our bodies. Conventional medicine definitely plays a part in things, but they cannot always save every aspect of our health. Medications and the like, only go so far sometimes. We are required, and need to, play the biggest role in our health care and in the state of our body's overall wellbeing.

We've become a population so used to taking some form of medication to try and relieve any symptoms and problems that arise, as we've learned to ignore the why or how things happened the way they did. Being a nurse in the industry for two-and-a-half decades, I've watched countless numbers of people *only* use the medical solutions offered to them, and do nothing for themselves. Their problems usually continued on, with new ones popping up, as they received endless grief from their body. They didn't have the understanding, nor the connection that they played a role in things. It's a huge disconnect that they either choose to have, or just know no better. Some would rather just choose to do nothing than to change things.

I know many people are sick and tired of being sick and tired. They're tired of the diseases and chronic illnesses they're riddled with, tired of being in fear, tired of luminating over how bad they feel, and are especially tired of watching themselves or their loved one's struggle and suffer on a daily basis. This puts them into constant stress mode and once again, living in constant stress mode leaves us weak, both physically and mentally.

I believe we're all smart enough to know better now, at least for the most part, to know what's good for us and what isn't. We all inherently know that our diet plays a huge role in how our health thrives or doesn't. We also know that if we added more fresh food into our diets (fruits and vegetables), we are in fact adding more nourishment, power, and support to our bodies and our cells. What we feed ourselves, feeds our cells, and our cells need us to bring in the nutrients that they need so they can work properly.

We know that smoking, eating a lot of fast food, sugary, fried foods, simple carbohydrates, processed foods, and alcohol, amongst other things, can burden our bodies. So, obviously when it comes to supporting them, we have to be mindful not to overdo anything for the sake of our body's outcome in the long run. We generally do not notice the effects that this stuff has on us right away, but it doesn't mean it isn't affecting us on an enormous level.

Our body also needs oxygen, sunshine, adequate rest, and movement. We weren't built to sit down and be indoors on a screen all day. We were meant to move, get outside, be in nature, and get fresh air and sunshine in order to live and thrive. To be able to exercise outdoors *and* in the sunshine and fresh air, is quite a powerful combination. I know there's been a lot of fear around being out in the sun, but just know that we need sunshine for at least for five to fifteen minutes a day. And without sunglasses or sunscreen. We need the sunlight to get into our eyes- not directly looking at the sun, but through the light it gives off. It's necessary for certain processes in the body, especially in making Vitamin D which we need in order to survive.

Movement is greatly necessary. It's good for our muscles, especially our heart muscle, as well as that it helps to keep our bones strong. We need to keep things moving for our lymphatic system, our heart, our lungs, as well to help oxygen pump around our body at a greater, deeper rate. Movement assists our internal organs, giving them a gentle massage of sorts, which helps move things through and out, with our digestive tract as an example.

A lot of the time our bodies begin to break down and get weak because we don't give them enough of these things, and to top it off, we feed them crummy food. There are some elders that prove all of these to be useful as they understand the importance of eating healthy, getting in sunshine, getting adequate rest, and exercise. The longer we care for our body, the longer it will allow us to do so.

Now let's talk about the make-up of our body.

Our body is made up of trillions of cells, approximately forty to seventy trillion. I like to think of each cell as its own little person, and that's because each and every one of them is its own living being. It eats, poops, works, reproduces, serves a unique purpose in the body, and eventually dies. Everything in our body besides the fluids, is made up of cells, and even the fluids of our body *contain* cells. All of our organs, hair, skin, nails, eyes, bones, teeth, muscles, all of it, is made up of cells.

These beautiful cells of ours work diligently and communicate with one another to ensure that everything is working efficiently and staying in proper balance. Every cell's entire life is dedicated to keeping us alive. They control what goes on in our physical body. Of course, all that we

21

give to our bodies and whatever we put them through, can either make life easy for our cells or make things difficult for them. The truth is, our cells do not get the credit they deserve. They're forced to work in whatever environment and conditions that we create for them, while doing their best to rebalance and repair things. They can only do so much when the conditions are less than ideal.

I like to break our body down to the absolute core level of what makes us up, so that we can understand our bodies as deeply as possible. At the core of all that we are, we're made up of atoms. Atoms are made up of particles of light and energy, which ultimately means that we are also made up of light and energy.

The atoms within us and around us, are constantly moving and vibrating which create vibrational patterns that are otherwise known as *frequencies*. I find it exciting to think about ourselves in this way; knowing that we're made up of light, energy, frequencies, cells, and water. It's such an expansive perspective around who and what we are. What our bodies are.

Still, most of us don't think to look at ourselves on all these levels. We focus so much on the physical pieces and parts, that we forget about all of the other aspects of our make-up. One of those being the energetic side of us. We literally have an energy field surrounding our physical, cellular structure known as the Human Energy Field. We're in fact made up of an endless supply of energy that acts as a conduit of reception and release.

This energetic field is affected by so many things in our environment. Our emotions and words even affect these fields, as well as the traumas and experiences that we go through, both physically and psychologically.

External frequencies can cause changes to our cells and energetic fields, which obviously involves our health and wellbeing. Some of these frequencies can affect us in a negative way, such as those of microwaves, cell phones, and other devices that emit harsh frequencies. However, we can also *use* frequencies to intentionally affect our energetic fields and physical bodies, and we'll get more into that a bit later, but it's essential to know that we can create a lot of positive changes and results from utilizing frequencies. Our energetic field feeds our cells and even affects the electricity within our body, which several organ systems, such as our heart and nervous system, use to function.

Let's also not forget about our DNA, which we mentioned a bit earlier. Our bodies were designed through our DNA, which goes back thousands upon thousands of years. Our physical features, characteristics, functionality, health stature, even our strengths, weaknesses, patterning, and responses in life, can all be linked to our DNA.

DNA is a molecule that holds genetic instructions that are passed down from generation to generation, where we inherit our ancestors everything and carry the familial torch, so to speak. It tells our body's cells what they're supposed to do, how to grow, how to live, how to survive, and how to reproduce. Unseen to the naked eye, DNA holds our genetic coding, memories, and all of our ancestors' experiences.

It is amazingly self-repairing and is highly responsive to frequencies as well. Believe it or not, our words, beliefs, thoughts, and emotions have a profound vibrational effect on our DNA and its coding. And of course, that which we eat, ingest, and take in from our environment physically, also have a huge effect on our DNA.

Some of what harms our DNA are free radicals, cancer-causing agents, gene therapy drugs, chemicals, negative frequencies, and traumatic events to name a few. When we make positive changes to our health both physically and emotionally, it all gets translated into our DNA whose codes can transform and will then pass on to future generations. We can also repair our DNA if it's been weakened or messed with, as it's never totally locked into to the weakened state that it's gotten into.

Knowing all of the angles of our bodies will only open us up to a greater level of understanding ourselves, and what our bodies need from us. When we have this enhanced level of awareness, it helps to assist us in having a stronger handle on things when challenges arise. Having the knowledge that we're more than meets the eye and not just this physical body, will only help guide us towards making more educated and loving decisions for ourselves.

Recreating the perspective around our bodies and moving beyond the limitations set in place for us, gives us strength to be able to go past our familial and societal boundaries. We do not have to end up like our family did. We do not have to inherit their diseases, weaknesses, take on their struggles, poor health, or poverty mindset. We don't even have to keep their beliefs as our own. We can change them all.

If our family and ancestors fell onto hard times, suffering, and ill health, we can use the information to our advantage by learning from their mistakes and shortcomings. We can consciously make more elevated choices that would in fact create a greater, healthier, more empowered outcome. Regardless of the limited thoughts we've been told about our genetics and heredity, or even what we've been told about our bodies from the modern medical industry, we can still transform things, hands down. We do not have to surrender to these limitations anymore. We can see our bodies as the beautiful and powerful miracle that they are.

It's also important for us to start tapping into our intuition more.

Our intuition is that beautiful voice inside of us that helps guide us through life. It brings things to our attention, amplifies the answers we need to hear, and serves us on making the most empowered choices for ourselves. When we tune in and listen to our intuition, we're usually guided to make the most enlightened decisions that will benefit us.

When we're utilizing our intuition, we might find ourselves deciding that we want to start exercising more, change our eating habits and diet, or change the way we speak and think about our bodies and ourselves. We get better at recognizing toxic people, situations, and the things in our life that we need to let go of. All from quieting ourselves enough to listen to the internal voice within.

Listening to this inner guidance can take us to new levels physically and emotionally. We become more in touch with taking care of our body in ways we hadn't thought of before. Following our innate, internal guidance system usually leads to greater outcomes than we could've even imagined.

Our desire and willingness to make changes will always help us to build up our confidence. Ultimately, we all want to create a greater state of health for ourselves, a stronger body, a better life. Now we've finally come to a point in our life where we realize that we don't have to settle for what's being handed to us anymore. Our bodies deserve better than they've been given over the past few decades.

Knowledge gives us power and strength. It helps to create a better understanding on how we can embody a more fulfilling and healthy life for ourselves. No one's health story or journey is the same as another, nor are there any that are perfect. We each have a unique experience that we go through.

It comes down to someone in our family making the changes, ending the cycles, healing the old traumas, and strengthening our genetic line, and that would be us. Changes don't have to be overwhelming, it's just one step at a time, because even small changes have a powerful impact. The new decisions that we make for our body, and the effort we put forth in wanting more for ourselves and our bodies, sets much more into motion than we realize.

When we decide that our wellbeing and health are one of the most important things to us and we acknowledge that we will no longer have to accept being sick and unwell all of the time regardless of what limitations or challenges we encounter, we can transform almost anything. If only we viewed our bodies as the sacred temples and amazing organisms that they are, we would automatically treat them better and in turn, love them more. We just need to remember that the connection to ourselves, especially to our bodies, is the most important thing of all.

The fact is, we're coming back around to all of this and how wonderful and powerful is that? I have to admit, it makes me feel so lucky for the times we're in. There are so many amazing people helping to bring forth powerful healing techniques and information around our bodies with each and every day that passes. All that's been left behind and forgotten is coming back into the light.

There's new technology that is coming around that is going to, without a doubt, change our lives. So, in the meantime, it's up to us to make the best choices we can for ourselves and make the necessary changes that we need to, so that we can return to the perfect and natural state that we are meant to be in. Our body has a beautiful way of regenerating itself, so everything we do for its benefit will only contribute to the goodness in our lives.

It's important to remember who we are. As a human being, we are a magical, atomic, energetic, light filled, self-healing, regenerating, living organism. We are the creators of our outcome. We have the ability and the strength to transform our bodies and recreate our lives on whatever level we choose to. We can make healing our body a beautiful and humbling journey, or we can make it a miserable one. In the end it's up to us.

It's time that we acknowledge the power that our bodies hold and take better care of them from this moment forward. We know that giving our bodies better food, rest, exercise, and loving, supportive words will ultimately create a better outcome for them, and they deserve nothing less than that. In time we will see that our devotion and love for them grows.

Taking good care of our bodies raises our vibration, which attracts so many unexpected blessings into our life. Tell your body that you love it, adore it, and cherish it, and that you are always here for it, no matter what.

No matter what we've been through or done to it in the past, no matter the disconnection that we've had for however long it's been, there's nothing stopping us from changing all of that, today. We can move forward in this very moment and do things differently. It's time to return back home to ourselves.

Our body will always love us, unconditionally. It's time we do the same.

HOMEWORK:

1. Note all of the aspects of what you think, believe, or tell yourself about your body. Highlight the positives of where you support and love your body, take notice the negatives.
2. If you have any negative thoughts or beliefs about your body or your health, how can you work to transform them? Write down that which you would rather say, think, or feel instead.
3. Write out a list of ways in which you want to start supporting and loving your body more in ways that you've already been doing.
4. Practice telling your body that you love it. It doesn't have to be aloud, but it's great if you can. Connect into it, think about it, and really feel it. Try to do this at least twice a day.

UNDERSTANDING A FEW VITAL SYSTEMS

N ow that we talked about the connection we have with our bodies, let's discuss a few of the systems within them that are worth knowing about. Of course, all of our organs and systems are essential and wonderful to know about, but these are a few of the underdogs who I think deserve our attention, especially in the times we're in.

I will try to keep it simple as best as I can, but know that no matter who we are or where we're from, we are all capable of understanding the systems within our body. It's true that we don't have to have a degree to understand that which is inside of us, in fact, we are meant to understand know all parts to us, as well as to be able to hone in on them.

The truth is, the more we have an understanding and relationship with the parts of our body, the easier it is to make connections and changes that we need. We can feel more confident in our ability to take better care of ourselves, especially when things aren't at their best. This greater awareness and knowledge, helps to create a deeper understanding and connection with our body.

Please know, it's not about memorizing complicated words and the workings of the body. It's about understanding their purpose, their potential, a little about how they function, and ways we can support them. When we agree to wanting to know this, we open ourselves up to receive the information and can take it in almost effortlessly over time. It only empowers us so that we can make better choices and decisions for ourselves.

So please, do not worry if you don't remember everything to a tee, just reading about these systems will help you to formulate your own personal understanding in the way that you need to. Once you know a few things, you'll know them, and you might even surprise yourself at how much better you understand things. By learning some of this, you'll create a new neural pathway that will help you understand the wisdom of the body through a different lens. Imagine the value you will feel within yourself and your body once you start learning a few things.

I would love nothing more than to cover all of our amazing systems in this section, as they all deserve our time and attention, but that would be a book in itself. I just wanted to give you a small glimpse of a few of the vital systems, that in my opinion, are essential to cover.

Again, every part and system of ours is super important, so feel free to go out there and do some research on your own, especially the other systems and organs that grab your interest. It's only ever good to have a better understanding and deeper connection to your body.

OUR PH LEVEL

The pH level is the chemistry of the body and its environment, otherwise known as the acid and alkaline level of the body. The pH level in our body has a huge effect on everything that happens within it, especially in regards to our cells.

The pH level can either create a good environment where our health will thrive, or it can create an environment that allows for sickness and illness to take place. Most of us have heard about this somewhere in science class back in grade school or high school, but I'm going to bet most of us don't remember too much about it.

We definitely didn't learn about it in terms of whether people lived sick and miserable, or healthy and strong, but this is seriously good for us to know.

The pH balance of the body is insanely important. The body cannot exist in the extreme of one side or the other for too long. In our modern-day lives, the balance has seemingly become harder to maintain. Most of the foods and drinks that we ingest are on the acid side of things. This includes our meat, dairy products, alcohol, breads, sweets, processed foods, and so much more. Alkaline foods on the other hand, are basically all of the wholesome, fresh, raw fruits and vegetables gloriously grown out of the Earth.

Depending on what we consume, use, and are exposed to, determines how acidic or alkaline our body's environment is. However, our chemistry is not only influenced by what we consume, it's also influenced by our stress levels and lifestyles. Especially when we're in an overly acidic state, our body is working hard to rebalance its chemistry and keep things from getting out of control. In fact, it's always working to get us there especially because of the diets that we consume these days. Our body ends up having to pull and utilize various minerals from other areas in an attempt to restore its balance.

The western medical establishment has a diagnosis for an overly acidic condition called acidosis. Acidosis is when the body cannot remove the excess acid well enough to balance things out, causing buildup and an overload of acids in the body and its systems. Generally, when this is the case, the body has likely been overly acidic for quite a while to have gotten to that point.

With acidosis, the excess acids that are left behind cause oxidative stress which is basically harm to the cells throughout all systems and organs of the body. Our kidneys, lungs, liver, lymphatic system, and bowels work the hardest to rid the body of excess acids, mainly the kidneys and the lungs. However, if they've been overwhelmed for a long period of time or are not in the greatest shape, it's more difficult for them to process and release the excess acids. They then get bogged down and overloaded with acids which end up collecting somewhere within our cells.

Unfortunately, it's not just our food and what we take in that creates an imbalance. Most of the products that we put onto our skin and even the pollution in the air that we're breathing in, are on the acid side of chemistry.

Stress also increases acid levels in the body. When we stress out, our body releases hormones that are supposed to be moved through and out of the body naturally, however, these hormones become a waste product (metabolic waste) which if not released properly, will stick around and cause a higher acid levels and congestion in the body.

Our body has to work so much harder to function when it's in an overly acidic state. Talk about stress! Acid is corrosive, which means it causes inflammation, destruction, and break down. An acid acts like fire, burning, inflaming, and basically will eat away and corrode whatever area it's in. Considering everything in our body is made up of cells, which are delicate on many levels, acid can and will strongly affect them, causing them to breakdown, malfunction, and essentially make them sick and unable to work properly.

Of course, having acid buildup in our body may not be quite this severe, however, if in this state for a prolonged period of time, things will begin to show us signs of stress and break down. The delicate structures within our body like our organs and vessels are very much affected by a long-term acidic condition.

Sugar is one of the most acidic substances we ingest. When someone drinks sugary, and especially caffeinated drinks, the body releases a burst of energy that we know as adrenaline. The sugar and caffeine trigger the body to release the hormone epinephrine which increases the acid level in the body. Adrenaline and epinephrine are the energy boosters and fight or flight creators.

In order for our body to buffer or balance out these acids, it needs a remedy and the number one remedy to buffer the acid is calcium. Calcium is an alkaline salt. The body grabs calcium from other areas and parts of the body, the number one place being the bones and the parathyroid. When calcium is removed from these and other areas of the body, it can then cause a series of other problems such as bone density issues, weakened parathyroid, and cause problems in other systems such as the cardiovascular system, the heart. The heart needs calcium as part of its electrical and chemical functioning. A lack of calcium can also cause decreased functioning of some of the endocrine glands, parts of the nervous system, and so on. When the body is being pulled out of balance chemically like this, all of the organs and systems are affected.

Acids will end up in our bloodstream flowing through our body, circulating around affecting our cells and their environment. In medical terms, this is called metabolic acidosis. These high acid levels *destroy* cells due to the corrosive nature.

A highly acidic environment also creates *oxygen deficiency* which happens to be a highly, unideal environment as it creates grounds for disease and illness to take hold. There are also some organisms that absolutely *thrive* in an acidic environment such as many types of bacteria, viruses, fungus, parasites, and cancer.

Removing the acids from our bodies definitely *deserves* our time and attention. It can be a bit overwhelming to take care of because embracing a new way of eating isn't always the easiest. We can at least take a good look at what does create more acids and work from there.

Increasing alkaline foods and decreasing stress are two easy steps we can take. It takes a little bit of time to adapt to and learn new ideas around eating a highly alkaline diet, as well as how to cleanse out the acids and heal the body, but it's well worth the journey. Letting go of a good portion of acid forming foods is never easy for those of us who are so used to incorporating them into our diets, so patience with oneself is necessary.

Detoxing and expelling acids from the body can be quite a birthing process, but without a doubt getting rid of these excess poisons in the body will by far help our bodies to live and function more freely and healthily. It will indeed help to keep us away from disease, even heal from it, and make it more difficult for breakdown to occur, as well as put a stop to those unfriendly organisms that are thriving inside of us and doing damage. We will talk more later about how to work the waste and acids out of the body, as well as these organisms. We truly don't want an environment that's favorable to all those critters and organisms because they consume our nutrients and slowly move us into a bad state of health.

An overly acidic condition of the body also causes aging to progress much more rapidly. Dr. William Howard, a brilliant man from about a century ago, brings this point across in his book 'A New Health Era'. As he states, the accumulation of acid in the body is cause for almost all diseases and illnesses. It's hard to accept this because we never hear this from the medical world (and I've been in the industry for over 25, never hear of it), but it makes absolute sense the more you think about it.

Almost every one of the people that have come through my hands during my career, who were suffering from all sorts of illnesses and diseases, in my eyes, could've been educated and helped around this concept alone. A large portion of them were highly acidic. Food, cleansing methods, and herbs are the major ways out of an overly acidic condition. Herbs are the alkalizers and the healers of the planet. We will talk more about food and herbs later on.

THE CENTRAL PROCESSING SYSTEM: THE GUT

The gut is the system in our body that is the key processor and assimilator. It is otherwise known as the digestive system, which includes the stomach, the small intestines, the colon, the pancreas, the liver, and the gallbladder. It processes more than just our food; it also processes what we use on our skin, what we breathe in, and even the situations, emotions, and traumas that we go through.

It is yet another system that is constantly working hard to break down and process everything we put into it, not only to our body, but also our mind. It keeps what's beneficial for us (nutrients) and disposes of what isn't, or at least it tries to. Our gut is our nutrient absorber and our main waste remover. It's also where our instincts lie and decision making can come from.

When we are being created in our mother's body (as an embryo), our gut is the second system to develop. The two systems that grow before everything else are the spinal column and the gut tissue. From the spinal and gut cells, all of the other glands and organs of the body are created which means, all of the organs in the body are innately and directly connected to the spinal cord and the digestive system.

We have approximately 31 feet of small intestine and our colon (large intestine) is about 8 feet long, equaling approximately 40, or so, feet of intestines. That's a pretty long journey for our food to travel. It's not a wonder how some of the food we eat never makes it out of the body. Our body has a lot of work to do during this process; breaking down the food we brought in, taking the nutrients out of it, and then moving and pushing what's left of the food through the intestines, so it can exit the body.

The small intestines have little hairlike bristles along the walls called the villi, which help move the food along with contractions of the intestinal wall. If we eat too much and have a lot of extra waste lying around (so many people do), the villi have a difficult time doing their job. Any chemicals or pharmaceutical drugs we take in, can damage these villi.

If the colon wall is caked up with leftover waste, it cannot pump the waste through properly, because it does not work as well. Then things really begin to get left behind and cause build up throughout the system, which in turn causes a host of other issues. Both the small intestine and the colon are made up of smooth muscle and it's important that those muscles aren't suffocated and congested by old waste. They need to breathe and be able to work correctly in order to remain strong and help us absorb the nutrients and properly process the food we eat.

As expected, the lining of the gut wall is quite delicate. Like everything else in the body, our intestinal system and its lining is made up of cells. The small intestine walls are where our nutrients get absorbed, through the pores in the lining. These pores can become clogged, and when they're clogged, they are unable to absorb the nutrients for us. The pores become constipated and much of our nutrients are lost.

However, we can overcome and change this situation, by working to get rid of or pull out the matter that is congesting the intestines with fresh fruits and vegetables, as well as by using drawing agents like herbs, charcoal, and something like bentonite (however this needs to be used with caution and lots of water).

We can absolutely unclog parts of our body with diet, herbs, and various cleansing techniques. Our kidneys, liver, and gallbladder, are again, a part of our digestive system and can easily become congested and clogged up, as they have tubes within their structure that are there to filter debris out of the body. These tubes can easily get impacted by waste and thick, sticky substances causing back up and malfunction of the organ.

Sometimes when they become congested, stones will form in these areas, which is hardened, calcified matter that ends up creating weakness and failure of the organ's functioning, not to mention pain and illness. The liver will end up with sticky, tar-like buildup in its tubes which creates massive congestion and an overload of toxins, affecting the gallbladder and overall digestive system as well. Our liver is the main detoxifier in the body. Sugary foods, high fat animal products, refined carbohydrates, fried foods, alcohol, milk chocolate, and full fat dairy products are all products that cause build up and the congestion in the liver.

Unless we've eaten a clean diet our entire life with perfect bowel habits, things likely aren't at 100%. I'll be honest, we all have a few leftovers in there somewhere, although I know people don't want to believe me, but after treating hundreds of thousands of people during my career, and having had a colonics business, I will say chances of having a perfectly working GI/digestive system at this time in society is rarely the case. Of course, never to discount those who do have a beautifully working and healthy GI system, but I'm here speaking in general terms, especially within the US population.

Many people do not know that a large part of our nervous system is laced throughout the intestines. The intestines are lined with over 100 million nerve cells. Scientists have labeled it our *enteric nervous system*. It has a direct link of communication to the brain and spinal cord, so that means our gut affects our brain and its functions.

This even includes our moods. At this point in time, we've probably all heard about this gut-brain connection. The gut and the brain send signals back and forth to one another for many purposes which affects more areas of our body and life than we realize.

90% of the body's serotonin is produced in the gut and found in the lining of the gut. Serotonin is our chemical messenger that stabilizes our moods helping to create the feelings of happiness and well-being. It also plays a role in our digestive process and bowel function.

The body releases serotonin at a quicker rate when it needs to move an irritant or toxic product out of the gut. If the body releases serotonin too fast, it can cause nausea. Serotonin also helps the body with sleep, assisting the body with melatonin production while working together with dopamine to improve our sleep quality. Serotonin gets released into the blood stream and is absorbed by the platelets in the blood, which also plays a vital role in wound healing.

Serotonin plays a huge role in our overall wellbeing, and 90% of it is produced in our gut. If our gut is not functioning properly, it can lead to a disruption in serotonin production, and undoubtedly, many issues will begin to arise. Continuously high levels of serotonin can eventually cause bone weakness and low levels can cause depression, digestive problems, and sleep issues.

Science has also found a certain type of bacteria in the brain that is connected to the gut, which is suspected to influence personality and mood. That certainly brings some perspective to light, especially for those who suffer from mental illness. I've worked with thousands of people suffering from mental health issues throughout my career and just giving their mental disturbance a diagnosis name is not going to be as helpful. Yes, when it comes to the medications they use for them, but they aren't working on or dealing with the root cause which could in fact be gut health.

Although I wasn't taught about this in school, it makes so much sense to me now. Knowing what I learned through my care for all of them, of course there were life events and traumas that brought them to this point but also, every single one of their diets was poor. Sadly, diet is not acknowledged as being a part of the problem when it comes to the mentally ill, nor is seen as a solution. And to boot, the food that is actually served in hospitals is without a doubt, unhealthy and only contributing to the issue.

It seems a large number of people suffering with mental illnesses have big time gut problems. I bet working on cleansing the body, dietary changes, and the reestablishment of a healthy microbial balance could correct a lot of things for some of them. Of course, along with the nurturing emotional and mental therapy.

As I vaguely mentioned, a huge number of people have pounds of leftover waste inside of them that has never left their body. People love to argue with me on this topic which blows my mind considering the constipated and overweight condition of the population. I like to use Elvis as an example. He was said to have over 40 lbs. of poop in him when he died. Those peanut butter, banana, bacon sandwiches and pain pills literally killed him on the toilet. Pharmaceutical drugs, especially narcotics, absolutely ruin the gut, by constipating, drying it out, and wrecking the nerves and organismal balance.

Speaking of organisms, there are several organisms to be aware of that happen to love our leftover waste, such as bacteria, fungus, and parasites. Yes, parasites exist outside of third world countries, even though it's something we were taught that really didn't exist here in the US. After endless research, I found out these critters are quite intelligent and stealthy. I've asked some doctors that I worked with their opinions on parasites in the body. Their response was that they do not exist in first world nations. In truth, their schooling doesn't focus much on this. Regardless of their opinions, I still studied parasites at great length. They are quite fascinating, and unfortunately, they can cause a host of serious issues within our body.

Parasites find the human body a wonderful home with everything they need to not only survive, but thrive. Our body provides quite a wonderful environment for them to live a long, fulfilling life. They even find their way around the body, and aren't limited to the intestines.

We can ingest these organisms through our food and water, especially meat, fish, and even unwashed fruits and vegetables. And no, our stomach acid isn't necessarily going to always kill them, unless we have a perfect, healthy gut environment and pH balance. Most people's internal environments are somewhat off, considering the diet and chemicals we take in on the daily, and especially if we already have digestive issues, weakness, or a chronic disease or two.

Parasites are mind-blowingly intelligent and know how to survive and adapt in almost any kind of environment (except for a highly oxygenated and alkaline one). They feast and feast, breed and birth thousands of their kind, and in turn cause a number of underlying health issues. This ginormous issue gets missed by the modern medical industry, and in my 25 years as a nurse, I've never once treated anyone for a parasite, not a roundworm, not a fluke, tapeworm, pinworm, nothing. I've only heard of children being treated once in a while, but apparently wasn't a thing for adults.

Certain medications such as antibiotics and chemotherapy can also cause imbalances in the gut, as they not only kill the bad cells and organisms, but they also kill the good bacteria and some of our necessary and vital cells. This causes a weakness in the balance of the system making us vulnerable to a long list of health issues. We need a good balance of gut bacteria reinstated in order to literally survive physically and mentally, and we'll talk a little about that in just a moment.

I'd like to also point out another unfortunate issue within the gut which is fungus. It's more present in people than we realize. Fungus grows rapidly especially when it has its favorite food to feast on- sugar. Of course, eating sugar itself is a source, but let's face it, it's in just about everything these days. Also, plenty of other foods break down into sugars, such as flour products, grains, and dairy, as well as that sugar is added to all kinds of prepared and processed foods.

Fungus will find its way to other places in our body, and not just remain in our gut. It ends up in our bloodstream which of course, travels around the body, where fungus can then get to places like our liver, lungs, and the brain. There are deposits of fungus found in these areas. The most well-known fungus found overgrown in our body is Candida which is found in any warm, moist area of the body. We see it show up physically often times the mouth, the female reproductive region, and in the bowels. People can have bowel movements with white, yellowish exudate, which is fungus. When it shows up for our eyes to see, it's highly likely that the candida is systemic, meaning, it's very much overgrown and unfortunately, flourishing in the body.

Fungus is linked to digestive issues, respiratory and breathing problems, brain fog and memory issues, neurological disorders like MS, fibromyalgia, reproductive issues, even cancer, and the list goes on. Fungus interferes with oxygen and nutrient absorption which eventually causes a variety of issues within the body, creating an imbalance which becomes quite difficult to diagnose or find the solution for. For whatever reason, there are not many pharmaceutical drugs that can help get rid of fungus, especially when it's become systemic.

Medications and drugs, whether it be pharmaceutical or street drugs, leave behind a residue in the body, especially in the intestines. Sometimes the body is in a state where it cannot fully get rid of these chemicals, so buildup occurs in certain organs such as the kidneys and brain as well as getting trapped in the leftover waste in the gut.

Generally, people taking medications already have a number of issues and imbalances happening, so it's highly likely that their intestinal system is not working as well as it should. I know there are a large number of people out there taking handfuls of medications several times a day because their body isn't working properly and is in a less than desirable state, so it's understandable that most of those people also have gut and bowel issues.

Somewhere along the way people have been given the permission and thought that one bowel movement every day, or even every few days is considered *normal*. It's the thinking that you're just getting older and things are slowing down, not because of your diet and hydration, nor about the condition of your organs and systems. Even if someone poops once a day, you can be sure that not everything that went in, came out. This has even become more common in children.

We can all be an honest judge of ourselves and what our body has been up to, in regards to this. After 3 big meals and snacks during day, what do you expect should be coming out and how often? There's old science that used to show one meal going in, one in the middle processing, and one on its way out. So, the theory is that there should only ever be 3 meals in there processing at once. Somehow, we lost sight of this truth.

The products that we use on our body get absorbed through our skin. So, what does that have to do with our gut? Well, the products get absorbed through the skin and into our bloodstream, which then finds its way into the gut. So, our lotions, sunscreens, shampoos, body wash, deodorant, makeup, the chemicals from our laundry detergent, even the petrochemicals that make up our clothing can be absorbed into the skin, into the gut, and the rest of our systems.

We will talk more about chemicals in a bit, but it's important to note that even if you didn't eat it, it can get into your gut via your bloodstream through the pores of your skin or even through the air that you breathe. Although the amounts may be small, the daily use of anything chemical will eventually have a detrimental effect, even if a very subtle one. There is a build-up that happens. Many of these chemicals also disrupt the endocrine and nervous systems, which we will discuss in a moment.

It's a no-brainer to know that what's going on in your gut directly affects your overall health, your mind, your thoughts, your actions, and even your emotions. If the gut is overwhelmed and out of balance, chances are, your life will be off as well.

A variety of physical symptoms that indicate gut and bowel issues can be fatigue, brain fog, memory issues, nausea, constipation, diarrhea, indigestion, weakness, pain, poor wound healing, sleep problems, along with gut diseases like Crohn's disease, colitis, and irritable bowel syndrome. These are generally caused by diet, stress, nutrient imbalances, medications, and even organisms causing issues to the sensitive, delicate interior lining and balance of the digestive system.

Did you know that 70% of our immune system also lies in our gut? The immune system includes the lymphatic system (which we will talk about next) which is lined throughout the intestinal system. It keeps track of the organisms and bacteria in the gut to the best of its ability. If there are negative or bad organisms present in our gut, the immune system sends in immune cells and antibodies to help take care of any bacteria, viruses, fungus, or parasites who want to make a home in there.

In 1985, a wise man by the name of Dr. Norman Walker passed away at the ripe old age of 99 years old. He was the first man to invent a hydraulic vegetable juice press. He is also well-known for his concepts and scientific theories around food and health. One of his biggest theories was that cooked food is dead food, because the food's vitality is not retained, *meaning the necessary enzymes and amino acids in the food are no longer present.* He believed eating a mostly raw fruit and vegetable diet (including lots of juicing) was both nutritionally sound as well as that it starved cancer. He was adamant that the source of all life was already available to us. Eating vibrant, fresh, natural, healthy foods that contain natural enzymes help our bodies digest the food easily and absorb the nutrients from the food properly.

Understanding all these connections empowers us to make better decisions about our health and what we choose to ingest. Truly, what we eat affects everything. Unfortunately, we have been allowed to devour just about anything and everything in sight whether it's real food or fake. They've even allowed "edible" plastics into our foods, not to mention other unsound and unsafe ingredients.

Then we're so used to throwing everything in at once, one food right on top of the other, totally unconsciously, because we're unaware of how it will affect us. We weren't taught anything about this. We just figure that our body takes care of everything without fail. Of course, this is not totally our fault for believing this to be the case, as we were never taught that combining certain foods could cause a problem for our digestive system.

People can argue about it, but it's a well-known fact that different foods require different enzymes to break down. The enzymes necessary for breaking down a carbohydrate are different than the ones used to break down a protein or a fat and so on. This constant overload eventually puts stress on the system, overwhelming it, and in turn creates difficulty in the breaking down of food and the absorption of its nutrients. It overloads the pancreas and liver, as well as the stomach itself.

Some quick and simple food combining knowledge is eating either a starch or grain with a vegetable, or eating meat or protein with a vegetable. It's the starch and grains combined with meat and protein products that overwhelm the system enzymatically. Surely, the body is amazing and can handle a lot, but it's the continuous overdoing of it all, that creates difficulties for the digestive system and all of its components. As an FYI, another big food combining rule is that most fruits should be eaten alone, especially melons. Though as I will mention below, a few can assist in digestion.

We can support our gut in lots of ways, besides transforming our diets, adding probiotics and enzymes can be of help. We can take a supplemental probiotic daily, either in capsule form, or some people like food versions of probiotics such as Kefir which is a liquid version of a high probiotic yogurt.

Fermented foods like sauerkraut and kimchi contain enzymes and probiotics that are helpful for your gut, as well as drinks like Kombucha. Enzymes can be taken before meals to assist with digestion and are available in capsule form. Papaya, pineapple, and apples are helpful digestives, papaya enzymes are sold in tablet form, as well as Bromelain which comes from pineapples.

Bitters or a bitter herbal drink is taken in other countries prior to a meal to stimulate digestion and help keep the food moving through the system well. They can even relieve symptoms such as bloating, gas, and sensitivities to food allergens. Some of the bitter herbs used are gentian, barberry, artichoke, and dandelion. There are herbs that also stimulate digestion such as fennel, ginger, cardamom, dill, and lemon balm. Charcoal is another agent that helps with bloating, gas, and toxins in our food.

Of course, cleansing out the system is the number one way and the key for a healthy gut from the bowels to the liver. In my eyes, it's hands down something everyone should do several times a year. Clearing out the congestion in our digestive organs will relieve a lot of the burden that is put on the other organs and systems. There is also great significance in doing a liver flush, as most of us already have all of the ingredients needed for it. I will list a few books in the back that are my go-to for liver care.

THE GREAT LYMPHATIC SYSTEM

When we hear about our lymphatic system from the medical field, it's usually because of a problem that is going on with, or a problem that *includes* it, most of the time being cancer. Unfortunately, the lymphatic system doesn't get a lot of attention beyond that, but its significance is vast and worth talking about even if you don't have a diagnosed problem around it.

The lymphatic system is part of our immune system and is a network that runs throughout the entire body just like our nervous system and circulatory systems do. It consists of lymph nodes, lymphatic vessels, and is connected to the other immune system organs such as the thymus gland, the spleen, the kidneys, and the bone marrow. The lymph nodes generally live in clusters that are laced throughout the body, even found in the head, around the brain. These vessels and nodes are found in the neck, arms, legs and torso as well as that they are found laced throughout the intestines, the liver, kidneys, pancreas, spleen, reproductive system, and spinal cord.

The lymphatic system is important for several reasons. It is known to maintain fluid levels in the body. It absorbs fats from the digestive tract, releases white blood cells to assist on attacking invading organisms, and is also a transporter for cellular waste products and dead or abnormal cells.

Our lymph nodes produce fighter cells, and they also filter and clean the lymphatic fluid. The wastes from within the lymph system are filtered through the kidneys and are excreted in the urine. Filtered lymphatic fluid transports immune cells that are produced in the lymph nodes back into the bloodstream to help fight off invading organisms.

The lymphatic system is a complex system that works to cleanse, strengthen, and protect our body.

It's easy to get a backed up lymphatic system, because it doesn't have a pump to move things along like the circulatory system has with the heart. Once it starts getting clogged up, issues begin to slowly arise. The lymph system is the *cancer cell remover* of the body and works with a team (spleen, thymus, bone marrow, lymph nodes) who help to produce the cells that *kill* the cancer cells. It is also the garbage disposal for all of our body's dead cells, so it's important to realize the massive significance in its continuous flow and movement.

When a lymph node swells up or becomes hardened, it's because of stagnancy or a buildup. A hardened lymph node causes a blockage that slows down or stops the flow of the lymphatic fluid movement in that vessel. It's like if a blood vessel were to be clogged, it stops the flow to the area. People may then find pain, swelling, and calcification (hardening) of the nodes in the area. If left untreated, this congestion can lead to what is usually diagnosed as cancer of the lymph node or system.

A stagnant lymphatic system is definitely a cause for concern as the body is no longer getting rid of all the dead and unwanted cells and their debris properly. And if your kidneys are clogged up too, they are unable to filter out the lymphatic waste, which is definitely going to be a problem at some point down the line.

It's a good idea to be more attentive to our lymphatic system and to do things to keep it healthy and moving. We can do simple things during our days to help keep it moving or to get it moving better. Dry skin brushing every morning before your shower and every evening is ultimately very powerful. Rinsing off at the end of a shower with cold water, stimulates the lymphatic system. Cold plunges stimulate the lymph flow. Bouncing on a rebounder helps to move lymph, and even happens to be the equivalent to jogging, so it's a two for one. Castor oil packs can soften hardened lymph nodes and are a genuine life-saver.

When it comes to food, grapes are a master fruit for the lymphatic system, as they are the powerhouses that help break up lymphatic stagnancy (especially the seeds). There are many herbs that help to break up and move congested lymph such as chaparral, poke root, plantain leaf, red clover, parsley, white oak bark, along with many others. These can also be used to help fight infections that the lymphatic system may be having a hard time with. Let's not forget that we do need our kidneys to be in good working in order to be able to help filter out the lymphatic waste.

As I briefly mentioned, one of the most perfect foods on this planet that assist with cleansing out the lymphatic system are grapes. The darker the grape the better, if seeded is available, even better. Grapes are known as "the queen of fruits" because of their powerful abilities and actions. They are considered one of the most potent of all medicinal foods. The juice of grapes is considered "the nectar of the gods" and "vegetarian milk". Here's some more info on this delicious fruit:

- Powerful cleanser, assists with acid overload (acidosis), constipation. High magnesium content.
- Excellent detoxifiers against battling acidosis, helping to detoxify kidneys, liver, the gastrointestinal tract, and the blood.
- Eliminates poisons from the system.
- The ellagic acid in grapes were found to scavenge carcinogens (cancer-causers) as it moves through and out the body.
- The skin of grapes contains an anti-oxidant called Resveratrol that protects against cancer, heart disease, and other health conditions
- The simple sugars of the grape can be easily utilized by the cells for their metabolism.
- The **seeds** of the grape contain tartaric acid which helps break down hardened deposits and mucus from the system. Seeds can be irritating to those with colitis or ulcers.
- Excellent blood builders due to its high iron and magnesium content.
- Grape juice combined with a nut milk "furnishes the system with new blood of the purest kind and is an excellent remedy for anemia" (from *Whole Foods Companion -book listed in reference section*).

Since I mentioned that the kidneys need to be unclogged, and before I close out on the lymphatic system, I will mention a powerful food for unclogging the kidneys and breaking up the built-up waste within them. And that wonderfully, powerful food is watermelon.

Watermelon is the most hydrating fruit, made up of 92% water and it contains powerful enzymes that help break up the gunk that's clogging up the kidneys. I know people view eating only one fruit for a meal or just fruit seems crazy and unhealthy, but this is where a meal of just one thing is powerful and healing beyond measure. Here's the benefit of eating one of nature's tastiest, water-filled, and powerful cleansers:

- Excellent cleanser and detoxifier for the whole body
- Breaks down inorganic minerals stuck in the body, dissolving them. Helps to flush out toxic deposits in the kidneys
- Releases tension on the blood vessels and arteries, assisting with blood pressure
- Great for heart health due to its high content of **lycopene**. Lycopene works to protect your cells from damage
- Nature's safest diuretic, very quick ability to wash out the bladder
- The rind has highest organic sodium in nature as well as that the green outside has a high content of chlorophyll. Good for juicing. Rich in nutrients
- Contains an amino acid called citrulline, which helps relax blood vessels and improve blood flow. Helpful with sleep and for the muscles, especially the heart
- Contains an amino acid called arginine, which helps increase blood flow and oxygen to the brain. Helpful with brain cognition and function, including mood
- The seeds are a potent, dense source of magnesium, zinc, and iron (so don't spit them out, chew them up)
- Helpful for mental depression due to the magnesium and high Vitamin B6 content

Of course, there are other powerful foods and herbs to assist the kidneys such as cranberries, lemons, apples, grapes, berries, cabbage, celery root, mushrooms, seaweed, buckwheat, juniper, basil, nettle, dandelion, parsley, and burdock root. We can talk more about the healing properties of food in a little while, I just wanted to give you a glimpse of some impactful foods that can have an empowering effect on the lymph and kidneys.

THE POWERFUL AND MIGHTY ENDOCRINE SYSTEM

This mighty system of glands in our body, play a huge role in how well all of our other organ systems run. In my personal opinion, this is one of the most important systems in the body. It is sometimes known as the *hormone system* because these glands are the parts of the body that create and release the hormones that are needed to coordinate all of the different functions within the body. The endocrine system is made up of the hypothalamus, pituitary gland, pineal gland, thymus gland, thyroid gland, parathyroid gland, adrenal glands, pancreas, prostate, and ovaries. Let's take a peek at what they do and what it looks like if they are in trouble.

Hypothalamus: Known to be the king gland, located in the brain. It's the main link between the nervous system and endocrine system. It receives information from the nervous system, communicating with the pituitary gland who then sends messages to the other glands in the body as to what is needed.

The hypothalamus assists with our growth hormones, as well as our dopamine production (the 'feel good' neurotransmitter). The hypothalamus helps to keep our body in balance assisting with body temperature, stress, and everyday bodily rhythms. It plays a large part in our mood regulation, sleep, sexual function, hunger and thirst.

Weakness in the hypothalamus affects height or body growth in childhood and can cause premature or delayed puberty. It can also lead to headaches and visual issues, including the loss thereof.

Pituitary Gland: This tiny gland is so important and powerful, and is the main growth gland. It sits right below the hypothalamus within the brain and works directly with it. The pituitary controls other glands such as the adrenals, thyroid, ovaries and testicles. It is responsible for

45

letting the other glands know when they're needed, signaling for them to get to work. It produces our growth hormones and plays important roles in sexuality and fertility.

Weakness in the pituitary gland would mainly cause growth problems, but being that it is the master to the rest of the glands, weakness in the pituitary gland can cause problems and weakening of the other glands. There may be neurological problems when this gland gets weak, as well as a generalized underactivity of the main bodily functions.

Pineal Gland: This small, pinecone-shaped gland sits right in the middle of our head yet gets very little mention other than for its use in creating and releasing melatonin. However, this gland is quite powerful. Scientists and experts have stated that the pineal gland is more powerful and complex than the brain itself. It creates a hormone known as dimethyltryptamine, or DMT. DMT is released during birth, during dreaming, and near-death experiences. It assists the pineal gland in creating and releasing melatonin. DMT and melatonin bring about a sense of peace, relaxation, and a meditative state. Keeping this gland healthy is very important for sleep, as the presence of delta, theta, and gamma brainwaves activate the pineal gland.

Sunlight and bright light also help in activating the pineal gland. Historically, before modern medical knowledge, this gland was widely recognized as the third eye, believed to have the ability to access dreams. It played a significant role in the dream state, particularly in Egyptian culture. In ancient knowledge it was spoken to be the *seat of the soul*. The Buddhists knew it as a symbol of spiritual awakening. In Hinduism it is known as the seat of intuition and clairvoyance. Ancient Greeks believed it to be the connection to our thoughts. For thousands of years both Eastern and Western beliefs believed this gland to be our connection to the spiritual world.

Pineal gland weakness affects one's sleep state, as well as the connection to their dream state. DMT and melatonin stop being released when the pineal gland hardens from buildup, which is caused by certain chemicals ingested such as fluoride and heavy metals. Iodine can help push heavy metals out. Staring into complete darkness activates hormones, that assist on breaking down the buildup around the gland. Sunlight and bright light activate it, however *blue* light from screens cause damage to this gland.

Adrenal Glands: These two walnut sized glands sit on top of each kidney. Another superior gland(s) with a very big job. The adrenals are best known for the 'fight or flight' response when we are in a dangerous, traumatic, or stressful situation where they release adrenaline and epinephrine to either help us get away quickly, or stick around and take on the threat.

They also release cortisol which helps to relieve the body of inflammation and aids the immune system. The adrenals help regulate metabolism and blood pressure. They speak directly to the autonomic nervous system which controls breathing and heart rate. The adrenals also have a direct effect on and some control over the thyroid and parathyroid.

Imbalances or weaknesses in the adrenals can cause some chaos in the body. Adrenal weakness can lead to nervous system issues such as anxiety, restlessness, and nervousness. Weakness in this gland can create overwhelm, fatigue, body aches, poor appetite, susceptibility to infections, breathing problems, heart arrythmias, and digestive issues.

Adrenal weakness will affect the thyroid and parathyroid, as they both take cues from the adrenals. If the adrenals are overworked and stressed out, they will cause the thyroid to put out extra hormones causing thyroid weakness. This is also true for ovaries and testes, as adrenal weakness affects their functioning as well.

Thyroid Gland: This butterfly shaped gland is found directly in our neck and throat area. It is the key to our metabolism, temperature control, and the rate and strength of the heartbeat and respirations. It sends signals to the body to produce more muscle and skeletal cells.

Many people suffer from low thyroid function, sadly the percentage is increasing. This low function or weakness is when the thyroid is not making enough of the necessary hormones needed for the body. Symptoms of an underactive thyroid include: bone loss, hair loss, brittle fingernails, cold hands and feet, dislike of cold weather, heart arrythmias, heart attacks, depression, muscle pain, weakness, connective tissue weakness, scoliosis, slow metabolism, weight gain, constipation, dry skin, fatigue, obesity, hot flashes, spasms, cramps, and growth issues.

The thyroid can also be overactive and produce too many thyroid hormones where a person loses weight, suffers from a rapid heart rate, nervousness, irritability, fatigue, shaky hands, muscle weakness, and an enlargement in the neck otherwise known as a goiter. The thyroid is weakened by toxins in our environment such as pesticides, radiation, and other various chemicals, which are also found in our personal care products and foods. Certain medications such as beta-blockers, diabetic medications, pain killers, anti-seizure meds, anti-depressants and anti-psychotics actually contribute to weakness of the thyroid.

If the body is in a constant state of inflammation due to diet, especially due to the intake of a lot of sugar and animal protein, the thyroid becomes taxed. Pituitary and adrenal disorders can cause thyroid issues, as well as not getting enough iodine in your diet. Pregnancy can also cause weakness in this gland as well as in the parathyroid.

Parathyroid Gland: This gland actually consists of four disc-like glands that are embedded in the thyroid gland. Both the parathyroid and thyroid play a large part in the use and absorption of calcium. The parathyroid secretes its own hormone which works to control calcium levels in the body. This hormone known as the parathyroid hormone (PTH) helps maintain calcium levels in the bloodstream and the tissues, as well as controlling phosphorous and Vitamin D levels. Calcium affects the connective tissues in the body, as well as the muscle tissues of the body, being a key factor in the contraction of the heart muscle.

Tiredness, fatigue, and brain fog are among the symptoms of a weak parathyroid. Again, connected to the thyroid, many of the weaknesses in the thyroid affect the parathyroid. Calcium levels are affected with this gland's weakness, as the parathyroid helps to control the absorption of calcium. A lack of calcium for the body causes weakness in the connective tissues which include the walls and lining of the organs and vessels, as well as the bones.

Decrease in calcium levels can contribute to mental health symptoms such as depression. Low parathyroid function affects the heart muscles and vessels, intestines, bladder wall, blood pressure, the immune system and the nervous system. When the parathyroid is weak it may respond by becoming overactive increasing the production of the parathyroid hormone, which then causes an *increase* in the calcium levels in the blood, known as hyperparathyroidism. High calcium levels can cause blood pressure issues, heart arrythmias, kidney problems, and can also be an indicator of cancer.

Thymus Gland: This gland is part of the endocrine, lymphatic, and immune system. It is located in the center of the chest, behind the breastbone, in between the lungs. The thymus gland is considered the master gland of the immune system. It secretes the hormone thymosin which assists T-cells in maturing. T-cells are the white blood cells known as the *natural killer cells* of the body. They kill damaged cells and pathogens like cancer, viruses, fungus, and parasites. T-cells are created by stem cells in the bone marrow, then travel to the thymus gland where they mature and head to the spleen.

The thymus also produces the hormone thymopoietin which affects the rate at which your skin ages. You can help activate the thymus by tapping a few fingers on the area of the breastbone in front of it. You will also notice that this tapping invigorates and energies you instantly.

This is one where weakness is not seen through symptoms like some of the other glands. A person can be born with a genetic or chromosomal issues that affect the thymus gland which will present as childhood illness such as immune system problems, developmental underdevelopment, and a range of disabilities.

If issues arise as an adult which likely coincide with immunity problems and other weaknesses, there can be symptoms such as shortness of breath, weight loss, night sweats, wheezing, chest pain, coughing, fatigue, and overall lowered immunity. Myasthenia gravis is associated to thymus weakness and also labeled as a cause to thymus gland enlargement and disorder.

Pancreas: The pancreas is both an endocrine (actually an exocrine) gland and an organ of the digestive system. It releases the hormone insulin, which regulates blood sugar levels. The pancreas also releases pancreatic digestive enzymes that we need for the digestion of carbohydrates, proteins, and fats.

Pancreatic weakness can show up genetically as cystic fibrosis. Weakness of this organ is generally created by dietary choices. Pancreatitis can occur which is the inflammation of the pancreas generally caused by high sugar, chronic alcohol intake, long-standing digestive and liver issues, parasites, or can be caused by other toxins or organisms. Poor dietary habits are indeed taxing on the pancreas, overworking it to exhaustion. Cancer can also show up in the pancreas.

Ovaries: These 2 glands are found in women and are located on either side of the uterus attached by the fallopian tubes. The ovaries produce eggs and the hormones estrogen and progesterone, as well as relaxin and inhibin, which are responsible for female body changes, menstruation, fertility, and everything to do with childbirth.

Weakness in the ovaries can show up as growth of cysts or tumors, ovarian fibroids, fertility issues, hormone imbalances, menstruation issues, difficult menopause, and cancer.

Testes: The testes are the 2 glands found in the scrotum on males. The testes secrete testosterone which is primary male sex hormone, and categorized actually as a steroid. Testosterone is necessary for male growth like deepening of the voice, hair growth, and increased muscle strength and size. It plays a role in bone density and acts to increase exercise endurance and energy. The testes produce the sperm that are responsible for male fertility. Healthy testosterone is essential for the whole body's cellular health.

Issues with the testes are sexual organ and fertility issues, growth problems, erectile dysfunction, muscle development issues, low testosterone levels, metabolic problems, and cancer.

WHAT CAN WE DO FOR OUR ENDOCRINE SYSTEM?

A good place to start is to let go of using some of the products that are hard on our endocrine glands which are known as *endocrine disruptors*. This is a well-known scientific term for chemicals that actually harm and damage our endocrine glands. They interfere with the body's hormones causing developmental and reproductive issues, as well as brain, nervous system, and immune system difficulties.

Sadly, they are put into just about everything we use these days. These chemicals are commonly found in our everyday personal body care and household products and are found everywhere; in schools, homes, workplaces, in the polyester clothing we wear, our food and water, as well as plastic bottles and containers (BPA and phalates), liners of metal food cans, detergents, flame retardants (in fabrics), processed food and beverages, toys, building materials, lawn care and garden products, sunscreens, automobile interiors, and so on.

Other insults to our Endocrine system are heavy metals, which can also be found in our personal care products like in women's make up. Heavy metals have even been found in baby food, formulas, and baby products. Arsenic and lead can be found in household products, water supplies, food colorings, cosmetics, perfumes, fragrances, petrochemicals, non-stick coatings, carpets, furniture, bed foam, soy products, and in pesticides/herbicides (like atrazine used on corn crops). There are also heavy metals found in the air nowadays that are being released for various reasons.

Diagnoses, medically and scientifically linked to these known disruptors are: ADHD, Autism, lowered immunity, metabolism problems, premature puberty, change in sex characteristics, reduce reproductive abilities, increase bodily fat, kidney breakdown, cancer, and changes in sensitivity to insulin. Endocrine disruptors are also linked to cancerous tumors, birth defects, and other developmental disorders. Websites with good information on these disruptors and their effects on the body (here in the US, where most of these disruptors continue to be utilized) are EPA.gov, NIH.gov. There are studies and Ted talks by doctors on www.endocrinedisruption.org.

Now that we know this, let's talk about what we can do to support the Endocrine system besides doing our best to use less, toxic products. Did you know that the best foods for the endocrine system are berries? Berries are one of nature's most powerfully packed, nutrient dense, fast foods. Berries contain anti-oxidants, polyphenols, high amounts of essential vitamins, quercetin, resveratrol, rutin, and anthocyanins which all fight cancers and free radicals. Berries have anti-inflammatory properties. They tone and strengthen the Endocrine glands. Other foods and supplements that feed and nourish our Endocrine glands are:

- Greens and green superfood powders that contain ingredients like wheatgrass, alfalfa, moringa, spirulina, chlorella, barley grass, spinach, sprouts, broccoli, kale
- Mineral rich foods or supplements- seaweeds- Kelp, Irish sea moss, Shilajit, trace mineral supplements
- Citrus fruits
- Avocados, Bananas, Dates
- Nuts and seeds (such as pumpkin seeds, flax seeds, hemp seeds)
- Goji berries, Ginseng
- Beans, lentils
- Garlic
- Sweet potatoes, potatoes
- Mushrooms, especially Reishi, Cordyceps, and Lions Mane
- Selenium, Vitamin D, B-12, Zinc
- Animal products: pasture raised eggs, wild-caught salmon, sardines, grass-fed beef
- Herbs such as Astragalus root, Parsley root, Schizandra Berry, Dandelion leaf, Saw Palmetto

The Nervous system is a super powerful system that also deserves recognition. It runs so many parts of our function including breathing, heart rate, movement, thought, and so on. It's vital and has other systems that it works with.

Dr. Joe Dispenza notes how the nervous system is the greatest pharmacist in the world, it makes greater drugs than any drug in the pharmacy. There is data that suggests that when you put the blood of an advanced meditator on a uterine cancer cell or pancreatic cancer cell, 70% of the mitochondrial function of the cancer cell is diminished. Our nervous system does way more than we ever thought it could. It's worth looking into further.

HOMEWORK:

1. If you want to get a bit of an idea of what your pH is like, there are pH test strips to test urine or saliva. What foods can you add to your diet to balance out your pH if your diet is too acidic?
2. Do you have any problems with your gut and intestinal health? Can you think about and identify anything that might be a cause for this problem? Stress, foods, medications?
3. What steps can you take to improve your gut health?
4. How connected are you to your gut feelings? Have you noticed them, ever make a decision based on them? Do you feel like you should hone in this more?
5. Do you have or have you had any lymphatic issues? What steps can you take to improve the health of this system?
6. Do you have a diagnosed endocrine gland problem? If not, do you have reason to believe that any of your endocrine glands are stressed out or not working at their best? What can you do on your end to help support these glands and this system with your diet, avoidance of things, or actions?

FOOD iS yOUR MEDiCiNE

M ost of us think nothing more of food than in the fact that we eat it simply to give our body energy to survive. While this is mostly true, there's a lot about food we really don't think about. We've been so lucky to have food put here upon the Earth to help nourish us and to take care of our bodies. It's already ready to go, in perfect form to feed the essential needs of our body. It works in harmony with our body on every level, chemically, energetically, and biologically. It is indeed, our medicine because it keeps us nourished and everything in our body working well.

However, the food of today is not what it once was. Unfortunately, much has been lost so we need to be wise and get to know a lot more about food than we once thought we ever needed to know. At some point soon, we need to make some serious changes to what's been done to our food and return it back to being strictly nourishing and health promoting, and to its original state. There's been tons of manipulation and chemicalization done that is very much causing us harm.

For the most part we can choose whatever we want to eat as we have total control over what we put into our mouth. We have a variety of choices, some being healthy and good for us, many others, not. If we can find a healthy balance in our diets, wonderful, but unfortunately, in our present day, it seems many of us have lost control or the knowledge around food, and what or how to eat it.

Our health can thrive because of food, or fall into ill health because of it. We know for most of us, at least here in the US, that our choices are endless. We even have an option to eat and include foods into our diet that aren't healthy for us. These unhealthier foods can open us up to possible disease and health issues down the line. Poor nutrition and unhealthy diets stress the body and lead to weakness. However, if we choose mostly wholesome, nutritious foods, disease and health problems are less likely to manifest.

With all of the foods out there made available to us today, it's easy for us to make those unhealthier choices. There are so many kinds of foods created now, many of which do not even come from natural food sources. Even the foods that are grown from the ground have been changed, altered, contain chemicals, and lack the nutrients that they once had because of industrialization and over-farming. Chemicals are added to increase crop growth, size, and speed up the timing.

There's a lot being done to our food that is quite literally, detrimental to our health. It's very important for us, at this time, to be more aware of what we eat and actively work on making healthier choices so we can live longer and enjoy this beautiful life. We want our food to support our body and its cells, because our body is this living, magnificent vehicle that we need to be able to do all of the beautiful things we want to do in our life. Food is meant to nourish and support our bodies, but unfortunately, it's become more complicated, less nutritional, and highly modified, and we're losing control at the helm of it all. The food industry has changed the way food is and unless you grow your own, we are at the hands of this industry's decisions.

We all know that the foods that grow out of the ground are always going to be the most health-promoting ones for us, due to the fact that they have the highest content of naturally occurring vitamins, minerals, and fatty acids that support our body's optimal wellbeing and function. Some foods even have other beneficial aspects in them that are medicinal to us, such as having cancer fighting properties or ones that strengthen our immune system, and other organ systems. There are many ways earth grown food can positively impact our bodies. Good food helps us to fight off disease.

Then there are the foods that hurt our body. Many of them have little to no nutritional value, and a lot of them even contain ingredients that our bodies either can't use or ones that can actually cause harm to our body. These foods are unfortunately highly chemicalized, sprayed, genetically manipulated, and highly processed. Unfortunately, the industry has tainted and contaminated our food on one level or another, making it challenging to avoid these issues entirely. This has affected not only conventional products but also wholesome, healthy, and even our organic food.

Fast-food hamburgers, for example, have chemicals added to enhance flavor, improve the texture or appearance of the food, preserve it, and sometimes as a more cost-effective alternative to using natural ingredients. It's not just one flavoring for that charcoal grilled taste, there are a lot of chemicals added just for that one *flavor*. You're not just getting ground up beef on a bun. The buns themselves even have many additives to ensure 'freshness' and a soft consistency that people desire.

Unfortunately, we've forgotten about the concept of our food as our medicine, as it's not talked about or taught, and certainly hasn't been a significant part of the health care philosophy, if at all.

Knowing what we know now, if food and the diet was the first thing that was looked at with someone who was struggling with health problems, it would change the trajectory that person's healing outcome. Whether it be the diet they were eating, or in adding foods *to* their diets, food would have an absolute impact on their recovery and healing process.

Thankfully, there's been a lot more attention being put onto it right now, studies are being done within the nutritional sector of the health industry, due to the growing interest around nutrition and food, and its impact on our health. Everyday people like you and I are beginning to realize that it's a bigger piece to the puzzle than we've been lending credit to.

What we're learning is just a rediscovery of old knowledge that's been around for centuries, if not thousands of years. Our ancestors understood food was nourishment that could help the body heal itself, just as well as they understood the wisdom behind plants being medicinal. It's so good that we're starting to recognize this, recognizing that many of our solutions are in the foods we eat.

Some foods or diets can help relieve us from disease or illness, and some can send us down the harrowing road towards disease and illness. People are starting to connect the dots and truly see that what we eat is affecting our health in big ways. All things edible aren't necessarily good for us to eat, so now our realizations are creating an empowering movement towards taking our food more seriously. The more we desire to find out what's in our food, the more moves we can make to create better choices for ourselves.

The American Society for Nutrition is the first organization that I noticed working with nutrition as an actual solution to people's health problems and part of the plan for them. They are currently creating programs that consist of *medically* tailored meals, *medically* tailored grocery lists, and what they call "produce prescription programs". (I pray this will become the **main** part of every doctor's health plan, eventually.) How empowering to receive actual instructions and a shopping list from your doctor?

In my eyes, the foods in the hospitals and healthcare institutions should only be healing, health-promoting, nutritious foods, because those struggling with their health need all the help they can get. And a lot of the time, diet and nutrition are part of the reason why they aren't well.

Seeing the sadness around the food offered to the sick throughout my career was a big let-down. It's why I decided to get into nutrition, the holistic side of it, in hopes I could incorporate it into my care. It wasn't well received at the hospitals I tried to make something happen in, but I did what I could on the side with my patients.

If it were up to me, the first thing I would do for hospitals would be to create a healthy menu with a variety of wholesome foods for the patients to ingest. Then I would start a garden on the grounds or maybe even on the roof of the facility. The cooks of the hospital would use the freshly grown ingredients in the food that they created for the patients. The foods that would be offered would only be nourishing and full of vital nutrients. As an added benefit, the patients would be able to participate in helping to care for the garden so that they could learn about growing and eating healthy food.

This would be so therapeutic and immersive, getting them to engage in this would help to create a deeper connection for them, as well as that they would gain a new found appreciation for healthy, earth grown food. Tasting something one helped to grow, is not only a physical, healthy experience but also a spiritual one. Going through this process would also create more of a desire and the motivation to go home and continue eating healthier, cleaner foods, and perhaps even starting a garden of their own, growing food for themselves.

Another beautiful thing we could do in the healthcare world would be to create home-based programs. These programs would help people to learn about food, its connection to their health, and how to prepare it, all while in the comfort and familiarity of their home environment. The effects would be more powerful and in turn help them establish new eating habits within their home, for themselves and their family, giving them tools that they can use in their everyday lives.

These home sessions would be created to help that person work through whatever layers around food that holds them back. There's a lot to our mindset around food. The process would go at a comfortable, steady pace to ensure it be long-lasting and that the knowledge and tools are retained. This would create a solid foundation for them to work from, independently and with the ones they love.

As part of the in-home education, we would take a look at what's in the pantry and their fridge, see what they're used to eating, and get their kitchen organized and clean to a place where they can start fresh. Imagine how great that would be! Then, together, we can discuss simple and powerful information about food, exploring its benefits or drawbacks, acquiring a wealth of beautiful knowledge along the way. Even during the clean out process, a lot can be discussed perhaps triggering questions or things they might have wanted to ask, or hadn't even thought about. This type of positive and supportive program would be very rewarding for them, creating a new momentum or enthusiasm, feeling proud of themselves for trying new things, making changes, and reaching goals. It would be so very empowering. It would also be to help them learn how to be creative in the kitchen.

A vital part of the program would be going to the grocery store, doing a grocery store tour, to get them familiar with things they never knew about and to find options, alternative to the ones they've been so used to eating. It's such a rewarding and eye-opening activity- the act of walking through a grocery store and getting to know about different foods and trying new things is so profound for most people. There would definitely be approximately three trips to the store together to really get things set into place, because their mind will be transforming and changing with time as they move through their transformational food journey. They would have a new mindset by the end of the program, which in my perspective needs to be about three to six months long depending on where they're at.

Of course, there would be simple recipes and weekly cooking sessions where basic skills are taught and where the motivation is built, as well as homework. This sets people up to be empowered in themselves, realizing the healing potential that food has on them, and how being a part of creating it, as well as eating its goodness, makes it medicinal for them on so many levels.

There would also be cooking classes out in the community, which there are some of those already, but there would be a lot more of them, as well as an actual building or section of the hospital built specifically for this purpose.

In my opinion, both of these are absolutely vital to the healing and wellbeing of every person who is ill with something. If they aren't able to participate due to disabilities or age, the family or a surrogate would step in for this.

There would also be a medical healthy food delivery service like some of the ones already out there, but would consist of *only* healthy, healing foods, even juices and smoothies. Doctors would order whatever one or a combination of these that's most appropriate. Food education and counseling would probably be prescribed for again, at least three to six months. This would be ideal for those who are homebound and very ill. There would be someone to assist with emotional support as well.

Let's talk about what's in and on our food a bit again, as well as to how it's being made, and some of the practices that occur to produce it. The food we eat either nourishes our body and keeps it healthy and youthful, or it weighs it down, ages it more rapidly, and creates grounds for illness to occur.

The thing is, some of the food, even healthy for us, is loaded with unnatural ingredients. Unless you buy food from a local farm, it's tough to avoid the chemicals sprayed, and of course, this includes our fruits, veggies, grains, and animal products. There are chemicals and drugs that are used on and in them, for production and because of mass industrialization.

There is also genetic modification which many believe is amazing so food can be produced at massive, quick rates, but there's always a kicker to something like that. Turns out GMOs have been proven to be harmful. Many countries have banned and continue to ban these foods, as it has been found that these foods are linked to cancer and other disease forming in the body, as well as causing mutations in our own genetics and DNA.

One very popular item we eat is flour. It's in practically everything, kind of like sugar. The quote *"the whiter the bread, the sooner you're dead,"* has stuck with me for years. We as a people, have known for quite some time now, that highly processed, refined flour is **not** the biggest friend to our digestive system, especially our intestines, liver, and pancreas. To boot, there's a growing number of people becoming gluten-intolerant, diabetic, and developing diseases such as celiac disease.

A study was done on rats who consumed white flour as the main part of their meals on a daily basis. It was proven and shown to cause diabetes in these rats, all of them. Popular medical websites will even tell you that processed white refined flour can lead to diabetes, heart disease, and obesity, so they are highly aware that this stuff causes enormous health issues within our bodies.

The flour of today lacks the nutrients it once had, due to the over farming, soil depletion, pesticides, herbicides, and genetic modification of the crop. It's nothing like what it was a hundred or two hundred years ago. It's become devoid of nutrients so they have to add in, or *fortify* the flour with synthetic nutrients to replace the ones that were lost.

The finer, powder form that flour now comes in, wasn't always the way it used to be processed. Unfortunately, these finer particles are actually much harder on our body. This powdered form has a tendency to make it easy for the flour to stick around, considering the fact that it's in the body with a temperature of 98.6+ degrees while it attempts to travel through forty plus feet of intestines.

We all know from when we were kids making paper mâché, that when flour is combined with water, it becomes sticky and glue-like, and we used it for art projects. Think about this combination trying to make its way through all of our intestines without getting stuck in the turns, curves, and ridges. A friend once referred to it, for lack of a better term, as "clogger-upper" of sorts.

White sugar is also an unfortunately harmful substance for our body. It's highly acid forming due to all of its processing, which then creates zero nutritional value with added chemicals. Actual sugar cane in its raw form *has* nutritional value, with high vitamin and mineral content. The refined sugar we buy off the shelves, is the stuff that weakens our immune systems especially, is not good for our kidneys, our lymphatic system, and is terribly hard on our pancreas and liver. It is yet another vehicle to take us down the road to diabetes and heart disease. Sugar is big time linked to cancer, as cancer feeds off of sugar as one of its favorite food sources.

The process of refining both white flour and white sugar is quite extensive and requires several chemicals including chlorine, bromates, peroxides, polymers, biocides, and colorings for that white look. It's unfortunate the stuff that is used and said to be needed to prevent bacterial growth and shelf stabilization, is also very harmful to us.

In 1933, Dr. William Howard published the book *A New Health Era,* where he discusses that self-poisoning by accumulation of acids in the body being a major cause of many illnesses. He states that disease, no matter in what form of expression, is greatly caused by the accumulation of acids in the body. It doesn't help when we have a buildup and accumulation of food left lying around; this only contributes to elevating the acid level in the body. Old waste carries a very acidic pH.

Balance is essential. If we don't have a high percentage of alkalizing foods in our diets and eat mostly acid forming foods, it's easy to understand that the balance will be off, keeping us stuck in the acid side of chemistry which as we know is corrosive and problematic. Acid is hard on the body. The endless food choices that we have these days makes it quite difficult to keep things in balance. Most people's diets lean more on the acid side of things because most of our sustenance is based on dairy products, meat, seafood, fish, poultry, bread, pasta, crackers, cereals, grains, coffee, alcohol, soda, processed and boxed foods, junk foods, fast foods, fried foods, sugar, candy, baked goods and so on. The fruits and salads or vegetables are usually considered snacks or sides.

This has to be an average of 60-70%, if not more of most people's diets. All of the main foods in our meals are acid forming. If we've eaten a highly acidic diet for several decades or more, it's not hard to see that this will have a direct effect on our body essentially causing stress on it and health issues, especially when our body has been sitting in a highly acidic environment for prolonged period of time.

And as I mentioned earlier, we actually age faster with a highly acidic diet, and the accumulation of acids in our body creates pain, inflammation, and a host of other issues. Things don't work quite as well as they used to.

A lot of people have asked me, "well, what am I supposed to eat then?" I know it's difficult to see yourself filling up on vegetables, a big salad, or a bowl of fruit, but the truth is, you can. You just have to start by adding more of them into your diet bit by bit, eventually eating bigger portions. Of course, we have to begin somewhere. It's not as hard as we make it out to be, it's our mindset that actually keeps us from believing this to be possible. We indeed need to work on this, but the truth all around is that we can make a huge salad with a side of roasted root vegetables and walk away stuffed and satisfied! We just have to get over the initial hump and resistance that's been built.

One healthy food in, pushes one less healthy one out. Once we start feeling better, experiencing less pain, and losing some of the excess weight and waste we've been holding onto, our desire for the unhealthy foods will change. We'll even find ourselves thinking about and even craving the more, healthy foods.

How we combine our food has a large effect on how our food affects us as I mentioned briefly when talking about the gut. Some foods truly do not process well together, especially when we combine all of the kinds, which believe it or not, is so easy. We just need a three-course meal at a restaurant that gives us that icky feeling, some indigestion, and a feeling of fullness to realize this.

As I mentioned earlier, each type of food requires different enzymes to break them down and there is overwhelm for the digestive system when things don't mix well. The enzymes that break down carbohydrates are different than the ones that break down fats. The enzymes that break down meat products are different to the ones that break down dairy. Natural earth grown foods often already have enzymes available within them that will help with digestion such as papaya, mango, pineapple, ginger, miso, avocados, apricots, and kiwis. This also makes these fresh foods super easy on the body to digest, especially when eaten alone. Great cleansers.

When foods are constantly combined over and over again, eventually it causes overload and stress mode for the stomach and digestive organs. Things don't break down as efficiently anymore; the digestive process has slowed down, causing increased stress on the digestive organs. This slowdown leads to a myriad of complications, issues, and illnesses related to the digestive organs.

Our body needs a break sometimes, especially if it's getting this continuous influx of food all day long. All of its hard work in trying to get everything broken down and moved along takes a lot of energy. It actually consumes excess energy that the body could otherwise use to assist other areas of the body in repair and other functions.

There is something we can do occasionally or even on a daily basis to help relieve our body of all of this strain and stress. It's something we've all heard about by now, but perhaps something we don't know much about, and that is fasting. Fasting has been around for thousands of years, and for good reason. Fasting gives the body a much need break with a chance to cleanse and help heal itself where necessary without the interference. The body needs breaks, end of story. Luckily, it gets some digestive rest during our sleep cycle, however, some people eat fairly close to bedtime so the body then never gets the break it needs. It has to work on digestion on top of its usual repairing that it does while we're asleep. Our body does its best healing work while we're asleep.

Intermittent fasting in particular, isn't so overwhelmingly difficult to do if it's timed right. You can fast for 16 hours with 8 hours to eat, or 14 hours fasting with 10 hours to eat. Essentially, you're sleeping for about 8 of those 14 hours, so 3 hours of not eating on each end of the day, makes it seem pretty doable. This gives the body more time to take care of the things it needs to do, and no, you won't starve or deny your body essential nutrients, especially if you eat healthfully during the eating time period.

Now let's talk about labels. When it comes to eating packaged foods, start taking a look at the ingredient labels.

We've been taught to check labels for the amounts of calories, sugar, carbohydrates, sodium, and fat content, so much so that we've forgotten to look at the *actual* ingredients in the food which are more of what we need to be looking at, in my opinion. This reveals more of the truth about what it is that we're consuming.

Some products may have only a few ingredients listed, while others have thirty or more, many of which we can barely pronounce. They have a lot of chemical names that we seem to blindly trust is okay to be in our food products. Sometimes, we might even notice that it's hard to find any actual, real food ingredients in some of this *food*, which really makes you think twice. Checking the ingredients and being aware of what's in the food we're buying and eating will ultimately increase our awareness, guiding us towards making healthier, more honorable choices for ourselves and strengthening us in both body and mind.

Some of the ingredients are busy making us unwell without our knowledge, and even unhappy because a lot of these artificial foods and ingredients have a huge and direct impact on our gut and nervous system, which affects how we're feeling and how we're doing mentally. Afterall, our gut is directly linked to our nervous system, brain, and our moods. If we eat a lot of processed foods with preservatives and chemical ingredients, we are damaging our bodies and messing up our mental health. Becoming aware of what ingredients are and doing our best to avoid the especially terrible ones, will only help our health both physically and mentally in the long run.

It's been proven time and time again that a poor-quality diet (processed, chemicalized, and high acid producing foods) has a direct link to chronic disease, especially heart disease, diabetes, and cancer. There are so many studies that have been done and information out there to prove this, it's a wonder how these foods are even allowed to be available to us when they are proven to cause horrific health issues.

There are some popular studies that have been done on reversing disease through diet and through healthy eating, such as in the books *The China Study* by Thomas Campbell or *Reversing Heart Disease* by Dr. Dean Ornish or by Dr. Caldwell Esselsytn (both with the same book name). They contain studies, testimonials, and dietary instruction to help give someone the necessary knowledge to be able to do it themselves. There is endless proof that it is possible to heal our bodies through diet and nutrition. Of course, this goes for many other illnesses as well, as there are tons of beautiful books out there on disease and diet, especially in regards to cancer.

Doctors every now and again mention diet changes to their patients, perhaps by telling them to stop eating certain foods, or that they need to limit certain things like salt, sugar, or fat. They might even tell them to add more protein to their diet, but it generally doesn't go much further than the mention of it.

Usually, they recommend that the person see a dietician or nutritionist for more information and to discuss food around their disease-process. However, I'd say that more than half of the people fall away from the recommendations. I've seen it time and time again, have even been there myself. It's quite difficult for some of us to change our mindset and taste preferences around food when things are so deeply embedded. People need more than one or two discussions or handouts about food to make lasting, lifelong changes.

If someone has eaten a certain way for the last 50 years and is pretty set on the way and the things that they eat, they may have some issues adapting to new types of foods or ways of eating. They need a lot more time, and a lot of patience to bring in the necessary changes. They need to understand and embrace the information at their own pace and through their own choices.

Our eating habits and choices are influenced by a multitude of factors occurring on various levels. These include aspects such as our childhood and upbringing, education, physical and emotional well-being, psychological perspectives, and financial circumstances, whether prosperous or lacking. A lot of us also have emotional attachments to food.

You can always tell someone to stop eating a certain food and start eating another, but as I've witnessed with my patients and even with myself over the years, many of us don't find ourselves following through and making the changes permanently. The state of our lives and the conditioning we've experienced over the past several decades regarding food significantly influences us and our ability to adapt to changes later on.

A lot of people face challenges on an emotional and mental level when it comes to food. There might be a few things they need to process in order to make some of those changes. Some people have reasons why they eat certain foods and not others. They might have had a bad experience, or were highly influenced by family members around what they ate. Many of us have different connections to food that we wouldn't even relate to it, nor think about.

Trying new foods can be difficult for people. It can feel like they're losing control over a part of their life because believe it or not, there can be a host of control issues around food. And, there's just the resistance some have towards certain foods, even fresh fruits and vegetables. We've either been that person or know someone like that.

Children, especially, can use food as a form of control or as an emotional tool when they struggle with their environment, traumas, or difficult relationships. Some of us may have grown up in less than happy circumstances, maybe being underfed or feeling like we didn't deserve food, because food was withheld as a punishment. Children typically have limited control over their lives, and in times of struggle, they may turn to food as a means of asserting control. This behavior often persists into adulthood, yet the underlying reasons for their food-related issues remain unnoticed.

A lot of us have learned to use food when seeking comfort or dealing with our emotions, whether we are happy or sad. We eat to comfort ourselves and soothe our nervous systems when we're undergoing stress and use it as a form of emotional fulfillment. A huge part of the food journey as you can see, connects back to our childhood. Childhood is the core of our being on most every level, including our food and nourishment levels. It's beneficial to reflect on our relationship with food during childhood and as we grew up. This reflection can help identify patterns and habits around food, offering insights into areas that may require attention and resolution in order to make positive changes. Writing things down is very helpful.

People have so many circumstances that revolve around food, and working through them is greatly necessary to be able to develop a healthier relationship with food and nourishment going forward.

This is why just being told what to eat and what not to eat won't always work for people. It goes deeper than that. Dietary changes need time, support, and patience. It's vital we process our emotions around food to make lasting, healthy changes.

Our chances of eating healthy and sticking with it are more likely if we move through some of our emotions around it, feel supported, and have the guidance through the changes. We also need to be given the time to adapt to making these changes to our diets. Learning about how whole foods, like fruits and vegetables contain life-giving energy and essential nutrients to keep our bodies healthy and strong, is vital. The more we get to understand and apply the health concepts and connections to food, things essentially click in more naturally. When someone realizes that they can improve their health by changing one food out for another, it feels easier.

Knowledge and guidance help create lasting change.

For those of us who are eating less than healthy diets at this moment, please know that it's okay. There is no judgement here and essentially, we're all doing the best we can with the knowledge we have. The good news is that you're here now which means there's a part of you that wants to make some changes. And, we can make changes to what we eat at any point in time, at any age. Most of us who have less-than-ideal diets have had these for generally a long period of time. It's beneficial to know that there's always room for change and transformation.

The best thing we can do for ourselves is to not hold onto the past or hold our past eating habits and difficulties against ourselves. The worst thing we can do is feel disappointment or resentment around it, as this only holds us back. We can start at any moment to create better, more loving food choices for ourselves.

I fully get that we may sometimes find that it's easier to sit in the unhealthy choices that we're used to, but deep down, most of us really do want to make better choices. We actually *want* better for ourselves. We may savor the tastes and feelings some foods give us, but as we work to re-empower ourselves and our food choices, we'll find that it's easier to make choices that serve us better, even finding foods that are healthier to match those tastes and feelings. We come to realize more easily and naturally that many of the old foods we're so used to are actually making us sick or tired, something we may not have realized or made the connection to prior to this.

It's also good to know that we don't have to give up *everything* right away, and that patience with ourselves is key. It's a big process and we can either take it seriously and go at it full-on or we can move ourselves steadily through to ensure that the changes remain. The exception to the speed or urgent need for change would be if we're on the teetering edge of an illness, or in a make-it or break-it situation, then it would serve us to dig in deep and more seriously so.

A great way to start making some changes is by doing a general assessment of what we are eating. Making a list and journaling about the foods that we eat the most, capturing our favorite foods, and looking at any attachments we have to them, is a great start. Of course, not everyone has attachments to food, so maybe it's just a matter of taste and habit. Doing this will help us record and observe what our diet looks like, how we're feeling around it, and may bring up things we might need to look at on a deeper level and process around it. We can even journal about the joy, accomplishments, and wonderful changes we're seeing in ourselves because of our new consciousness around food.

We can then start to figure out what more we can do to improve the quality of our eating habits and choices. We even end up being more willing to find healthier versions of foods as replacements knowing that small steps make huge strides.

And as time moves along, we blissfully find ourselves feeling motivated and pulled more naturally towards making new and empowered food choices for ourselves. Our willingness to try new foods will increase. We begin to start feeling better physically and clearer mentally, which just makes it so much easier to make those healthier choices.

There is also a renewed sense of self-love and a new found joy that comes along with this. It can actually end up being easy for us to change our eating habits and food choices, because we weren't even happy with how it was going in the first place. Or, we were just so tired of feeling miserable and had wanted this change for a long time, we just didn't know how to do it. Sometimes all we had to do was give ourselves permission to let go of the old foods and patterns so that the new ones had room to come in. We just had to realize that we deserved better and it was okay to want more for ourselves.

Having others there to support us and guide us can be hugely impactful especially when we're just starting out. If doctors prescribed these changes with the classes or programs, a lot would change for people. Most unwell people would do well with support and someone to be there for them along their journey. Someone to help create personal, realistic dietary and food goals towards their success and healing. For myself, personally, I needed someone to guide me or I wouldn't have ever made the changes I was able to make. She was my support system even when I had setbacks, she was gently and lovingly there to boost my confidence and help me get back on my feet.

Learning about food puts the power back into our hands so that we can make more informed choices and decisions about what we put in our mouths and into our bodies. We can take the responsibility in creating better states of health for ourselves with the ability to navigate our way around all of the poor food choices and products that are still out there being offered. With some guidance and support we can create new food standards for ourselves.

Any of us can make changes to the food we eat at any point in our lives if we have even a smidge of desire for it. I've met people in my career who changed their lives through their diet reversing disease in their later years, and I mean sixties and up. I knew a couple in their mid-sixties who were tired of being sick and unwell so they finally decided that they were going to change their diet. They slowly began to let go of inflammatory foods like sugar, dairy, breads, and processed foods and replaced them with tons of fresh and fermented foods.

They filled their plates up with more fresh fruits and veggies and ate tons of kimchi and krauts (which help break down old matter). They let go of thinking that their health was destined for sickness due to their age or where they had gotten themselves. They let go of their doctors telling them that heart disease was a condition that was irreversible. They essentially got over the mindset that they were too old and set in their ways and instead, created a whole new level of living their life.

When we possess a burning desire to get off the path of insufferable illness, it sets things into motion. We discover a newfound courage to establish goals and educate ourselves more. And through this, we come to understand more about food's potent medicinal properties thus feeling more blessed and humbled when we're consuming them.

We feel more grateful for them. This amazing planet has all of the essentials that we need. It was designed that way. The earth's nutrient-rich foods and their powerful properties were put here to nourish, invigorate, and heal our body.

There are endless amazing books out there full of wonderful information about food, and one I treasure so very much, is *The Whole Foods Companion* by Dianne Olstad. It's an absolute goldmine of information that speaks on the origination of the food, right down to its medicinal properties. It's inspiring to read about food and finding out about the benefits and impact they can have on our health.

There are so many powerful and positive aspects to food. We can make the connection to eating them and how they will affect our body, giving us more power to work through our physical issues. Knowing there are medicinal aspects to the food growing out of the ground, changes everything. How beautiful that we are finally moving into the realization that food is powerful in our lives.

Did you know that how we speak to ourselves, how we feel about our food choices, how we feel *while* we're eating, as well as while we're preparing our food, all make a huge difference in how the food translates in our body? What we think about and focus on affects so many angles of our life, a huge one of them being our body's response to the food that we eat.

We spoke earlier about Dr. Emoto's studies on how our thoughts and words have an impact on our bodies, the same is true when it comes to our food since so much of it consists of water. How we speak or feel about the food we're eating influences the way it is received or interpreted in our body. If we dwell on how unhealthy the food is or constantly remind ourselves of its negative aspects, we are essentially adding those thoughts, emotions, and energy into the mix.

The same can be said if we're thinking about how amazing and healthy the food is that we're eating. Something I heard that resonated strongly for me was that even if the food we're eating isn't the healthiest or most pure of foods, we can bless it and embrace the emotion that it's going to nourish and feed us. This can actually change the vibration of the food to impact us more healthfully. Believe it or not.

Our thoughts linked with our emotions have been proven to be powerful enough to transform so many aspects of our lives, this includes the food we eat and that which we put into our bodies. Some people are unable to find or afford nourishing foods, so this is a way to add to our food's potential and create positive effects.

The mental and emotional state that we're in while we're eating, has an effect on our body and how it processes the food we feed it. If we are eating in a moment that is free from stress and we're in a relaxed and good-spirited state, our body will receive the nutrients at a greater capacity. If we're in a state of distress, anger, sadness, frustration, or fear, our body has more difficulty digesting and receiving the nutrients. Our nervous system is affected, which also affects our body's ability to assimilate the food and its nutrients.

Most of us can agree that if we are sad, angry, or depressed, our eating habits and food choices can become affected. When something life altering occurs, good or bad, we can notice how it affects how or what we eat. We might find ourselves unable to eat anything or that we eat everything in sight. Sometimes, we use food to cope with our grief, sadness, and pain, or deprive ourselves as a response to feeling empty and lost. Our emotional needs can guide our eating habits and food choices, without a doubt. An example is when life is stressful or challenging, people may often turn to sweets, seeking both their sweetness and the endorphins released by sugar, which momentarily helps elevate our mood.

Understanding these aspects shapes our awareness of both our food choices and our behavior while eating. We could be eating the healthiest meal on the planet, but if we're in a rush or stressed out, we absolutely lose some of the benefit and nourishment of it. Distractions that take our focus away from the act of eating also have an effect on our digestive process and our absorption of the nutrients. For example, if we are part of an intense or negative conversation, watching a horror film, or involved in something overly distracting and stressful, this can absolutely have a negative effect on how our body processes the food.

When it comes to preparing our food, this too, is important. When we prepare our food with feelings of love and gratitude, strange as it may sound, that vibe projects into the food we are handling and creating. Like when grandma made that food that she so loved to make for us, we could almost feel the love she put into it.

What we are feeling, speak, and thinking effects our food while we're preparing and cooking it. It's good to take notice of where we're at emotionally and mentally while preparing a meal. If we're not in the best mindset or head space and we're stressed out or frustrated, it's a good idea for us to do something to reset our mindset and emotions to move into a better state of being before we begin to prepare the meal. When we switch over to a more positive mindset and emotional level, we can learn to create our food with intention. It may even become a form of meditation or prayer when we do this consciously. We can intentionally put good vibes and loving intention into our food while chopping, stirring, and cooking it.

We even can literally say things like, *"thank you for this beautiful food"* or *"this food is nourishing and healing"* or whatever resonates with us, if that sounds like something that works for you. Whether or not we actually state those things, we can always move ourselves into the feeling of being grateful for the food, as well as for all of the reasons we have to be grateful in our lives, because it's only ever empowering to do. Giving thanks and being grateful in itself, nourishes and feeds our bodies on so many levels.

Food can inspire us and invigorate our senses. It stimulates the bliss hormone, known as *dopamine*. When we are in a state of enjoyment, dopamine is produced. Add to that a feeling of celebration and gratitude, what an amplified blissful feeling. We get to feel elated both by the food itself and through the experience of enjoying it.

Physically, it's beneficial to observe the effects certain foods have on us. At times, we consume food without much awareness – we eat it, it goes in, we feel satisfied, and that's the end of it. However, on other occasions, our bodies might react differently to the food we ingest, manifesting symptoms like stomach pain, indigestion, diarrhea, or nausea. These reactions often indicate that the food doesn't agree with our system or may even reflect our current emotional state. It's good to note how certain foods make us feel, identifying which ones may cause us grief, and which ones make us feel like a million bucks.

Having a journal or notebook to keep track of things, a food diary of sorts, is so helpful if we want to follow the progress we're making, or notice the common feelings and symptoms that come up for us.

As we become more aware and conscious around what we eat and how we're eating it, we begin to form a new connection and perhaps some new thought processes around food and eating. It helps us to notice patterns we have, things that don't agree with our bodies, and helps us gain the perspective we need to make long lasting changes.

It's always important that we refrain from being hard on ourselves no matter what we notice or what occurs, setbacks and all. None of us are perfect, and it's okay that our diet and food process has ups and downs. Being upset and disappointed in ourselves will only hold us back and keep us stuck. Once again, acknowledging that we fell off track, but getting back up is what brings us closer to success.

Every human should learn about the goodness around food and what it truly does for us. On every level. It's so important for us to be educated around its nourishing and healing properties, as well as how to grow it and appreciate it, so we can work towards creating a better outcome for our health and for those that we love.

Embodying and working through all of these aspects around food, can bring great transformation that not only affects our health in a positive way, it also affects our mind and overall life as we know it. Know that your greatest potential is yet to be realized as you move forward with more consciousness and love around food and your body.

HOMEWORK:

1. What foods do you eat that you wish you could give up or know that they aren't the healthiest for you?
2. What symptoms does your body give you when you eat foods that aren't the best for you?
3. How do you feel when you eat foods that are wholesome and healthy?
4. What changes can you make to your food and diet? What small step can you take today?
5. Take notice of how you feel and where your heads at when preparing and eating your food. What changes would you make to this?

BONUS QUESTION:

1. What foods did your ancestors eat? Where did your ancestors come from? What are the native foods to those lands, what was grown and commonly eaten?

THE LESS CHEMICALS THE BETTER

We've come into a time where chemicals are an everyday part of our lives on just about every level. They're unavoidable, as they exist in so much of what we eat, consume, and use on the daily. We can find chemicals in our food, water, air, homes, schools, work places, cars, clothing, medications, household items, and everything in between.

Most of us aren't very aware of this. We've gone about our lives trusting that what's out there and made available to us, is safe. We've been taught to believe that there are people looking out for our safety, monitoring what's allowed in our food, products, air, and water to ensure that nothing harmful is put into them. We don't even think twice about it; we blindly trust it all.

Well… it turns out, and unfortunately so, this isn't exactly the case. We actually *are* exposed to things that we shouldn't be.

The truth is, we're taking in and are exposed some rather harmful, toxic chemicals and elements. We eat them, drink them, breathe them in, apply them to our bodies, clean with them, clothe ourselves with them, and even them give them to our children and our pets. The thing is, we don't see it because we trust things are okay for us. Why would anything that's offered to us, be toxic?

We don't have to look back very far to see that there *was* once a time when chemicals weren't overwhelming our lives. They weren't even considered as something to be put into the things humans consumed or used. There was a time when chemicals weren't purposefully put on our food and in our water. If you look back a century or more ago, the difference in the state of our food, air, and water is incredibly different.

I always wondered how these chemicals came into play in such a massive way. How, in almost no time, thousands of chemicals were figured in as safe, useful, and purposeful for humans to use and ingest. As though it would add to our lives in some way, they began showing up everywhere.

When I started to research these chemicals that I was finding in my food products, toothpaste, and cleaning products, I found that most all of them are man-made, produced in a lab, or the by-products and waste products of different chemical and elemental industries. Being the nurse that I was, it seemed like something to be concerned about. I mean with all of the suffering, sickness, cancer, and disease I witnessed for over two decades, literally watching people's bodies falling apart, I began to wonder what else was causing this to happen to people.

Over the last fifty years or so, the world of convenience has expanded quite massively. We have such a variety of practically everything in life, and so much is offered to us. We have the ability to make choices on so many levels, with just about everything at our fingertips. We've been graced with all kinds of foods, products, and material items that have added richness to our lives. It's been a blessing without a doubt, but unfortunately, as with anything in life, there are usually a few downsides to things like this.

The food and that products that *do* contain chemicals are supposed to only contain what is considered a *safe* amount, so as not to cause harm. However, anything that needs to be put into a *safe enough* dose or amount, is likely unsafe to begin with. Common sense to me is that if it's harmful, let's just keep it out of things we humans consume and expose our bodies to.

Since there are *so* many of these chemicals in everything these days, it only feels right to me that we at least raise our awareness, and if we're feeling brave, our concern. It seems logical to put some attention onto it, especially when people's health is at stake. None of us would initially be aware of the harm that's taking place from any of these chemicals because micro and macro amounts aren't usually felt. But, it's what we *don't* know that's something to think about; what some of the long-term effects of these chemicals are.

Remember, our bodies are pretty delicate structurally, being made up of cells and organisms and all. So, it's easy to see that chemicals can and likely will, directly affect and have an impact on them. In my nurse mind, I know that the body cannot possibly handle a constant influx and bombardment of this stuff over a long period of time, without suffering some sort of consequence. There's no way it knows exactly what to do with each and every one of these chemicals, and many at once no less.

Again, these chemicals are not naturally sourced. We're not talking about the stuff of the Earth, even if they are made up of some of them, the stuff we're getting is more complicated, chemically.

We've all taken a chemistry class in high school at some point, and we know how things can get complicated. We were taught not to mix certain chemicals together for good reason. The reaction they might have could be dangerous, if not toxic or explosive. Now, don't get me wrong, I'm not stating that all of these chemicals that are added to our food and goods are all explosive and toxic when combined. What I am saying is that some of them are generally a bad idea to combine, and worst of all, hard on our physical/cellular and electrical body.

Even if these chemicals are consumed in the smallest and tiniest amounts, which is how they include them in things, at some point, it's going to be a burden. Especially, with the weakened state that some of our bodies are in, there will undoubtedly end up being some form of accumulation in the body, which can only cause problems.

There have been a few chemicals along the way that have gotten some attention due to concerns around them. Some have been connected to certain health issues and problems, even studied greatly, however, they aren't always taken off the market. Many that have been found to be harmful to us, yet have found their way to stay in the game. Aspartame is an example. They're still out there being used by us, and sold to us.

The truth is that none of us know what kind of problem these chemicals can cause. Most people aren't overly concerned, as we don't usually see immediate, direct effects taking place. The small incremental doses that are included in these formulas and products are small enough that we don't notice anything. Most of us, once again, feel that if it's something that's been approved of and is allowed to be out there on the shelf, it must be safe to obtain and consume.

Afterall, we have different agencies in charge of making sure our safety and health are a priority when it comes to what gets put into our food and products. They are specifically there to make sure that what is available for us to consume and use, is not harmful to us. We understandably, trust that we're being protected.

The truth is, and I'm sure you'd be very sad to know, the agencies aren't actually testing them. They put their trust in the companies who produce the products and chemicals, who do their own set of testing, but the approving agency doesn't do their own.

How we can help ourselves is by having the awareness. We can at least know that when we ingest these chemicals, our bodies are so spectacular that they handle them all pretty well considering. They work hard to try to process them, protect us *from* them, and move them out to the best of their ability, through our urine, sweat, bowel movements, and breath. This is a wonderful aspect of our body, although they cannot always expel them.

Unfortunately, some of these chemicals actually get stuck inside of the body, especially heavy metals. They get built up in the body and actually trapped inside of the lining and tissues of our organs, and deposited into our cells, particularly fat cells and weakened cells.

Our body does its best to protect us and works hard to excrete them, however sometimes it can't. It's dealing with putting out so many other fires, and has so many other issues that it only has so much energy to be able to do this. Some of these toxins are super difficult for the body to remove altogether.

I heard someone recently speak about the enormous amount of chemicals that a woman, in particular, is exposed to just in her morning routine alone. It was up towards about three-hundred chemicals, give or take, in total. A lot of women a ton of different products throughout their routine of getting ready for the day, such as shampoo, conditioner, soap/body wash, shaving cream, hair styling products, skin care products, lotions, deodorant, perfume, make up, toothpaste, mouth wash, and even dental floss. They all contain a number of chemical ingredients within each of them.

Some contain more chemicals than others. Makeup as an example, contains quite a few toxic ingredients, one of those being heavy metals. Studies have been done linking makeup and its ingredients to certain reproductive issues, as well as cancer of the breast and organs of the reproductive system.

When any of these products are applied, as with anything put onto the skin, they get absorbed into the body and end up in our blood stream, even if it's just in *small, tiny* amounts. The liver and the kidneys work to eliminate them, however, some of these chemicals when used on a daily basis, or over used, can stick around and largely affect the endocrine glands, aka the hormonal system in the body.

Heavy metals especially, which are known for getting trapped in the cells, cause damage to the cell membranes and to our DNA. They attach to the cells and prevent them from performing their functions, and to boot, heavy metals are one of the most difficult ones to remove from the body.

As we are ultimately aware, the body is a biological, living organism and chemicals and metals have a massive effect on it. External chemicals can interrupt or wrongly affect the naturally occurring chemicals and processes in the body.

Some medications are made with the intent on correcting chemical imbalances within the body, but the truth is that we need to fix the issue that is *causing* the chemical imbalance, only using the drug as a bridge for a short period of time to get us to the other side of things. Unfortunately, when the issue is not fixed, the body then becomes reliant on the medication to maintain itself, which ultimately weakens the body even further. The drugs cannot artificially keep things going forever if there are issues that are creating these imbalances that aren't being resolved. It only causes things to fall apart further.

If there are chemicals being built up in the system, just correcting the imbalance without removing the excess chemicals will only make the issue worse. It's important for us to remember that this beautiful living organism that we live in is sensitive to some degree. It's affected by chemicals and we need to be mindful of just how many of them we are allowing in.

As we know, our bodies work hard to get rid of poisons and toxins that it encounters. Part of how our body deals with some of these overloads and in order to correct the imbalance created by these, it will pull minerals out of other areas of the body, to try to reestablish a balance in its chemistry.

Often this imbalance is continuous, which causes the body to be constantly working on trying to adjust the issue, eventually making it more difficult and more taxing on the body and its systems. Eventually, it pulls other systems out of whack while doing this as it reaches for and borrows minerals and salts from other cells. It looks to buffer out and even out the imbalances with its own chemistry. This just ends up causing further disruption, weakness, and essentially breakdown and dysfunction.

However, we can interject and do some things about this. Even if we're exposed to these chemicals and are still living in the world as we do, we can help ourselves in many ways. Obviously, by using less and choosing less toxic products, we help ourselves enormously. But we can do things purposefully, such as eating certain foods and taking different supplements or botanical remedy to counter and buffer these things out more easily.

The natural chemistry of whole, earth grown foods, can affect our body chemistry in a *positive* way, especially with herbs. Naturally speaking, and as we know, most of the food grown on the planet contains beneficial nutrients, vitamins, and chemical components that our bodies can easily access, use, and ultimately need to maintain a good state of health.

An apple as an example, being on the alkaline side of chemistry, contains calcium, phosphorous, magnesium, potassium, beta carotene, folic acid and a bunch of Vitamin C. It has malic and tartaric acids that help break down food, remove impurities from the liver, and help stop the growth of disease-producing bacteria in the intestines. The chemical components of an apple are highly beneficial for our body. It's an alkalizer, cleanser, and nutrient rich food.

It's no wonder why there was an old saying, '*An apple a day keeps the doctor away.*' However, these days, the soil has been largely depleted and has been highly tainted by what's being sprayed and added to the food growing, i.e., pesticides and herbicides. An apple today is 1/16th of what an apple was forty plus years ago in nutritional value. Meaning, we would have to eat about sixteen apples today to receive the same nutrients that one apple brought to us back then.

Other foods like processed foods, fast-foods, and mass-produced industrialized foods, including animal products, also contain loads of chemicals. Some may argue that these mass-produced, genetically modified, and processed foods have only been a blessing to us, as they've been a saving grace for feeding enormous amounts of people, making food available to almost everyone. They've also been how food prices at one point in time, were cheaper, though that's not even the case anymore.

They have the ability to feed a large number of people, but to what detriment? Unfortunately, those of us who eat them are just adding more chemicals and insults to our bodies.

Processed foods generally always contain chemicals to help keep them "*fresh*" and preserved, or even added to enhance the flavor and taste of the product. Mass-produced food, even if it's fruits or vegetables, have chemicals found in and on them. Many fruits as an example, are sprayed with pesticides to protect the crop from insects and such other invaders. They are picked unripe, sprayed again with chemicals to preserve them, packed into boxes, and shipped around the country or sometimes even the world. These post-chemicals are used for preservation of the food and to repel bugs, ensuring the food makes it to the store shelf intact and able to sell for weeks to months on end. However, this is not good for us in the long run.

They also add other chemicals like colorings and wax to fresh fruits and vegetables, to preserve them *and* to add to the appeal, so that we will want to purchase them. So, that shiny, red apple you bought might actually be colored, but even if not, there is definitely a wax coating on it, and who wants to eat wax? I've even seen videos of potatoes being painted red.

We can see the abundant availability as a huge blessing and benefit absolutely, but when do we realize what's going on and happening, is it really a blessing? Why the colorings? I'm very sure it can all be done on some other level and that we would still buy an apple if it's fresh and available for purchase. We don't actually *need* it to look extra colorful, do we? And the fact the colors of the fruit are lessened is because of the deficiency and loss of nutrients that come with the food being grown at massive levels, and the depletion of the soil.

There have also been toxic chemicals found in many items that come from overseas, a lot of them being food items. Candy, pickles, crackers, rice, seafood, as well as tons of others have been found to be tainted with formaldehyde, illegal dyes, heavy metals, plastics and many other toxins. Plastic has been found in rice, literally some grains being made of plastic. Our recycled plastic is bought by another country and then reconfigured into our products, including our food.

Here in the US, we have a fairly new practice for the past few years of sending our own home-grown, slaughtered chickens over to China for processing. As stated by popular media sources on the internet, it was stated that chickens will be raised here in the US, or Canada and Chile, which are the other two countries approved by the US to produce our poultry, then sent over to one of four approved poultry processing plants in China to be processed and exported *back to the US* for our consumption. This is all approved by our governing agencies here in the US. My question is, why wouldn't we just process them here, saving money and time on something perishable and easily spoilable? What is China doing processing our food that we actually raise here ourselves? Doesn't make sense to me and it sets off a huge number of red flags for me. The one thing I do know is that they're allowances of toxins is a lot looser than ours here.

Many other countries that produce these chemicals or products for us, don't have the same regulations on their exported products. The US allows for a certain percentage of toxins *over* the allowable limit to be placed into the products that come in from overseas. Why the limit if they're allowed to go over it? Many people also do not realize that even our pharmaceutical drugs, baby products, and just about seventy five percent of the products we use are produced in these countries. Sadly, if there are chemicals that are harmful in the products, the people making the products are exposed to all of that as well.

There are literally a handful of corporations here in the US who control pretty much all of our food and beverages. No matter how many brands you see on the shelf, there's about 10 companies who now own it all, with about two huge companies that own all of them. It's been an absolute since the twenty twenty event; all of the big food corporations survived, left to shelve all the grocery stores with their products. Sadly, the smaller more, mindful companies either shut down or were bought out. The big corporations bought out all of the popular organic and independent brands, as well, so the ones that we see on the shelves, that we once felt safer in consuming are now owned by the same corporations.

When you look at the ingredients in those products, things may look sort of the same, but it's been found that they are not, because, well, we didn't memorize what the original product contained, we just trust that it's the same. Turns out, these corporations are using cheaper, more chemicalized ingredients, as there has been evidence showing this from scientists who have actually been looking into these products since they were bought out. It's not all as naturally derived or healthy as it is supposed to be. Cancer causing agents, known endocrine disruptors, as well as other toxins, are being snuck into our products, even the ones that have been labeled organic and natural.

Some of the food items on the shelves that are considered to be edible, and are there for our consumption, should not even be considered as food, nor offered in my opinion. A lot of these food products have little to no natural ingredients in them, instead are made up of processed by-products and ingredients with no nutritional value. They have even recently turned plastic into ice cream... you can't make this stuff up.

There are bulking and foaming agents added, chemical additives, preservatives, artificial colorings and the list goes on. So many artificial and chemical ingredients are added to these food products that at this point in time, you can even taste some of them. When you start cleaning up your diet and eating cleaner foods, you actually begin to notice and taste these chemicals more profoundly.

Many chemicals are added in micro and macro levels, and as stated earlier, the body doesn't respond like there is a full-on threat at first. Macro amounts are indeed small but, it's like a frog in boiling water, going undetected, and when eventually noticed, it's too late. People are just so unaware that this stuff is harmful to them especially because if it's on the shelf at the grocery store. Why would something that is offered as food be harmful to us?

Especially, when there's a cartoon animal drawn on the package, attracting children, we would *never* expect something harmful to be in something put out there for children. However, popular cereals, breakfast items, ice cream, and snack foods contain terrible chemicals like propylene glycol, food colorings, and hormone disruptors that are linked to neurological issues, cancers, and other health problems in the body. These chemicals are also a reason why obesity in children has become so prevalent.

Here in the US, they allow a chemical know as glyphosate to still be used as an herbicide which is applied onto and around our crops and food. It is the most popular weed killer in the US with a brand and company that is widely known and monopolizes the pesticide industry here in the US. This chemical is banned in other countries, as it has been proven to cause cancer. Glyphosate gets into our food, saturates into the soil, and even finds its way into our water supply. This is a well-known harmful chemical that builds up in the body and can easily be linked to cancer. (Cancer rates around the world are the *highest* in the United States.)

Glyphosate kills the good bacteria in the gut, is shown to cause leaky-gut syndrome, and is linked to kidney disease. Not to mention, people have become gluten intolerant and it's not about the wheat. Glyphosate also kills the bees which many people don't realize that we rely on bees to live.

Health agencies state that this chemical is *essential* for food production mainly fruits, vegetables, nuts, corn, and soy by blocking the growth of weeds that grow around it. It blocks the enzymes needed for the plant's growth, basically stopping the weed from growing. They've then had to make the food crops modified to be able to *not* be affected by this product, and this isn't a good thing.

This is just *one of many* pesticides, insecticides, and herbicides used on and around our food that have harmful effects on our bodies. And recently, they've come to realize that we've noticed this and are now replacing glyphosate with a similar herbicide which does the same damage. We will begin to see packaging stating it's *Glyphosate-free,* but just remember, they have 20 other herbicides and pesticides sitting waiting for use, that do similar things.

Other countries like Europe as an example, ban so much of what we allow here in the US. That's right, they ban their use. They ban genetically modified food, tons of the chemicals and -icides that we still use, as well as corn syrup and other insulting stuff that's put into our food. We can even see it in products that are seemingly the same being sold in the US and other countries, except the ingredients are vastly different.

You can have two identical products like ketchup or a soft drink. There are chemicals and other substances added to the US version that do not exist in the European version. Ketchup as an example made for the US, contains high fructose corn syrup *and* corn syrup, which is not allowed in the European version. Popular orange soda here in the US has no orange juice in it and again has corn syrup and food colorings added, where the European version contains regular sugar and orange juice, with *no* food colorings or corn syrup.

Corn syrup is a whole topic of its own and is something that is linked to diabetes and heart disease. Our body cannot process it, it's cheap to make, they use GMO corn that is loaded with atrazine (a highly toxic herbicide that is harmful to our Endocrine system) and we sit here and consume it. It causes obesity as well, and it just so happens that America is the most overweight country on this planet.

Heavy metals are another part of things, as I mentioned earlier, that are placed in our products and cause serious issues to our health. Heavy metals are harder to detect and cause a host of problems. They hide out and eventually can become a burden as they buildup in our bodies. They create an underlying toxicity that modern medicine does not detect. They don't think about it as an issue, nor do they test for them as a possible, potential threat that's causing chaos in our body.

One of the places toxic levels of heavy metals have been found recently was in dark chocolate. Just when we think we're doing good for ourselves eating dark chocolate over milk chocolate. We've known that there are anti-oxidants, magnesium, zinc, iron and other minerals in dark chocolate, as well as that it is said to be good for heart health. However, 28 of the most popular brands were recently tested and *all* of them had toxic levels of lead and cadmium in them.

Heavy metals are not our friend. Once again, they stick around in the tissues of the body and stress out the liver, kidneys, brain and nervous system, and lymphatic system where they also like to accumulate. They are found collecting in the soft tissues of the body and are indeed linked to cancers and are terribly difficult to remove.

Aluminum is a common ingredient found in deodorants, and it's really in a hundred other things as well in small amounts. We use it to cook our food believing it's safe. Aluminum is linked to breast cancer, prostate cancer, and Alzheimer's. Basically, cancer and brain/neurological diseases. Aluminum is also found in vaccines due to the fact that aluminum helps to break the blood brain barrier down so things can cross over and through to the brain. Our body has this blood brain barrier for a reason, to prevent toxins and harmful pathogens and organisms from *getting* to our brain, and to protect it.

Aluminum in one form or another, has been used in vaccines to trigger a stronger immune response as well, to help the vaccines work better, and this has been going on since the 1930's. Interestingly enough, the medical industry completely changed over during that period of time, something to look into if you're interested. Vaccine studies state that the aluminum is not readily absorbed by the body, however, it's labeled as a neurotoxin.

Throughout the last one hundred years or so, many other metals are being found in our foods, products, and homes such as lead, mercury, and arsenic. Research has shown that there are *no safe* levels of heavy metals that should ever be consumed by people.

There have been recalls on thousands of products that come here from overseas for containing unsafe amounts of toxins. There has been lead found in baby bibs and children's toys amongst hundreds of other items, including baby food where arsenic, lead, cadmium, and mercury were all found. Shocking, I know. We've likely all fed our children baby food at some point. Seriously, especially in regards to our babies, I'm sure we can certainly all agree that their products should be the safest, most non-toxic, and natural products out there.

In regards to heavy metals and doing our best to rid them from our body, there are foods and herbs that can work in our favor to remove them at least on some level from the cells that they're locked into. Cilantro is as powerful as it gets. Parsley, celery juice, chlorella, spirulina, garlic, barley and wheatgrass, blueberries, seaweed, lemon, turmeric, ginger, and radishes all help remove the metals from the cells. Fully chelating and removing metals needs to be done with, and alongside a qualified doctor, which is mostly naturopaths who work to on helping to remove metals and other toxins from the body. Starting with the herbs and foods however, will without a doubt help out tremendously.

Our water is another area to think about when it comes to chemicals. This of course, varies greatly depending on where you are in the world, because there are still people in the world today who don't even have access to clean water. Those of us who do have access to water don't even think twice about it and we take for granted that's it's basically sent right to our homes. Because of this, we wholeheartedly believe that it's perfectly healthy and safe for us to use and drink. However, there's more than meets the eye with our water. And it's only gotten worse over time...

It's pretty hard to believe it, but some of the medications people take, still remain in our water supply regardless of the filtration being done. Water treatment facilities do a marvelous job trying their best to remove everything that they can, however, they can't get *everything* out. This is proven by water testing that's been done around the US. Drugs like anti-inflammatory drugs, fever-reducers, antibiotics, hormones, mood stabilizers, heart medications, narcotics, even the most recent injections are being found in *already treated* and filtered drinking water that arrives to the sink in our homes. Antibiotics in the water help to create drug-resistant bacteria, which is bacteria that no antibiotic can treat.

The most popular anti-depressant has been found in large amounts in our water supply, *post-filtration*. This is known as a 'forever chemical' and there are around 12,000 of them that have been identified. They're found in pharmaceutical drugs, makeup, textiles, carpets, non-stick pans, dyes, clothing, dental floss, and much more, and they all end up in our water. 45% of US tap water was found to have some of these chemicals present, as well as some of the well water around the country, and my belief is that number is largely played down.

Especially, with all of the chemical spills and things going on in our present moment, this percentage, in my opinion, is definitely much higher. And being that cancer rates are super high in areas where certain industries make their products, like the petroleum processing plants in the Southeastern part of the US, it's a no-brainer to know that some of that toxic waste is running off into the land and water supply of the people who live in those areas.

Another toxin that is vastly present in our water supply, is fluoride. You see there are different chemical make ups of fluoride, one of them being *sodium* fluoride and the other being *calcium* fluoride. We've been told that fluoride is beneficial to us, especially for our teeth and to help prevent cavities. However, the version of fluoride present in our water and toothpaste today is the sodium fluoride version, which is actually a waste product of a phosphate fertilizer that is known to be toxic. It is *banned around the world*, even in some cities in the US it's been banned, and is actually classified as a *toxin*. There's a reason that there is a poison control phone number on toothpaste tubes.

Sodium fluoride has *no* health benefits, however... *Calcium* Fluoride, which is a naturally occurring earth mineral, *does* have benefits to the body. Calcium fluoride tones and strengthens the elasticity of joints, veins, vessels, and connective tissue in the body. It strengthens bones and enamel of teeth, as well as that it helps to repair the tissues in the body. Sodium fluoride, however, is a waste product and is toxic to the body, being especially hard on the endocrine glands, the pineal specifically, and is cancer causing.

So, having a good water filtration system at home is not only a good idea, but these days essential (I'll list some trusted brands in the back). There are many kinds but the idea is to remove as many chemicals, metals, and organisms as we can, because all of them can cause harm to our body. Fluoride, along with those forever chemicals are difficult to remove, but there are some filters out there that are created to remove some of these.

Reverse osmosis is a powerful filtration system and highly recommended if you can afford a system. The more popular water filters available at stores today, are very ineffective, except maybe to remove some chlorine and such. Good water filtration systems aren't necessarily cheap, but distilling water is the best way to go that doesn't cost much other than the initial purchase, and buying some charcoal filters every few months which aren't that expensive.

Distilling water even removes fluoride, because when you distill water, it removes all of the minerals and salts from the water, one of those being fluoride. Distilling water removes 99.9% of dissolved materials from the water. Distillation removes lead, arsenic, viruses, and so many other contaminants. Personally, I believe distilled water is the best way to go nowadays as we can get the necessary minerals we need from things like Irish Sea Moss, Shilajit, or Celtic Sea Salt. We can replace our mineral content, because wouldn't you rather have a mechanism that will remove as much of these chemicals and viruses from your water as possible?

Endocrine disruptors that were mentioned earlier are found in so many of our products. These disruptors are mainly parabens, BPA, dioxin, PFC's, and phthalates that are found in things like non-stick cookware, plastic bottle and containers, cosmetics, toys and fragrances, to name a few. Laundry detergent and fabric softener contain various endocrine disruptors as well. They are even found in the clothing that we wear, such as with polyester fabrics. Polyester is made from petroleum and you can look up more about it if you're interested. Of course, the best fabrics for us are linen, cotton, and wool.

There are innumerous chemicals found in our products that over prolonged periods of time, can cause harm to our endocrine glands altering our hormones and causing disruptions in our nervous system, immune system, and digestive system, as well that they are linked to cancer. They're found in our shampoos and hair products, bathing products, cleaning products, paint, everyday products, even in the fumes of permanent markers.

Xenoestrogens are also found in our water which happen to come from pesticides, plastics, and industrial waste. These are chemicals that mimic estrogen in our body and mess up our hormones causing infertility, cancer, and even gender changes. They're in our tap water, bottled water, and even filtered water. It's almost impossible to avoid them, unless we live by a natural spring or have an ionizing alkaline water filter. I'm unsure if distillation removes them, but I would love to find out.

See, these products don't cause an initial response within the body, however they end up posing great health risks over longer periods of time of use and exposure, because as with most harmful chemicals, they build up in the body. So, when disease or cancer hits, no one would even think twice about it being related to the products we've been using for over 40 years or the water we're drinking. Thankfully, we are becoming more conscious of this information so we're able to make better choices, make some changes, and move away from using the extremely chemicalized stuff.

It's better to be aware of these things than be completely oblivious. My strongest belief is that turning back to nature is the way to go. If we really wanted to, we could make our own toothpaste, deodorant, soap, and so on. I truly hope that more and more small companies will birth through during these times, bringing back natural and non-toxic products to the people.

Once we all begin to realize that so many things we use and take on are toxic, we will be flooded with the need for new, more natural avenues and products, as well as the knowledge of how to make our own. Want to be a part of the solution? I personally invite you to do so if you are feeling drawn to it.

At this point, we need to check the ingredients on everything. We can then make more informed decisions on what we will, and won't allow for ourselves and our loved ones. Sadly, we can't just trust what's on the shelf to be healthy and safe anymore, even if it has a label saying *natural* or *organic*. It's not easy to let go of some of the products and items we've been using a long time, trust me I've been there, and there aren't even much in the way of substitutes anymore. However, the next time we purchase health or food items, we can try our best to choose products with more natural ingredients and less chemicals. It's okay to go through this process slowly, as long as we have the awareness, small steps are always better than no steps at all.

There are a few companies who are being mindful and are making products with less of these ingredients such as Melaleuca and a few other ones out there, so we are moving towards this awareness and changes are coming.

Speaking of the label that states something is *natural* such as natural flavorings or just natural stated on the package, it's good to be aware that natural doesn't actually mean from nature, because in the game of the industry, there are all sorts of angles "natural" can be used in advertising. It's interesting, yet disturbing how the word natural can be utilized when it comes to labeling a product. There are unfortunately so many ways in which chemicals can be snuck into our food and products. Sadly, we have to be a lot more diligent these days in the purchasing of food, personal, and household products.

It can be stressful to hear all of this, especially if you haven't been aware of these things before. It's quite overwhelming to say the least. I've definitely come across more people than not, who argue against this in disbelief and think it's nonsense, however, the information is out there. There's been a lot of keeping this information hidden, but luckily where we're at a time where everything seems to be coming up and out, no matter how hard they try to suppress it.

The truth is, we've been practically handed these products and foods full of chemicals. We even spend our hard-earned money on them unknowingly. We've been fooled into believing things are safe when they're not. We think we're just sick because our bodies just get sick. Time and time again we find out that they always knew these things were harmful to us. Advertising manipulates our feelings, emotions, and thinking to a place where they get us to believe whatever they state and put forth. There's a reason why we have so many more natural or organic foods and products these days, but the unfortunate part of it is that they are much more expensive. So average, everyday people cannot afford them, and have to give into the more chemicalized, tainted, cheaper products.

All of these chemicals, toxins, and poisons harm our body's delicate organ systems and environment, whatever way you look at it. They are indeed partly the cause of some illnesses and disease states. Getting rid of, or limiting as many toxic foods and products from our life is a good first step to take.

When it comes to food items, it's best to try and stay with the cleanest, most wholesome, organic foods as possible. Even if it's organic, it's important to wash and soak your food to clean off as much of the pesticides, residues, and whatever else is on them. We can use baking soda and water, apple cider vinegar and water, fruit and veggie washes, or CDS if you know what that is. Growing our own food is the most ideal, of course, however, this is not always possible for everyone, but if you can, it's worth the effort.

Also, if we can't pronounce an ingredient, nor recognize any actual real ingredients in a product (especially food), it might be wise to keep looking and find another product with better ingredients to purchase. Essentially, the things that come from nature work best with our bodies, as they can be assimilated much easier by them. Stay as close to nature as possible.

We can even make removing chemicals from our life a chance to be creative, perhaps even making our own awesome, homemade goods and products which saves us both money *and* will make us feel good knowing what's in them. We might even find ourselves sharing it with our friends and family because we ultimately want what's best for them, too.

Maybe we'll even start our own company! We need small companies to come back, because it's the big industries and corporations who are controlling all of our food and products, are the ones who are putting all of these chemicals into them. It's time we take our power back and start creating products and producing food that's in its purest form, so we can start thriving and freeing ourselves of these burdens that have been put on our bodies.

HOMEWORK:

1. What personal care products do you use? This is anything you use on your skin or body. Go read the ingredients. Which ones could you let go of and change over to something less toxic? Make a list and if you have time, do a little research online. Online is usually a great way to get good prices on cleaner products, and you can buy in bulk.
2. What household products do you use that are toxic? Bleach can be available to use but does not have to be the disinfectant you use. Those harsh chemicals are harmful to breathe in and get on your skin. Which products can you begin to use instead? Tea tree based, vinegar & lemon, Thieves essential oil, etc. There are companies out there that are coming to the forefront that use natural and safe ingredients that do just as good of a job.

3. What other chemicals you are exposed to either at your job or perhaps where you live? Any production plants that off gas or put something out into the air? Farms? Take a moment to look around you and see what's going on. Awareness is key.

4. How can you cut some of these chemicals out of your life? What are you inspired to create in the way of natural products?

DiSEASE

ifty to sixty years ago, the percentage of people who suffered from chronic illness and disease, was around 7%. Today, that number is 60%. That's ***over half*** of the population that are suffering with chronic illness and disease. As a society, it appears that we've just become more unhealthy, sick, and disconnected from ourselves than ever.

People are struggling to take care of themselves, with stress levels through the roof, the food we're given is barely even good for us, so much is missing in the health care scene, it's honestly heart breaking. Personally, I find it mind-boggling.

Clearly, as most of us would agree, this is not how things should be going. Aren't we supposed to be advancing more with time? It's not hard to realize that there is now some very advanced technology out there, they talk about it every day, it's just never in regards to the healing of the body.

There are literally inventions that can open up portals and bend time (look up CERN). The point being, humanity should not be as sick and miserable as we are, half crippled and on forty different medications, it's just not right. But sadly, people have surrendered to this being the way it goes, giving into it and surrendering themselves.

The question needs to be, why aren't there technologies that help get people out of diseased states? Or rather, where are the technologies that can help us do that? I'm sure there's got to be a few.

However, being the good people that we are, we trust that we will be given an answer should they find one, so we sit and wait. We put our faith in them, hoping for the answer, or the invention, or the cure to come, sometime soon. We hope it's next month or next year, hopefully in enough time to save us.

I can't tell you how many hopeful patients I had throughout my career, who wholeheartedly believed, prayed, and wished for an answer, a solution, or a cure. They truly put their faith into the medical field and its science, hoping something would come save them before it was too late. And how much I wanted that to be true for them. But, sadly, most of them ever got their wish.

It breaks your heart.

There are so many people who die without a solution; sick, afraid, and suffering immensely and it's just not okay.

We deserve *so much better.*

It's understandable that many of us worry about getting sick and dying. We're bombarded by the news and the media which fill our heads up with so much chaos and fear-based material that keeps us awake at night. We're terrified of becoming sick, or even worse. We worry about something going wrong with our health on top of all of the other stresses we have going on in our life, trying to get by and afford to live. And medical care is expensive, no matter the insurance we have.

Between germ fear and obsessive thoughts around just about everything, it's no wonder we're so busy getting sick all of the time. People are totally overwhelmed, especially when it comes to taking care of their health.

We've learned to go to the doctor when we have a concern or a problem, or really when anything shows up. We go in hoping for an answer, and a solution. We just want to make whatever it is, stop doing what it's doing, and for everything to be okay. If we're lucky, we find out what it's called and maybe we'll get a pill or some kind of solution to sort of fix it. We just want everything to go back to normal, so we can go on and continue living our lives the way we want to.

We wholeheartedly hope the doctor can fix us.

And maybe they will.

But sometimes, they can't and things don't get fixed.

Band-aids only go so far when the issue is more than skin deep.

And, maybe the issue doesn't have a simple answer, so it's not going to fully go away with a medication, or a procedure or something. In fact, things may continue and even get worse, and before we know it, more symptoms show up. Then the fear really starts to kick in. This only renders us weaker and more stressed out, which only puts more strain on our health and mind.

The doctors do all they can with the tools that they have, but sometimes there's just nothing more they can do. They know that the body will try to work to correct itself, so they hope they've given us an adequate amount of solutions, and they honestly hope things get better for us somehow. Our emotions pour in, and we are left feeling somewhat helpless. We've been told nothing about what we can do for ourselves and how to help our body heal from this issue.

Obviously, something is amiss that needs our attention. The problem has been that the beautiful people within our medical profession, aren't always able to help people get out of the bad place that they're in. It's because *we* have a big part in our healing. There's only so far that their medications and procedures, even their knowledge, can take us when it's a real system or organ problem. They try their best to correct the issue and patch things up as best they can, many of them really do work hard to help us, but it's rare that they help us figure out a good *game plan* to get our body <u>healed</u> and back to a healthy state. And I'm talking about a game plan. Illness and disease require a lot of time, attention, and action, not just a quick fix.

If we don't get down to the core of the matter, things usually resurface later. Especially, if there are other weaknesses in different areas of our body, and things are still out of balance and unsettled in some area of our health, eventually something will pull us back out of balance. Unfortunately, often times it's in an even bigger way.

How to reinstate our *total health*, from the inside out, isn't really a thing in the medical industry. Reinstating one's health is kind of a big job. It's not easy to change things and give up the terrible foods and habits that we've had for years. The doctors don't work on the smaller, yet largely important details of the person's life such as their food, stress levels, activities or lack thereof, thought processes, habitual practices, even relationship and self-image issues, as they all have something to do with it. Not to mention the level of toxins that are found in the body, it's not often those are even noticed.

Ok, some of them touch on a few of these, maybe they put us on a low sodium diet, but that's not really working on one's diet in my eyes. Unfortunately, never in my all of my years have I seen a doctor create an all-encompassing health and healing plan with a patient. One where they work on cleansing and rejuvenating all the systems of the body, cleaning out the cells and making sure the eliminative organs are rejuvenated and in good working order. Basically, a guided plan with a timeline of all of the steps, stages, and goals of the process.

These plans would likely be at least a good year long and then some, to really get someone back on their feet if they're riddled with several chronic diseases, cancer, and the like. This plan would improve the quality of their health, and honestly, their entire life. However, this has yet to catch on in this industry.

Of course, that's not to say that there are *no* doctors out there who do this kind of thing, there might be a few, but it's a rarity, and it is something that is needed to be done by the majority.

Whenever we receive a diagnosis around some symptoms that we're having, it's generally got more depth to it. Meaning, the symptoms showing up usually aren't just a surface issue. It's not just a name of a disease. Sure, having a skin rash might just be from poison oak, but one that shows up out of nowhere with no direct cause, requires more than just a cream.

When symptoms show up, there's usually an imbalance, dysfunction, or something wrong that's going on within the body that is needing our attention and care. Often times there is a deeper cause or reason for what's happening that just takes some investigating to figure out.

We've become so blissfully unaware of how or why things happen to our body that we don't even think to look below the surface. We take the name of the disease, accept it to some degree and walk away. So many of us have lost touch with the fact that *we* can actually do things for *ourselves* when we're not in the greatest state of health.

To be fair, somewhere along the way we fell away from realizing our amazing potential, our body's healing abilities, and how to truly take care of ourselves. We forgot how to get our health back in order. The wisdom around food and nutrition, has been lost. All of this vital knowledge must have been rolled off a cliff at some point in time, and since then, we've evolved into being even more unaware of our physical potential and power. We've even come to believe that there's someone else who knows what's happening with our body, and it isn't us.

When our body has a bleep, we're supposed to go see a doctor. And yes, it's important to see our doctor, to have someone there to try and figure some things out for us, but we still need to understand what's going on with ourselves enough that we can figure out what it is that *we* need to do.

Doctors are indeed there for good reason. They're there to check on our condition, give us a name to our problem, and are wonderful at catching things we wouldn't otherwise want to miss. Of course, that's not always the case, sometimes they do miss a lot, but they do the best they can with the knowledge they have.

That's why it's so important for us to be on top of things for ourselves and know what to do when our body needs help. The connection we have to our bodies and how to take care of ourselves, is nothing less than vital. Even in the times that doctors do know what's going on, sometimes there's no direct solution for things, and it's a wait and see. Or, it's three to six months out to be able to see the specialist that we need, and in the meantime, we're not being told about all of the things *we* can do. And there is *a lot* that we can do while we're waiting for our next doctor's visit and testing.

Every human being is built with the ability to do things for themselves (except for the highly disabled, of course). We all have the capacity to hone in on what's going on within us and to start figuring out what we need to do. We even have an internal guidance system that gives us clues and signals, telling us what it is that we need to change, stop, or begin doing for ourselves. That is, if we know how to listen, because we all have an inner knowing, we've just gotten so used to ignoring it or shutting it out. We're never reminded of this, so we've basically forgotten that it even exists.

Having assistance, guidance, and support is essential, but that includes other people, like someone who can help us work on our diet, our activity level, or our mindset. While we're alone and perhaps waiting for the help, there's always something we can work on personally. There's an enormous amount of information out there on self-care, diet, and improving our health; it's all over the internet, there are tons of health and healing books, as well as many beautiful people out there sharing information on all of this stuff.

The fact of the matter is, we *always* have the power to make a change. We have the power to take something away or add something to our life that directly affects our health. Often times, we even know what some of that is, without even having to think twice. We're honestly all able-bodied enough to help ourselves, on one level or another. There's a lot we can do for ourselves that can instigate healing. We've just not been educated around this enough.

A disease name can be very useful, but not just because the doctor may have a remedy. More so, because it tells us what part(s) of our body is having difficulties. When we're told we have diabetes for example, we know that our pancreas is involved, and knowing that is powerful. (Along with our kidneys, digestive system, liver, and endocrine system). Just knowing that our pancreas is struggling to work properly, gives us something to work with. It helps tremendously to know what organs and systems are involved in our health issue, so that we can start working on taking care of them better.

We've come to the understanding and belief that some diseases are manageable, some are not yet understood, very few can be cured, and others are progressive and may eventually lead to death. There are so many chronic diseases out there today that are stated to be incurable, which makes it feel like there's little, to no solution in sight. But is that really the truth?

Chronic illnesses create chronic medication users. However, there are quite a few people that work to get *themselves* out from underneath all of their health issues and free themselves from having to take medications for the rest of their life, but they did have to work hard to get themselves there. These beautiful people prove that it's possible. And they are not unlike you or I.

The times I've seen patients come out of their chronic illnesses and off their medications (with doctor monitoring) they put in the effort, made the changes, especially with their diet, mindset, and activity. People can do wonders with their health through diet alone. People can change their lives if they have the determination and desire to do so.

These days, it seems like there's a never-ending list of disease and disorder names that just keeps growing. There are so many different disorders and diseases to each organ and system it's hard to believe, let alone keep up with. There are so many variations to system and organ weakness and malfunction, that everything gets overly complicated, which is how people lose their footing and have no idea what they could possibly do for themselves. When in truth, it all comes down to the same thing; the dysfunction of an organ or system, cellular difficulties, and the body being overloaded or burdened in one way or another.

None of us want to be labeled with a disease, nor do we want to have some problem for the rest of our lives. We really don't want to have to take a bunch of pills every day, nor do we want our bodies cut into. We would prefer wholeheartedly, to avoid all of that and live a comfortable, healthy, and disease-free life, crazy as it sounds.

It's safe, but sad to say, that we're at the most diseased time in history. The US is the most diseased country in the world. Nothing can match the level of sickness and weakening of the human body that we have going on in our population today. We also have never had the amount of chemicals and poisons thrown at us that we have in our lives and the world today.

It's not hard to understand why there are so many diseases plaguing humanity considering what's been happening to our food, our environment, and our mental health. Sadly, a lot of people by the age of sixty or seventy have at least a few weaknesses and disease processes going on, if not a long list of them. I understand why people are so caught up in the fear of getting sick, I really do. Especially when there are bugs and viruses being thrown at us on top of everything else.

The constant worry and obsession of getting some kind of untreatable illness, overwhelms most people, rendering them weaker. The endless fear of the unknown consumes us, so we become anxious or depressed, much of which is treated with a pharmaceutical. We then throw ourselves even further away from connecting back into ourselves, where we can actually figure out what to do to take care of things. Our bodies need our attention; they need us to strengthen up and take responsibility for ourselves, no matter how overwhelming the situation feels, and our mental health needs our compassion and some serous TLC.

The first thing that would be the most helpful is to move our energy and mindset out of fear. Big time. Most people don't realize that fear eats away at us, slowly and stealthily. It zaps our vital energy, our immunity, and overall weakens our body. Imagine if we took all of the energy that we put into fearing things and instead put it towards getting ourselves stronger and healthier. Which it turns out is a hundred times more powerful.

Fear drains us. Working on our wellness makes us stronger.

I often think to myself, why did we suddenly become so weak and susceptible to all of these diseases? How and why are we encountering this intense onslaught of problems, illnesses, diseases, and harmful organisms all at once? What happened that we're in such dire and desperate times?

What I do know is, that it doesn't need to go on like this. We need to rebalance our nervous systems, strengthen our health, and get our stuff together. We don't need to be living in this fear state that's been slowly infused into us. It's not natural for us on any level, the fear, sickness, disease... this is not how it should be, nor how it needs to stay. We can actually change the course of things.

We need to regain control of what's happening to our bodies so that we don't remain, or in fact become more vulnerable to the million elements that are out there that can cause further harm, disease, and basically cripple us.

Something we often hear when things are happening to our health is that *"these things just happen."* Most people just surrender to that statement, because we've learned to believe this is true, and it's easier than questioning things. But what we need is to get back to realizing is that there are *always* reasons that our health is having issues. It always involves an organ or system, or the general state of the body, even if an illness was brought on by a toxin or organism.

Finding the root cause to whatever problem or disease that presents itself, is vital. There is a reason why things aren't working well, so this gives us the opportunity to hone in. We can start by looking at our body's overall status. What things look like physically, externally, from the skin to the eyes, to all the beeps and bops of our external being. Without judgement, of course. Then we can start looking at the internal signals that we're getting. How well is our body handling everyday things like digesting food, expelling waste, breathing, and handling stress? Do we have chronic issues with these, yet just consider it to be normal?

The organs and systems that are involved when we're sick or ill, all have mechanisms as to how they work, as well as to how they can be helped. If we go to our doctor and they gave us a good breakdown of what's happening with our body, some of why it's happening, and we received information on what we could do in the meantime, we'd be in such a better place physically, mentally, and emotionally. We'd be more grounded and better equipped and able to help ourselves.

We've gotten so used to the process of handing everything over to someone else. We just drifted off into some other world ignoring our problems, sitting around watching reruns on TV, instead of paying attention and doing some of the work that needs to get done. We've come to learn that it was easier to do this, than to actually work on the issues ourselves. We kind of just figured this is how it goes and have since become indifferent. We eat and do what we want without even considering what it could be doing to us, then when things show up, we act totally unaware of how or why it happened.

Some beautiful people unfortunately end up with a list of diagnoses that's a mile long. It's almost as though they get a new one practically every visit. Not to mention, it ends up being twelve different names for the dysfunction of the same organ or system. To me it seems someone's not connecting the dots, because this organ has been screaming out for a long time, yet no one has been helping it.

My brain has always worked to see other angles and sides of things, which brought me to look my patient's diagnoses, surgeries, problems, and medications through a different lens. After about 2 years into my career, I just couldn't ignore all of the other things that were going on with my patients. I felt like their diets, what was going on in their lives and homes, their emotional state, their traumas, and even their level of understanding, was affecting everything about their health problems. I could even read their body language and felt their desire for me to know more about what was going on with them. They needed someone to listen to them and help them find a way out of this difficult time.

I picked up so many cues and had so many more questions, I couldn't understand why anyone else wasn't seeing this?

I got that things weren't always what they seemed. It wasn't just stones in their kidneys, urinary retention, difficulty breathing, or chest pain. There was a bigger picture at hand. Surely, we could work on resolving the physical symptom or problem, and need to, but more was needed in getting down to the deeper layers of what was happening.

Another thing that really stood out for me was when a person had this long list of disorders and diseases happening, how it affected them. Can you imagine just how stressful and disempowering it must feel to keep being told there's yet another problem that you have, or another diagnosis that you have accumulated? (You may actually even know how that feels.) Then we sit there, more powerless than ever, by yet another issue being added to our list, feeling *even* more helpless and hopeless, like our body is falling apart bit by bit with no end in sight.

This vulnerability further weakens the physical body and affects our immune system, endocrine system, and nervous system. When we feel so disempowered, it affects all realms of our being. It weakens our mental and emotional health, and even puts stress on the connections and relationships we have with ourselves and others. It effects our joy, the ability to do the things we love, as well as the everyday tasks and work that we have to do.

All of this lowers our immunity. The stress, worry, angst, sadness, fear, anger, and disappointment all lower our vibration and our physical stature. Every single part of us feels it.

Maybe you've been there, or are there right now in this very moment. In a place feeling really down about how thing are going, especially your health, with no direction to take, nor an answer in sight. Nobody has really helped you figure things out. Although you're maintaining, you worry about what's around the corner next or what else might go wrong, leaving you feeling overwhelmed, weak, small, and hopeless. I've seen this happen way too often to so many beautiful people.

I can feel their emotions and heartbreak so palpably, it's really humbled me to the core. As they have these realizations, they end up feeling like their bodies are useless or worthless, and they themselves powerless. This has truly saddened me to no end. And the help that they are offered, just isn't not enough. The help they need *isn't* offered. It's a huge loss in my eyes.

When we take a piece of paper and write down our endless list of problems, issues, and physical hardships, it's really hard to feel positive and good about it. Our health problems affect every aspect of our life. Of course, there are some people who live quite the opposite and maintain a very positive outlook, taking what comes day by day. Even when they are struggling physically, their attitude and actions are beyond what you would expect. They don't let their physical issues ruin their life or even to dampen their spirit. They may even step in and make some changes for themselves to ensure their health moves forward and not downward.

But for others, and for most, health problems can be the breaking point where overwhelm and fear take over. We have a harder time enjoying life when we're not feeling well. We aren't as funny as we once were, we don't laugh as much, we can barely take care of our daily needs, our stress levels are insane, and we've probably lost the motivation to do the things that we once loved to do.

With a long list of problems sitting in front of us and plaguing us, it can really feel impossible to turn things around. However, even with that long list, you would be surprised at how amazingly well the body responds to a new regimen and a new outlook. Instead of feeling like our world is ending, we can look at it and figure out what systems and organs are being stressed out, take our power into our own hands, and do something about it.

Helping ourselves in a time of ill health is vital. Even though we haven't received a ton of information on how to do this, it's a beautiful thing to know that there are many ways in which we can. *Many ways.* We just have to want to do it and start looking, asking, and receiving the information.

During my career, I didn't notice or hear of much advice being given to people around the things they could do at home, or within the natural realm of things, that would help them heal some of their issues. There was a doctor or two who did share a few things, and they happened to be a part of the older generation of doctors (those who went to school over forty plus years ago), where some of the home remedies or natural thought processes were still present. But unfortunately, it was few and far between.

There are so many simple things we can do and small changes that we can make that would improve our health and the state of our body, hands down. There are many reasons that illness and discomfort take place in our body, but the first thing we have to do is realize that we have the actual ability and power to do something about it.

When our body is giving us messages and is as sick as can be, it's trying to tell us something. It might be telling us to just do our best to rest, eat well and to let it birth out and detox all the stuff it needs to, like in getting rid of a viral load or build-up of toxins. It might be telling us to stop doing what we're doing, or that it's time to make a big change in some area of our life.

There are tons of messages that we often miss. We interfere on so many levels through our busyness, distractions, and consumption of things, so much so, that we lose out on the messages our body is trying its hardest to give to us. It's always trying to get our attention.

I know that it can seem a bit scary when we know we have to undergo big lifestyle or dietary changes. The hardest part is even knowing where to begin. Sure, it sounds easy to let go of alcohol or sugar, but as most of us know, it isn't always the case. Letting go of something can be overwhelming, and that's why it's important to look deeply at what's going on and why we're having a difficult time with it.

There are reasons as to why we do things or ingest things that aren't good for us. Sometimes it's an actual physical reason, like sugar and fungus in the body, or it's mental and emotional. Having an understanding, and honestly, some compassion towards ourselves, will have a more positive impact on how we handle it, as well as that it will help us towards making the changes and new decisions that we need to.

It's helpful to try and identify the reason as to why we're consuming certain things, especially when they have an emotional or mental reason behind them, like with smoking cigarettes or in drinking alcohol. Often times, its necessary to work on the emotional and mental aspects of why we do things or consume the things that we do, which only helps us in letting them go.

Doctors don't necessarily always know the layers behind why or what we're doing. They do their best and give their patients general advice like to stop smoking, get more exercise, or eat better. Unfortunately, they aren't really taught how to assist someone in restoring their health to its perfect, natural state. This process requires a significant effort on the patient's part, along with the recognition that aspects of their life beyond the physical realm are influencing them. Imagine having your doctor as a mentor and coach along the journey of working on yourself in all of the areas that need assistance.

Unfortunately, there's a huge disconnection.

There's been a lack of information put forth on the powerful impact that nutrition has on the body and illness, or how some diseases are actually caused by nutrient deficiencies. There's a lack of information around cleaning out and ridding the body of excess waste or toxins, and not much is said about how a person can work on themselves to help correct the imbalances and weaknesses that are going on within their body.

We also never really hear about how the body can regenerate, how cells can reproduce a better version of themselves, and that they can then recreate and rebuild a stronger, healthier organ or system. The natural processes of the body, especially its self-healing capabilities often seem to get left out of the equation, as does the acknowledgment of plant and botanical medicine. We've lost touch with all of this extremely valuable information and knowledge that goes back thousands of years. There's endless information that isn't being accessed around natural healing remedies and modalities that are out there, which could, hands down, save a lot of people from further suffering.

We never really think too deeply about how or why things are this way. We don't think about how modern-day medicine came to be, or how all of these diseases erupted onto humanity, we just accept that it is what it is. We believe that what is told to us is the most advanced and best routes and methods that are available.

We should all know that healing the body of disease really does involve more than just one solution and that there are layers to it. More importantly, that it is possible to heal from *almost* everything. It's not just a black and white situation and solution for the most part. Of course, there are some exceptions here, but disease is a something that can be broken down, looked at, and worked on.

Even if it was a virus that caused our body to respond with sickness, there's more than just a virus to deal with. There are systems involved, ones that we can strengthen and support. There are even so many things we can do, and different therapies we can use to help our body combat the organism.

People do find themselves nervous to branch out into the unknown, and understandably so, considering it's not promoted in the conventional or modern medical model. Using natural means or going at things by ourselves, feels risky, and it's definitely not promoted. It's totally unchartered territory. We're afraid that if we try to do something to help ourselves, or look into natural, alternative methods, we might end up worse off, and in a place where no one, and nothing will be able to help us, thereafter. Often times, natural and herbal medicine isn't agreeable, nor is it acknowledged much by our healthcare providers.

I will say that this cold shoulder that's been given to herbal and natural medicine world is beginning to warm up. There's a reintroduction of energy around natural healing methods and medicine that's catching fire. It's actually more like old healing wisdom is once again being accepted. More and more people are growing interested in learning about these natural methods and practices and are even willing to try them.

We're starting to delve back into great-grandma's recipe book for remedies around various health ailments such as colds, coughs, and other issues, as well as that we're happily doing some research of our own. Discovering other methods and remedies can be so exciting. A lot of us have already decided to take greater responsibility for ourselves and access more of this knowledge. We've started moving towards being more health conscious and open to things that can possibly help us.

We're working to change things around with our diet, exercise routines, and trying our best to incorporate other self-care techniques that we can do on the daily, such as meditation, lymph brushing, sauna sessions, or yoga. We are learning to do more things to strengthen our body's and its ability to heal itself. The information is flooding in and it's hard to ignore.

In recent years, doctors have even started to recommend some alternative therapies to their patients such as acupuncture, chiropractic, or massage therapy. It's definitely not everything, but it's a start. Insurance has even opened the door to pay for some of this care, which is a beautiful step in the right direction. This openness and acceptance have given people the permission to broaden their perspective and to realize that other therapies and medicine can also be helpful when it comes to regaining their health.

When it comes to disease or illness, as we ultimately know, the most important thing we need to do is get to the root cause of the problem. What area is being affected, is it an organ, or several organs that are involved? Is it a system or systems that are involved? Or is it a combination of things that aren't working well?

When we get to a place where we can look at things this way, we can find ways to help these areas and figure out what we need to do. We can work on things such as our diet, our actions, our thoughts, and by creating a new regimen for ourselves. Basically, we need to add goodness to the areas that are weak, so we can help our bodies with their healing process.

If we all knew the basics about the body, like where things are, and even just a short, general synapsis of what each part does, we would have a lot more confidence in our ability to step in and help ourselves when things show up. Essentially, by doing this, we're putting the power back into our hands. To know at least a few things, gives us the ability to identify with and recognize more of what's actually going on. With some basic knowledge, we're better able to take on and handle a few of the things that are going on with us. We end up having more confidence in ourselves, enough to try and figure out more of what we can do for our body.

We are all way more intelligent than we give ourselves credit for, especially with the one thing that's strictly ours- our body. We are with it every day, constantly around it, and we never leave it. Honestly, we're the ones who know our bodies the best and we should never shy away from learning more about them or listening to them.

When our body is thrown off by an imbalance or some sort of trigger, and sends us signs that something isn't right, this is our go time.

It's our time to hone in, connect to what's happening, and start really paying attention. Is there something we are doing or neglecting that's causing a burden or stress on our body?

Of course, there will always be a mystery or two that needs more insight, attention, looking into, and counseling, but if we don't at least do a few things for ourselves, we could end up in an even worse off situation. In the very least we can always do things to boost our immune system or give our body support, such as changing our diet or getting more sunlight and exercise. We can always do something to promote a greater state of health for ourselves.

Medications do absolutely play a part in things and they can be helpful, however, in all honesty they should for the most part, a bridge to get us over to the other side, not a never-ending solution. This is where a lot of things get messed up. Some of those medications bring along a whole other slew of issues for our bodies. They all carry a long list of interactions and side effects. Most of them don't just do just the one thing they're given out for.

What we really want is to avoid having to take so many of them, especially over long periods of time. More so, we want to create a desire within ourselves to be able to work on fixing the problem or the weaknesses at hand, trying our best to avoid creating new issues and problems. Especially, the ones that the medications may bring about.

We want to do more than just manage our diseases, we want to understand them and figure out ways we can help overcome them. As I've mentioned some already disease manifests for one or more reasons some being stagnancy, an overly acidic condition, toxin buildup, mineral and nutritional deficiencies, parasitic or organismal overload, endocrine dysfunction, a weakened immune system, poor liver function, poor digestive/bowel function, excess leftover waste, weakened kidneys, and a lack of oxygen. Basically, a system overload, toxicity, deficiency, and weakness.

When our body spends a long period of time in, or with any of these conditions, our cells and organs are not going to function their best, to say the least. These situations are all hard on the body, which makes it easier for things to break down and stop working properly. Our delicate cellular structure is vulnerable after so much heaviness and stress is put onto it. Our cells end up overwhelmed and having a difficult time breathing, eating properly, and doing their job because the conditions are too harsh.

If person's body is sick, there are reasons as to how it got there. When we send someone home without fixing the root cause of the problem, nor give them the support that they need to be able to work on their issues, it's only a matter of time until they're back in the same, if not a worse position. I've had many patients return to the hospital over and over again because the core issue and the condition of their body, was never truly addressed.

I like to talk about a medical diagnosis that's no longer used, called *auto-intoxication*. It's when we accumulate waste in our eliminative system and do not release it. The food then begins to rot and decay, off gassing and emitting poisons into the bloodstream, causing these toxins to circulate around the body.

This creates huge stress on the cells of the body, as the blood circulates to each and every system and organ. And, if there's a weakness anywhere in our body, these toxins will have a harsher effect on them. It weakens and causes stress on the cells. Some of the cells may become so overwhelmed that they might have a really hard time getting rid of these poisons.

Poor elimination and the accumulation of leftover food happens due to a variety of reasons. Insufficient exercise, a diet full of processed and chemically treated foods, poor intake of fresh, natural foods, poor water intake, trauma and emotionally difficult events, and many other stressors can end up causing the eliminative systems to slow down. When we are stressed out and in fight or flight mode throughout our day, our digestive system slows down its activity to be able to lend the fight or flight mode all of the energy that it needs.

Symptoms of an overly toxic body can be as vague, or as simple as feeling under the weather, tired all of the time, or generally unwell. Having leftover waste laying around, also turns into a feast for bacteria, fungus, viruses, and other parasitic organisms who are in turn, not kind to our bodies. Our bodies are then forced to work on overtime to buffer out all of the poisons, as well as deal with these undesirable organisms, on top of all of the jobs it already needs to do.

We need to give our body the helping hand it needs to release excess waste, rebalance its chemistry, and get rid of unwanted organisms when we're in a less than perfectly healthy state. Through my perspective and opinion, with the help of botanical medicine, cleansing techniques, and a clean diet, we can help the body move out of this eternal state of stress and misery and into a more peaceful, balanced, and healthy state of being.

There's been an unconscionable and excessive emphasis put on bugs and germs and how scary they are, but there's something people should know. For one, WE are an amazing organism in ourselves. A powerful, complex and strong one. Then, our immune system and the cells that it creates, when working correctly, are powerful beyond measure. It's built to take care of undesirable organisms and foreign cells that enter the body.

However, science seems to focus on one or two organisms, leaving out many others, who in fact are just as, if not more harmful to our body. People are so busy being afraid of viruses that they don't consider the other kinds of organisms that do our bodies harm and go undetected, that being parasites, worms, and fungus.

These organisms happen to be quite intelligent, no less. We spoke about them briefly earlier. These organisms are highly intelligent, they nourish themselves with our nutrients through the food we ingest, our leftover waste products, and even siphon out nutrients directly from our blood. Some such as the tapeworm will attach itself to the liver and take out the nutrients that it wants, especially iron.

Parasites love a warm, acidic, and waste filled environment. If they are well fed, they thrive. When they thrive, they reproduce. The influx and overproduction of these organisms create further burdens on our body. Even their waste products are toxic to us, their gas and urine alone can cause much havoc. They live off our leftover food that we have laying around, producing tens of thousands of eggs, monthly. They take up space in our body, creating a burden on some areas, the intestines being one of them.

The thing to know about these organisms is that they are stealthy.

They know how to exist undetected, without being noticed for long periods of time, because their species depends on it in order to survive. They do not want to cause too serious of an issue that they lose their host, so they remain under the radar. And if health problems such as anemia arises, they aren't suspect whatsoever, as they cannot be detected through the usual lab tests or x-rays.

Time and time again, I've seen innumerable people walk away from their doctor or the hospital without answers. To me all the signs are there, the bloating and digestive issues, the anemia, the nervousness and irritability. These are usually seen as separate issues, and definitely aren't looked at as to being created by one of these organisms.

Unfortunately, these undetected organisms create inflammation and an underlying infection in our body. If our body is aware of these critters, it's working hard trying to fight off these organisms. However, as mentioned, they hide in such a way that sometimes our body cannot even detect them, especially because they are well-known to cloak themselves under the heavy metals that are found in the body.

Have you ever seen a picture of a hookworm? When you look at them under a microscope, their teeth alone will give you nightmares. Do yourself a favor (or don't) and look up pinworms, hookworms, tapeworms, and flukes that are all found in the human body. Pictures are worth a thousand words. It's not to freak you out, rather to make you aware. There are even videos about them.

Worms have been known to be responsible for things like nutrient deficiencies, mental health disorders, respiratory problems, intestinal and skin issues, and even bedwetting in children. They even link up to our nervous system and create messages and signals that direct us to do the things they need from us, causing things like cravings as an example, so that we eat the foods they can get the most out of. And, it's not just worms and parasites that can do this, fungus, mold, and other organisms are just as intelligent. These parasites live in lots of different areas of the body, some have even been found in the brain.

Again, most doctors believe this is a third world nation problem and isn't an issue, at least here in the US. Their schooling doesn't cover it as a root cause of people's health issues, so it's greatly overlooked. Getting a lab test for parasites is rare, and frankly one stool sample isn't going to prove much.

Eating pumpkin seeds, raw garlic, onions, coconut, papaya seeds, sunflower seeds, cinnamon, cloves, oregano, thyme, sage, cayenne, kombucha, fermented foods, and grapefruit seed extract are all foods that parasites do not like. There are simple, herbal formulas that are available that help to eliminate parasites; however, the process generally takes a few months.

Studies show that parasites reproduce in cycles with the moon, being most active and reproducing during the full moon phase. Knowing what parasites can do to the gut, nervous system, and when you read a bit deeper, what they can do to our mental health, it's completely understandable why we have very intense occurrences during the full moon. Especially at the hospital, ask any health care professional how that day usually goes for us. Once you know what they do, it makes so much sense. Or at least it does to me...

There are plenty of books and online resources that can give you more details. There's a science labeled as Parasitology which reveals so much about these critters. It's not as though science hasn't already studied them fully.

When we have a weaker intestinal system and a low nutrient diet, we are more vulnerable to these organisms. I get that people think any organism consumed would die in our stomach acid, but considering the condition of people's bodies these days, and knowing how adaptive, strong, and smart these organisms are, there's no doubt they can find their way to survive. And they do. They know how to live and thrive inside of and on all living species which includes plants, animals, and humans. They have been around since before man, for hundreds of thousands of years, even millions of years. Parasites are survivors.

Now, let's take a look at another fun one, fungus. Our body naturally consists of some fungal organisms, as well as bacteria that are all necessary for the function and balance of the biome of our body. It's when these organisms overgrow because of an imbalance in our body, that they become a hazard to us.

If our body is in a well-balanced and healthy state, it will naturally maintain the levels and growth of these organisms, keeping everything in check. Our internal bacteria and immune cells are there to take care of this overgrowth, but only if we are in good health and our bacteria and cellular situation is in good standing. But, when we are filled with leftover waste, stressed out (which creates acids), ingesting a lot of sugar, alcohol, flour products, and processed foods, as well as taking a lot of medications, the fungus has the opportunity to get out of control.

An overgrowth of fungus in the body is not our friend. Throughout all of my years as a nurse, especially having worked hospice for 7 years, I saw endless amounts of fungus growing in, and literally on external parts of people. It is very well known that fungus can overgrow with the overuse of antibiotics, as well as with chemotherapy and radiation treatments, and the long-term use of steroids.

The overgrowth of fungus is not friendly to our body and in truth, can be quite invasive and difficult to get rid of. There are no medications that can completely rid the body of fungus. First of all, we do need some of them in there, but there are several different strains, some more beneficial than others. We also need to put in the work ourselves to help rid our body of this overgrowth. We cannot get things under control if we just continue eating all of the sugary, processed foods that we're so used to.

Well-known manifestations of an overgrowth of fungus are yeast infections, athlete's foot, jock itch, ringworm, vaginal yeast infections, oral thrush, rashes, and yeast that is noticeable in bowel movements. These however, are just indicators that there's a larger issue at hand. When any of these show up, it generally means there's not just an overgrowth in that area. There are a few medications available that are prescribed to help out, some doctors might even prescribe or suggest that the person take probiotics to reestablish the good bacteria in hopes to curb an overgrowth.

When fungus goes unnoticed and grows extensively, it can become what's known as a *systemic* infection. This is where the fungus gets into the bloodstream, becoming laced throughout the gut and intestinal system, and can even be found in and around the brain, the heart, the vessels of the circulatory system (causing many heart issues, blockages), the eyes, and even can affect the bones. Fungus can cause volume imbalances, blood pressure issues, brain fog, pain, and the list goes on.

Fungus is another organism that doesn't like oxygen. Ways to get rid of fungus is for one, to stop eating sugary, processed foods, simple carbs, etc. Lots of green juices and powders are a great way to combat fungal overgrowth as well as certain herbs like Pau D'Arco, Echinacea, Oregano, Aloe Vera, Tea Tree, and Chamomile. There are many anti-fungal herbal blends out on the market that have been created to combat fungal overgrowth. Grapefruit Seed extract and anti-parasitic herbs all help combat fungus as well.

Even if a disease has been stimulated by an organism or external toxin, there are several systems being affected and there's a lot we can do about it. These organisms may come in and stir things up, but if our immune system, nervous system, and digestive system are functioning properly, they will combat and address the issues. We can add support through good hydration to help flush things along and by eating wholesome, alkaline foods to minimize the hard work body has to do.

When it comes to the more common ailments and symptoms that we get such fever, runny nose, mucus, and so on, these are all ways that our body works to get rid of toxins and to let us know that it's working to fight things off. The body is literally activated to get rid of these things, hence the cold symptoms we might get. That's what the body is naturally supposed to do. Our body is not weak or sick, it's actually working quite hard to take care of business.

Our body is constantly working its hardest to try and put out the fires happening within it. It does its best to get rid of invading organisms, repair itself, recover from any damage that was done to it… it's really always working so hard for us. If we continue with the same substances, chemicals, toxins, and foods, and keep waste laying around, then *we* are a big contributing factor to a lot of the problems, imbalances, disruptions, and overwhelm that happens to our body that eventually turns into disease.

As we already acknowledged, the human body does not naturally fall victim to disease or illness. We're the most intelligent life form on the planet containing billions of cells with their own innate intelligence, and it's very humbling once you realize this. It also gives us power. We really don't give our body the credit it deserves a lot of the time, and it's so much more powerful than we think it to be.

I believe it's essential for everyone to first acknowledge the amazingness of the body and what can happen to it, especially on account of what causes disease to manifest. While it's vital for us to seek attention from medical professionals in certain situations, more importantly, we need to learn and be taught basic skills that support our health.

We can either think disease to be this complicated, complex, mysterious situation, or we can see it as a message that our body needs our attention and some help from us.

Every day we are given the opportunity to make changes to our health for the better. We all just need to be reminded of the essential ways that we can help keep our bodies healthy and free from disease. Different cleansing methods, healthy, whole food diets, the importance of purified water, getting in sunshine, exercise, fresh air, and how to move through emotions and stressors in a healthy way. Also, if we know how to keep as many toxins out of our life as we can, it would move us further away from disease and chronic illness.

It's vital for us to question why things are happening with our bodies, because it's kind of like us standing up for our body. Questioning how or why, connects us into our body and helps to expand our vision so we're better able to see what's happening. As I said many times before, we all have an innate connection and the ability to recognize what's going on with our body and what it needs.

The fear of helping ourselves is falling away, and as this fear is slowly released, we're taking our power back. More power in our hands helps us to make more educated decisions and better choices for ourselves. It helps us to see things more clearly. In essence, we learn to care more about ourselves, building up the trust we have in ourselves, as well as the strength that we need to create change.

Of course, it's important to consult with our doctor, but in the meantime, we can make better choices for ourselves through our food and daily habits. We can instantly give up toxic foods and products and switch to cleaner, more natural, and healthier ones. This knowledge is flooding out into the world right now, it's hard to ignore! And it's there because more people are asking and looking for it. We're all beginning to want to repair and improve our health so we can literally avoid and combat disease.

I like people to know that other medicinal practices around the world, ones that have been around for thousands of years, understand the body and sometimes see it under a different lens. Western medicine has its place and it's thought processes however, Eastern medicine looks at the body and health quite differently. It even can tell things by observing and assessing different parts of the body, from the iris to the face, to the tongue and the skin in order to get a good idea of what's going on *inside* of the body when someone is unwell. They also treat the patient with food, herbs, therapeutic modalities, and even spiritual treatments.

Health is also seen by other cultures as to involving all aspects of life, which includes the mental and emotional state, as well as spiritual practices and beliefs. It's powerful to understand the connection to all things when it comes to our health. There's so much more to health than in just breaking down parts, cells, chemicals, molecules, and atoms. We are made up of so much more than that. It's taken a long time for us to come back to the understanding that health and disease don't always just pertain to the physical.

There's a book called 'You Can Heal Your Life' by the one and only, Miss Louise L. Hay. This book is where I first saw the hyphenated version of the word disease as, **dis-ease**. *Dis-* means without, -*ease* means comfort and peace. Disease then means 'the body is without comfort and peace'. It was an instant connection for me. I always knew there was more to illness than just symptoms and labels, that there were stories and influences around almost everything that manifested within the body. Sometimes the bigger picture and details to a person's story can give us deeper insight into what's going on, and in turn help us to better understand what's happening, as well as what needs to be done.

Of course, this is not discounting the physical reasons at all. This is just another take on things, or perhaps an addition to what we may want to be aware of and consider when looking at someone's health problems and healing process.

We've all heard about people dying from a broken heart or from deep sadness, quite literally. Loss, hardship, and depression can create a rapid decline in a person's physical health. Depression can lead to poor appetite and nutritional intake, lack of movement, sleep disturbances, feelings of giving up, isolation, and serious life events.

There have been several cases during my career with a few elderly men who had just lost their wives, who had chest pain or a heart attack shortly after their wife's passing. Some of them even passed away. Sometimes emotional matters of the heart can cause physical disorders of the heart, as the heart cells are affected by deep sadness and emotion. This resonates with other organs and systems, as well.

Someone who undergoes a traumatic event can be so strongly affected that their nervous and endocrine system go into overdrive. A new onset of tremors, anxiety, heart palpitations, chest pain, headaches, breathing difficulties, even digestive issues may arise. Chronic or unresolved trauma can bring weakened systems into a worse off place, even leading to chronic illness if not dealt with.

Statistics show that two out of three people suffer from some type of trauma in their lifetime. Traumas usually shake us to the core. We either come out on the other side stronger, or our world is forever turned upside down. We all respond differently to trauma, so our coping mechanisms also differ, some of which will affect our body's physical state of being.

As studied by science, the most common symptoms caused by traumas and devastation are pain, lowered immune response, digestive issues, nervous system disturbances, muscle weakness, blood pressure problems, heart issues and weakness, fatigue, depression, anxiety, endocrine system dysfunction, as well as respiratory and breathing problems.

Trauma weakens the body's defense and coping mechanisms, because that person's entire being has been thrown into fight or flight mode. Some traumas leave people stuck in these modes, creating a new onset of problems and illness. Especially, in the case of chronic trauma, something as serious as heart disease or cancer may even manifest.

If someone incurs physical or sexual trauma it can affect the very part of the body where the trauma took place. These trauma victims can develop a host of physical issues and diseases in those areas either immediately, or later down the line. The initial problems can be in the form of a rash or infection. It's in adulthood that they may in fact develop more serious illnesses in the area.

Someone may have been struck in a certain area of their body during a traumatic event and the health of that area may suffer. Different ailments, dysfunction, or pain can conflict that area for a long time, even creating a *life*long issue.

Someone can be picked on or criticized about a certain part or area of the body, or their entire body as a whole. Besides the esteem issues that are likely going to manifest, mental and emotional abuse can also cause people to develop a host of physical issues such as immune, digestive, nervous system, and breathing issues. There is a suppression and lowering that can occur to parts of the body, especially the immune system.

Truth be told, criticism hurts us in more ways than one. We may take on excess weight as a form of protection, or develop a disorder such as anorexia, even try to hurt ourselves in some way because of the absolute distress that we feel. These traumas and responses can again, carry on further down the line and develop into bigger problems physically, especially if the emotional and mental sides of things aren't addressed. We will talk more about that a bit later.

If I haven't said it enough, it's vitally important that we work on our mindset and emotions when it comes to working through our illnesses. Healing from emotional or physical trauma can be some deep work, but it's so essential. One of the ways we can do this is through affirming our healing and stating what we do want for ourselves; release, freedom, to let go, and to heal from these issues. Speaking in terms of what we *do* want over what we don't want affects our outcome greatly.

It's more true than not, we bring about what we think about, so instead of focusing our energy on the problem we've been held down with, we can choose to focus our energy on where we want to be, and what we do want.

Let's take a statement like "My diabetes is getting worse and my body is falling apart." Maybe this is somewhat true or feels like an honest statement, but is it serving us to say it? Maybe we can work on what we're focusing on and replace these types of statements with ones that are more life affirming and positive. In this case we can change the statement to, "My body is getting healthier and stronger, and my pancreas and kidneys are healing." I know, it's not necessarily the absolute truth, but I can't impress enough just how powerful it is to say. Our thoughts and words resonate quite immensely into our cells and physical being.

When we actively work to speak more lovingly and positively to our body, and we do all of the things that we can to help it, without a doubt, we can *absolutely* bring about the changes and improvements that we need to much more easily. We can add power to our body and our health in doing this.

We always have the opportunity to work on connecting back into and feeling more love for ourselves, especially our body. If we're always so willing to hand everything over to someone else to make *all* of our decisions, think for us, take care of everything, and we do nothing to help ourselves, it's a total loss of power. It also amplifies the lack of love we have for ourselves. Without working on things within our own abilities, we're doing ourselves a huge injustice and just losing ourselves and our health, further.

Of course, everyone responds differently to a health crisis and many of us even go through a grieving process of some kind because feel like we've lost a part of ourselves or failed ourselves greatly. It's absolutely understandable, but staying in these emotions won't help us get out of it.

Getting through where we feel the most broken, fearful, and hopeless is probably the most impactful and important part for us to work through (with help, of course). It's from here that we can find our core strength, as well as the motivation that we need to move ourselves forward towards getting better.

No matter what our health issue or problem is, we need to work on it. We need to be there for ourselves, even if that means getting all of the help that we possibly can to help us through it.

It's ideal, even essential that we carve some time out for ourselves. Perhaps we can find a point during our day, maybe even several times during the day, to tune into our body, listen to what it has to tell us, and ask it what it needs from us. First thing in the morning and before we go to bed at night are wonderful times to listen in as well as show some emotional support, as these times are usually the most still and quiet times of the day, ideal for honing in and increasing our awareness.

As we get into the practice of doing this, we'll begin to notice that we *do* have a connection to our body after all. It may take some time to get there, but it's absolutely worth it, especially when we see our connection deepen with time. It will give us the confidence to be better able to support ourselves and do the things that our body needs for us to do for it. These quiet moments give us the opportunity to also express our gratitude for what our body does do for us.

Our body is always fighting the good fight for us, regardless of the condition we're in. It's always trying to fix things. It really needs our emotional support and love, as well as some kudos every once in a while. We can *always* say nice things to our body, thank it, feel happy that we have it. There are always little things we can do to support it and add to its healing.

When we *intend* better for our body and put in even just the smallest amount of work, it's tremendously beneficial for it. Speaking in the terms of what we *do* want over what we don't want, will affect our outcome.

It's important that we get into alignment with our bodies and its issues. We can deliberately build up a mental image of the physical state that we *want to be in,* or of the health we desire.

Speaking more lovingly and positively to our body will *absolutely* bring about changes and improvements to our health. Even if it doesn't seem so easy.

It's important to do our best to move fear out of the way when it comes up so it doesn't zap all of our energy. Finding reasons to be grateful for things in our life or the parts of our health that are doing well, is a great place to start. The more we emit the emotions and energy of gratitude, the easier it is to make the moves we need to, eat the better foods, and act in ways that promote our health.

Disease and illness require our time and effort. We can all work on our diet, mindset, movement, and make more positive, life-affirming changes. The motivation builds as we move through, our energy shifts, and we become so much more happy with ourselves than we ever thought we could be. It's a blessing to realize just how much we can actually do to make lasting, positive changes and impacts on our health.

I know this isn't the usual way of thinking in comparison to the present and century old way to think, but it's empowering nonetheless to realize that we can help to heal every organ and system in our body.

What it really comes down to is how we take care of ourselves. How we listen to our body, treat it, and speak to it. When we understand and realize that there is a connection, and that everything plays a part in how our health is doing, we're empowering ourselves.

I know that we cannot control *everything* just in doing these things or by noticing our emotional state, praying or eating healthier. There's no fix all. It's definitely a journey. There are always going to be unforeseeable and unfavorable circumstances that we cannot control. I will never discount the fact that some of our physical bodies just cannot turn things around, but if it's possible to at least try, why wouldn't we want to?

Our bodies are always ready and hoping that we will get things back into balance and work hard to get its health back. I've always believed that we have the opportunity to change our ways at so many points in our life, and at pretty much *any* age.

No matter how old we are, we can learn to free ourselves from our old ways of thinking and doing. Although it might prove to be a huge challenge, we can learn to move into a new direction and work towards getting healthier if we're willing and able.

Today we are very fortunate to have so much beautiful information coming to light as well as so many fantastic, wise people out in the world, who are there to help us take our lives back. There are so many wonderful teachers, coaches, mentors, counselors, alternative practitioners, even some medical professionals, such as doctors and nurses who are out doing all they can to help people. There are always people out there who can help us realize the amazing healing potential that we have.

Taking care of our health is much easier than we think and having people alongside of us, will help us make it through. When we have the support, we have more determination, motivation, and success.

Remember, ultimately, *we're* the ones in charge. We're in charge of what goes into our mouth, what we do with ourselves and our bodies, what we think about, and what we allow.

Everything goes hand in hand. It's time that we create a peaceful, healing environment for ourselves, and ensure that we keep a good balance in our lives mentally and emotionally.

When we're willing to truly take a look at ourselves and do some of the work, the rewards are epic. We can take baby steps as we need to, remaining kind and loving towards ourselves as we move through the harder times, to transform our health. It's always worth it. Regardless of the ups and downs, continuing to strive for good health has so many benefits.

There is so much more in life that we have yet to experience, and we need our health to be able to do the things we love. Finding our way back to health is a beautiful journey.

CANCER

Statistics show that in the United States alone, there will be an estimated 1,735,350 new cancer cases diagnosed this year, and by the time you're reading this, that number has likely grown.

There is at least one cancer death per minute.

We're supposed to be advancing with time. We spend trillions of dollars year after year *researching*, looking for clues, answers, *a cure,* yet after almost a hundred years of doing this, there's still apparently *no cure.* That's about how long the cancer industry has been around and raising money to figure out a way.

Hippocrates was the first to identify and name cancer. He used the word *carcinos* and *carcinoma* to identify tumors of the body. It was then translated into the word *cancer* which means crab in Latin. *Onco* was added to the mix, meaning swelling in Greek, which was associated to the tumors that were found.

This manifestation of disease has been going on in humans for eons of time. There have been sick people with cancer like illnesses for thousands of years. They just weren't doing autopsies until the 16th or 17th century so causes weren't always figured out. Tumors had been around for hundreds of years.

In the 1700-1900's cancer was seen to be caused by one of many factors: genetic and chromosomal dispositions and changes, physical injuries, chemical exposures, radiation, or pathogens, like other microorganisms.

These days, chemo and radiation have become the number one answer for practically all types of cancer. Sometimes there are surgeries performed to remove the tumors and parts of the body containing it. However, another group of pharmaceuticals are becoming widely used and popular, and they are called immunotherapy drugs.

I would love to talk about these, but I cannot be positive enough about them and I want to keep this from getting too heavy for anyone. Basically, most of the treatments that are offered are chemical in nature, even the biological ones they speak of, are all lab created, have side effects, are taxing on the immune system, aggravate the body further, weakening and negating the internal environment.

I hoped for things to come to light, beyond this stuff, I waited patiently to see if any of the more positive therapies and modalities would be added to care, like IV immune boosting vitamin and mineral formulas, oxygen treatments, or powerful cancer fighting diets, but it never happened. Just more drugs and acid creating treatments. Although, just recently, there is a new treatment for tumors that's been approved that uses sound and frequency to combat tumors. Things are starting to look up.

There's not a lot of attention put on what cancer actually is, other than that it's *bad or invasive cells*. Nothing much is said about what it likes, how it thrives, what it *doesn't* like, or what we can do to help get rid of it on our own account. We fully surrender all of our power over to the doctor, use his remedies, and pray they will work. Of course, sometimes they do, but many times, they don't.

I speak in these terms because I've been in and around cancer for over twenty-five years, seven of those years was working in hospice where I saw thousands of people pass away from cancer. My breaking point was my mother's recent passing; her diagnosis and the mystery around how they claimed it as cancer, the injustices in her care and treatment, and her eventual death.

I realize this is a very sensitive and heart-tugging topic that sadly, we can all relate to. At this point in time, every single one of us have lost at least one person we loved or knew to cancer. Maybe we've even had a brush of it ourselves, or have it in this present moment. It has certainly become the epidemic of the century.

It would seem that all the money and intelligence in the world cannot seem to solve this problem no matter how hard they try. In the last twenty-five years that I have been serving as a nurse, cancer numbers have increased dramatically. The kinds and types of cancers have grown into the hundreds, and the treatments remain relatively the same, just with newer formulas.

The cancer industry is a multi-trillion-dollar industry. This is crazy to me because from where I'm standing, there are reasons for and many methods and ways to handle cancer. Over the course of the past two hundred years, there has been tons of research done around different scientific methods that have literally eradicated cancer, yet they aren't supported by the current industry. Dr. Otto Warburg was one of the great ones to discover certain means to destroying cancer in the body with something as simple as oxygen therapy, but it's not being utilized, nor being shared.

The truth is, that if anyone ever stated or claimed that they found a cure or treatment for cancer that was outside of the medical industry's research and information, it would be stated as false, misleading, and that person would even face criminal charges, and jail time for giving false hope.

There was a recent article on cancer.gov that stated that they need *more time and more money*, as well as that they will *stop at nothing* to find a cure. It's hard to understand this since there have been billions put into newly named missions to fight cancer every year. If there were answers and cures, the whole industry would no longer be of value or necessary.

We sure have had some brilliant people, scientists and doctors, throughout time who have figured out *a lot* about cancer and ways to treat it, but all the information seems to get lost somewhere along the way, and usually discredited.

Recently, I learned that some women who are diagnosed with breast cancer are told to use organic make up, over traditional make up because of the *forever* chemicals that are in the makeup. Forever chemicals are huge cancer-causing agents and unfortunately, makeup is chock full of them.

The sad part about it is that these chemicals, amongst many others, aren't banned, nor is the information about their harm, broadcast to people. If these cancer centers and medical staff know to direct these women away from these destructive chemicals after their cancer diagnosis, why would they even be allowed to be given to people in the first place?

Being diagnosed with cancer is one of the biggest hits on humanity today. It's a huge eye opener, severely affects all aspects of our life, sometimes it even cripples us physically, it crushes our spirit, and may have us leaving this life way too soon. The fear is felt loud and clear.

Cancer is known to be cells that have gone bad. However, for the body to fall victim to these *bad cells,* or to have cells turn into cancer cells means there's a lot more going on. Things aren't in a place that they need to be, the person's body and health is weakened and susceptible, their immunity lowered, and their body is struggling greatly in order to have this occur.

The body is obviously having a difficult time being able to defend itself or take care of these cells gone rogue, and it's unable to fix the issues and imbalances going on, on its own. It's overburdened, likely has other organisms that are out of control, it's undernourished, lacking oxygen, and toxic. Cancer doesn't show up in balanced, healthy bodies where the internal environment is in a healthy place.

It takes form because the body has weakness, or has been bombarded by something else that's put a great stress onto it. Again, the reasons why body becomes weak and vulnerable to cancer is because of stress, malnourishment and poor oxygenation of the cells, a weakened immune system (which could happen for a list of reasons), a highly acidic internal environment, genetic weaknesses, or it can be caused by a direct attack of an organism, chemical, or radioactive element. There are new elements that are seeming to cause harm and stress to our body in the everyday things that we partake in, and on a *daily* basis.

There are many reasons as to how cancer cells are produced in our body, science has explained some of these, but the one reason a cell turns cancerous, is because of a mutation in the DNA of the cell. We are learning that there are a lot of reasons our cell DNA can get messed with, it's a list a mile long, and many being the chemicals that are in our food, water, and products that we consume. Even though they are well-known to cause cancer, they continue to be put right in front of us for our everyday use and consumption.

I've done a lot of research and reading over the past twenty years about cancer, all the theories, causes, reasons, and answers that have been out there. I've read many first accounts of people who went through and survived cancer and how they did it.

One cancer survivor, Chris Wark made it through his cancer with both modern medical treatment and in understanding that he himself had a lot of work to do. He knew it was going to require that he make some drastic and serious changes to his diet and lifestyle. At one point in his book he stated, "*Cancer is a divine tap on the shoulder. The way you are living is killing you*".

That spoke volumes to me. There's so much truth in that, because so many of us unintentionally create an environment for cancer and illness to take hold. We wear the makeup, eat the processed foods, smoke the cigarettes, drink the tap water, the alcohol, and carry tons of stress around. We add insults to our bodies and we don't take good care of them, at least as well as we should. I know this is hard to agree with, because the truth is, it's not all our fault. Why cancer-causing agents are even put in our food, makeup, and practically handed to us, is definitely something to wonder or feel upset about. It's not what we would *actually* want for ourselves.

Of course, as mentioned, there are other factors that can lead to cancer, but in general, it's the condition that our body is in and what we're exposing it, to that makes it easier to manifest itself.

Cancer like other diseases, is a way that our body is calling out for help. Like the other diseases, it needs us to listen in. Whether we need to let go of unhealthy foods, habits, stop certain activities or substances, heal emotional and mental issues and traumas, or let go and forgive things, it wants us to make some drastic adjustments and changes. It wants us to utilize the information we have around us, especially now that we know more about what is cancer-causing, so we can avoid it at all costs.

Our body wants us to eat healthier foods that will support it in fighting and getting rid of these cancer cells. It wants us to clean things out and do more to help support its environment and all of our systems and cells, who are trying their best to fight the good fight for us. We need to make moves around our food, our environment, our quality of life, right down to the things we think about.

It's a good time for us to take a look and see what we may have been overlooking, suppressing, fighting, or neglecting for a long period of time. We may have deep emotional traumas or things that have happened in our life that are festering inside of us. There has been a connection to holding onto past hurts or resentments that can creep into our physicality and cause an underlying stress and dysfunction to our cells and our body. Cancer and other diseases are a time for us to learn how to take better care of ourselves, figure out what's got an emotional and mental hold on us, and work to get a lot more serious about what we're actually doing and allowing into our life.

Louise Hay was the first person I heard mention how cancer represented on an emotional, mental level long standing resentment, deep hurt, a deep secret or grief eating away at the self, and carrying hatred around. Of course, this sounds ridiculous to many people, and isn't the *cause of it* altogether, but after working in hospice and going through cancer stuff with my mother, I couldn't deny this being a part of it.

Of course, this is not related to everyone, as some cancer is a direct result of physical causes, however, this sat with me quite significantly for the past twenty-five years. My mother was the perfect example of how true hate, holding onto hurt, resentment, and anger can manifest in someone physically. Of course, she didn't take care of herself either, but that was just a big lack of self-love that she never got through and something I witnessed in her my entire life.

Louise is well known for her new thought patterns to go with different illnesses, and the one for cancer, as many of them did, hit me quite strongly. It helped me to realize a lot of what we hold onto can show up physically somewhere in our lives. The thought pattern for cancer is "I lovingly forgive and release all of the past. I choose to fill my world with joy. I love and approve of myself."

Of course, cancer is a serious diagnosis that shouldn't be taken lightly, it's not just about some mental thought form or letting go of what it is that we are holding onto, but acknowledging *all of the different levels* is just as important as working on the physical aspect. All angles are eye opening and healing in their own way, for sure. What we are working with mentally, emotionally, and spiritually are all a part of any disease and healing process.

Cancer brings fear to the table, especially because there are no *cures* at this point in time, just a few treatments that bring people into remission. Within the medical industry, it's never stated that someone is *cured* from cancer, only that they're in remission. However, remission gives us the thought that it could possibly show back up again. It gives permission for it to resurface, so to speak.

This is unfortunate, in my opinion. Not only are there no life and dietary rules or changes prescribed or given to people, nor much of anything to follow after the body becomes free from cancer, people then move on living in fear of its return. This really does a number on one's mental mind from the very beginning, that carries on for far too long of a time. Where is the after plan and diet to follow?

You see, if in the meantime we were told to work on creating a better internal environment in our body so we can in turn heal and regain our physical strength and health, the truth is, the cancer would be less likely to show back up. If they gave us valuable information on what causes cancer, what to avoid, what fights it, and what to do to support our body, we would end up in a much stronger place and in my opinion, cancer rates and its return, would absolutely go down.

If only we were given life-affirming, valuable information *before* the cancer even showed up, I can imagine cancer wouldn't be taking hold of half of the population the way it is. There are tons of stories out there about people who actually got through cancer, and completely changing the way they lived their life and their perspective to remain cancer free, like Chris Wark, whom I just mentioned.

Some people do make it through with just the chemo and stuff, but most of the time, the people who aren't taught better ways of eating or living, fall right back into their old ways, usual dietary and other habits, and end up with the same results down the line. The cancer returns because they never changed anything. Besides, in all honesty, chemotherapy is highly acidic, to a pH level of battery acid. When our body is already in a compromised state, adding a highly corrosive solution into our veins although to kill off cancer cells, has damaging effects to our body's internal environment and our other, healthy cells.

Even our self-healing machine of a body sometimes needs our assistance and help to get it to a better place so it can fight off trouble and take care of us better in the long run, especially when the treatments we're receiving are creating a lot more stress on the body.

There are insults everywhere we turn, so we really need to work on being more aware and conscious of what we eat, use on our body, and surround ourselves with. Toxins and chemicals are found everywhere, and once in or on the body they are processed by the liver. Hulga Clark, naturopath and author, believed that all cancers began in the liver, and that deeply resonated with me, I understood it right off the bat.

Our liver processes everything that gets into our system and filters our blood. Our liver takes on all of the chemical compounds that enter our body and breaks everything down to be eliminated. If the liver itself is not working properly, the rest of the body takes a big hit. If the biggest detoxifier in the body isn't able to do its job some of the toxins and poisons we ingest or absorb will end up in unwanted places.

I fully believe that in the least, the liver needs a lot of attention in the face of cancer. Foods like lemons, dark greens, grasses, and herbs like dandelion are so helpful, as well as a good nutrient rich diet, less heavy, fried, sugary, and fatty foods, and intermittent liver cleansing will help care for the liver. This should be ordered by a doctor, but that's just me.

I also felt deeply that a dirty colon and digestive tract was a source for cancer to form and then spread to other areas. Or, the lymphatic system being clogged, the kidneys… actually, if any of the eliminative organs in the body are clogged up, backed up, and full of toxins, that will create a heavy, toxic situation that can cause a host of health issues and diseases, including cancer. When the body isn't able to get rid of the poisons and garbage, serious issues are going to happen one way or another.

Having worked as a hospice nurse for over seven years, I did witness some people go into remission through some truly amazing efforts and natural means done on their part. Some people choose to use both western medical treatments *and* alternative and complementary ones as well. There are endless accounts and testimonials of people, everywhere around the world, who have gotten rid of their cancer, for good!

There are also endless videos, books, websites, protocols, even clinics and centers who are focused on *healing* like the Gerson institute, the Hippocrates Institute, the Hope for Cancer Institute in Mexico, Dr. Morse's Clinic, as well as innumerous others all around the globe. They all delve into powerful plant medicine, alternative therapies, dietary changes, oxygenation, cleansing techniques, and all kinds of movements and specialized therapies.

The most important thing and easiest thing a person can do when they realize they have cancer is to oxygenate. Get outside and go for more walks, getting as much fresh air as possible. If you have a center or clinic nearby that does hyperbaric oxygen treatments, see if you can find a way to bring them into your treatment plan. In an ideal world, cancer patients would begin *right away* with hyperbaric oxygen treatments or some other form of oxygen therapy. Cancer does not use, nor like oxygen. An oxygenated environment is not a hospitable environment for cancer.

The next most important thing we can take care of right away is our diet. Firstly, the chemistry of the food is important. Cancer thrives in an acidic environment, and doesn't prefer a highly alkaline one, so giving the body primarily live, energy-filled, alkaline foods is huge. All of the acid forming foods, especially sugar, truly need to be let go of when it comes to cancer, especially if someone is in a late stage or dire straits situation.

It's vital to give the body a heavy dose of nutrients, as well. Cancers are also rooted in nutrient deficiencies, so nourishing, dense, rich fruits, veggies, and a whole foods diet, is essential. *"Every time you eat or drink, you are either feeding disease or fighting it."* -Heather Morgan

And lastly, cleansing must take place. We have to clean up our diet, but we also need to work a little more diligently on cleaning out the old stuff in the body, the toxins and leftover poisons. Enemas, colonics, herbs, and cleansing formulas can be used. Almost anyone can do some form of cleansing on their own, there is plenty of knowledge and wisdom out there about it. Finding a practitioner to help guide us or a colon hydrotherapist to work with us, is also great support and mentoring to have, if we can find it.

We have to get the toxins out, so the body has room to heal and get well.

There are many amazing therapeutic modalities, methods, and practices out in the world that have been proven as beautiful pathways towards healing from cancer. The medical and pharmaceutical industry's methods are indeed put at the top of the list on first defense against cancer, however, now that we're learning about people like Dr. Otto Warburg and other amazing doctors and scientists who've come up with easy, cheap ways to combat disease and cancer, we can begin to shift how things are getting done, so people can heal more easily.

I want to mention several insightful and well-studied methods below, just know that there are many monopolizing websites and groups out there who do not support natural methods and cures and do indeed, discredit them.

Afterall, you cannot promise someone a cure to a disease, especially not with cancer, because it's forbidden. Even if some form of therapy has been witnessed or proven to help someone, no matter how many people have used it, it is unfortunately considered false information.

In my perspective, there is no one cure-all, and each individual person has to do the work alongside any treatment or therapy. We always need to do the work, whatever it is we're facing, especially on diet, removing toxins, and working through any emotional traumas or unforgiveness that's being held onto. We can have the best diet on the planet, but if we don't work on the other layers of things, we may not end up in as good of a position as we could've been.

We're at the turning point in time where we have access to some of the easiest starts to getting healthier as well as to some of the hidden truths that have been pushed out of the scene. Dr. Otto Warburg's work alone is worth looking into. Of course, none of these are claims for cures. <u>I do not claim there's a cure, I am not recommending, nor prescribing.</u> This is just for people who are wanting to learn more, and need some avenues and information to look into.

Sometimes we have to find some of our own answers, because each and every one of our journeys through health issues, are unique. We need to remember that not everything is for everyone, but it's always good to get to know about other things and healing concepts and methods that are out there, because you just never know what might help you. And know, that there are tons of people out there who have been through it and made it out to the other side. You can always find them if you look.

Always follow your intuition and gut instinct, first and foremost. It will often lead you to the gold you seek.

- Dr Johanna Budwig's protocol
- RSO- Rick Simpson Oil Protocol
- Hyperbaric Oxygen chambers
- The Amazing Oxygen Cure
- Raw food: Fruits and/or veggies juices- Alkaline diet
- Fasting methods
- Detoxification and Herbs (Dr. Robert Morse, ND)
- Ozone therapy
- Quantum Healing: Frequencies, Rife Frequencies
- Dr Hulga Clark Protocol
- Hydrogen Peroxide Protocol
- Vitamin C infusions, Glutathione infusions, other IV high nutrition- vitamin and mineral infusions
- Gerson therapy
- CDS Oxidizing Solution
- The Breuss Cancer Cure

HOMEWORK:

1. Start a notebook or journal about your health journey. Write down the problems and issues you have currently and the ones you've gotten past. Note around when they began and what was going on in your life at the time.
2. What parts of your health most concern you? A certain organ system, a certain part, or a chronic issue maybe?
3. Write down any changes you've made because of your health problems. Whether you have or haven't made changes, write down some new changes you believe would be a good idea to make. Hone into yourself and listen to see what comes up for you.
4. Journal how you feel about your illnesses or problems. Notice if there are any emotions that come up for you around them.

"it's a mess, but it's a beautiful one.
That's the thing about healing. The end result is beautiful
but the process is anything but. Healing is messy. it is
confronting, confusing, conflicting, yet completely
transformative. There is no timeline, you will heal perfectly
when you are ready to.
Don't give up just as it gets messy, because that is when
the real work is done. Be patient and gentle with yourself
in the process. Tell yourself that it does get better, day by
day. Even if you can't see it or feel it right now.
Sometimes you need to reopen an old wound to make peace
with it, to accept that it is part of who you are, and to trust
that it does not define where you are heading."
                    – Charlotte Freeman

STRENGTHEN YOUR SYSTEM

During the last few years with the virus and pandemic happening, we have unfortunately gotten weaker in some aspects as a population. Mostly because, it took a hold on so many of us mentally, emotionally, but also very much, physically. Some people are still suffering. The fear around this virus unfortunately continues, new variants and other situations are in the mix, and a lot of people don't even know what to do for themselves anymore.

Too many wonderful people have spent their precious time worrying and scared of everything, instead of enjoying their life. Of course, something like a virus can occupy all of your awake time, even when you lie your head down at night. We can set our system up on a continuous cycle of worrying and draining ourselves physically, mentally, and emotionally. And about something we can't even see.

This time in history has been a big hit on us. Many lost their loved ones, their health, jobs, businesses, homes, hopes, dreams, and so on. Many fell into drug use, alcoholism, and even our children ended up on drugs to help with their depression and feelings of isolation. It's been a hard road for many.

So, what happens if this hits us again? Are we physically or mentally prepared for it? I will hope we don't have to get to that point again, we deserve to go up from here. Whatever level we're at right now, there are always ways we can improve upon ourselves. We can always work to improve our physical health, our emotional and mental selves, and take pieces of our lives back that we've lost.

We just need some information on how to stay healthy this time, how to get stronger, to realize just how lovely and powerful our body is, as well as how to take good care of it. We need to be reminded of how we can support our body and strengthen it in the face of any health challenge, such as during flu season or another viral hit. And of course, that our body is a powerhouse!

Unfortunately, there was very little, if any, information about wellness out there in the main stream world of things. We needed information about food, what to eat more of and what to eat less of. We needed emphasis put on how important exercise and movement is, and how to do it even while indoors. We needed to hear how important sunshine is and all of the beneficial methods of how to stay well and stay strong in the eyes of a health adversity. Keeping our health in check is necessary in these times, and frankly, always.

Instead, we find ourselves coping with prescription medications, alcohol, a poor diet, and drugs. We are only adding to the burden. However, so many people have reached to these to manage dealing with the chaos and fear. It's not a good place for people to stay, and wouldn't it be so great if we had content on TV that promoted working our way back to health.

These substances not only kill our spirit, motivation, and inspiration, they kill the body. They lower the immune system and hinder the body from being able to fight to the best of its ability. The gut is destroyed by these substances and we know how the gut plays a big role in our mental health and immunity. Too many innocent, good people were hit hard by this pandemic, suffering endless loss, exhaustion, health issues, and heartbreak. Too many became addicted to substances to cope with all of the hardship and loss.

We just need to be equipped with more knowledge. Stuff that's not overwhelmingly complicated and easy to apply. It's time we find more positive and health promoting methods to keep ourselves stronger. We all deserve to have access to empowering interventions and methods that will keep us strong in the face of any challenge.

As we become wiser, we are better able to help ourselves in and through different situations, how to take better care of ourselves, and in turn, each other. This way, we can get through other health scares and events. We can share what we learn each time as we go, and lend our strength to one another, instead of feeding into fear. Next time we will respond better, because we will know better, and hopefully have more tools to use so we can move our lives forward with strength and more fearlessly.

The first thing we need to identify, is the fact that fear weakens us, especially over prolonged periods of time. We can use our fear of something as a tool, as it's meant to get us out of a bad situation to begin with. Why not allow it to ignite a fire beneath us which will help us create and act in a way that promotes strength and health, instead of weakening us.

The present fear state people have been in, is the kind that is a slow burn. They aren't even aware they're in it anymore, as it drains so many areas of their life. They've learned to almost ignore it, as it silently drains their vitality, energy, and health from them. Fear puts our body into survival mode slowing everything down, including our immune system.

TV shows and news need to promote tools and resources to help people keep themselves healthy and strong. Imagine having cooking lessons, health talks, exercise classes, meditations, and other therapeutic lessons on during these stressful times. So many people would participate, imagine the outcome.

If this was the case, people would feel more supported and better able to handle whatever it is that arises in their life. There are hundreds of beautiful ways to remain strong and healthy in the face of fear. Any kind of fear. What an advantage it would be if we could all learn what to do at home that would assist our bodies and minds during a stressful time. It would move us out of fear if we were told how powerful, strong, and resilient our bodies are, not to mention we ourselves as a whole, are very powerful.

Essentially, we need to work on this by educating ourselves on a few things and taking on a few new tools that will help us navigate through our health and life circumstances should anything come up for us.

The first thing I want to say before talking about some good stuff we can do, is that *you are stronger than you think you are*. We are all capable and strong on one realm or another, and then some. Most of us under-notice just how amazing and powerful we are. We have been undermined in a way, but that doesn't have to be the case anymore.

Knowing how powerful we are is a vital part of surviving pretty much anything in life, it doesn't even just have to be related to a virus or organism. At this point, strengthening our system is related to anything that comes our way. We're all hit with life issues, job, family, and health stresses of all kinds throughout our life. So, this applies to all things.

We are all stronger than we ever thought we were!! We can always change how we think of and see ourselves.

Let's start with a focus on breathing, because it's something we can all relate to. The truth is, we can all use a little more of a conscious connection to it and practice more gratitude towards it. It's not too often that we notice or acknowledge our breathing, but it's obviously a big part of our life. Focusing on our breathing can make such a huge difference in so many areas, especially in regulating and strengthening the body and mind. Breathwork has gained popularity and is designed to help us adjust our state of being, to be better able to let go, and even to alkalize our bodies.

It's an *immediate,* wonderfully effective, easy tool that helps us break out of fear before it gets too out of control. We don't have to know a special method of breathing, just as long as we know how to take deep, slow breaths. Deep breathing is revitalizing. It calms down our nervous system and gives our systems a break.

You can try to breathe within a certain number of seconds, for example using what's known as the box breathing method. It's breathing in and out to a count of four, with holds on each side of it. First to take one deep breath in and out. Next, inhale to a count of four seconds, then hold the breath in for four seconds, exhale to a count of four seconds, and then hold for another four seconds. This slow breathing cycle calms and brings us back to our center, as well as that it nourishes our nervous system.

We can fill up our chest cavity to give our lungs good expansion and oxygenation, or we can breathe into our belly, bringing in nurturing, deep oxygenation and a sense of security. Several cycles of slow, deeper breathwork will reset our entire system. All that we were fearing will feel a little less overwhelming, giving us more ease in moving forward more constructively and less fearfully. We feel more balanced and confident when we're at ease.

We then find ourselves looking at situations and scenarios that are in front of us from a different perspective, finding that we have more control over things than we once thought we did. Deep breathing is literally a game changer. Our focus can then shift onto something we actually *want* and desire to create in our lives. We have more time and energy for the good stuff. Breathing opens us up. It's how we take in life.

It's not difficult to find some of the glorious, beautiful people out in the world who are sharing the blessing of breathing practices and information. Online is a world of resources, of course YouTube and other video streaming platforms have a wonderful number of practices and people to learn from. It's free, easy to follow, and ultimately so nice to have in the comfort of our own home. There are studios in different cities and towns with in-person yoga and breathwork classes, which is great if you want to join in with others. This sometimes has a wonderful effect on us, being around other like-minded people who are wanting to heal and be healthier. Breathing exercises take so little time, yet have such a powerful impact.

Another great method and information to know about, is how healing the vibrations of sound can be. We all know how music can impact our mood and energy. A wonderful tool that has a profound healing effect on us, and that we can do at any-time and anywhere, is humming. Humming has been shown to reduce fear and strengthen the mind and immune system. Sure, it may sound silly, but it has indeed been proven scientifically to have quite an impact on the physical and energetics of the body.

Humming creates a vibratory resonance that benefits our nervous system, blood pressure, stress levels, immunity, and sleep. It increases our lymphatic system movement, releases endorphins (happiness chemicals), assists in melatonin production (for sleep), and even creates new neural pathways in the brain. The foundation of our nervous system is strengthened. Humming can sound like whatever it is we choose for it to be. Changing tones and being creative with it is easy and fun.

Let's chat a little about our creative space. Our creativity contributes to our health, strength, and well-being. How many of us actually spend quality time expressing our creative side on one level or another? When was the last time we allowed ourselves the time and space to create something? Of course, some people are lucky and work on projects and fun, creative stuff in their days, but not everyone does. People don't think about it pertaining to much of anything other than a hobby or past-time. We don't realize how healing it can actually be for us.

So, I want to bring forth how absolutely life-changing and healing it can be for us. There are truly no limitations as to how we can express our creativity. It can be through art on any level of course, but it can also be through physical movement and expression, a project, shifting things around our home or space, cooking a creative meal, designing our garden, or we can even find a creative way to clean our house or play with our children. It's unlimited, the ways we can use our creativity.

Creativity is an expression of our soul, it's about who we are and how we feel. It empowers us in the difficult times or can bring more light to the most joyful ones. We get to release everything, even sadness, fear, or loss. We get to expand the joy and the happiness within us, as well as our immense gratitude we hold for life itself. Art is highly therapeutic and helps us to reconnect to ourselves in a way that the other parts of life don't always allow for us. Art helps us find our way back to ourselves on so many levels.

Most of us as children, were more deeply connected to ourselves in our younger years and able to access our creative potential much easier, before all of the feedback, rules, and opinions came in. We had wonderful imaginations that kept us in that creative flow. However, life happened, we had to *grow up,* and many of us lost our connection to it.

Perhaps though, we've gotten to a point in time where we've begun to realize just how important it is for us to have this in our lives. Even if it's been over 30 years since we found ourselves being creative and artistic, it's never too late to do something. My ninety-year-old grandmother-in-law took her first art class when she was eighty-six! It only ever benefits us, and it very much may benefit others, as well.

It's never too late to tap back in. You'll be surprised at what arises when you choose to access this hibernated part of you. You'll be surprised at what you remember about yourself or perhaps find out about yourself all these years later. Have a little chuckle with yourself for feeling like you are 6 years old again. It's a great feeling.

Art is an ageless therapeutic modality where people of all generations, from young children to the elderly, can find some relief. It allows a space for expression when words are not enough or what's needed. Where feelings and emotions can be released.

Creating art is deeply therapeutic for the nervous system, the heart, the emotions, and the soul. It strengthens our immune system. It enhances our value in ourselves and the desire to connect with ourselves more. It can birth us into a new direction, help us to break through barriers and stuck energy, as well as transform and help heal different parts of our life.

We can find ways to express our creativity in the *everyday* things of life, as a safe place to express our emotions, including our fears. We can be creative about cleaning our home, rearranging things, changing the décor or arrangement. We can make ourselves some new curtains or build a table, or just add our own personal touch to something we already have. When we live in an environment that is more "us" and to our liking, an atmosphere we enjoy being in, we end up living a healthier existence. Our health literally responds to these kinds of things. It's how we take care of ourselves and let go of the external stressors that are placed in front of us.

Creating a healthy meal when we're stressed out and worried about a health scare, is very empowering. While making the meal, we can consciously make an effort to focus on how much the food will nourish our body, and keep us healthy and strong. It can be a meal that we create to support ourselves. We can infuse love into it, feel gratitude for it, or anything that adds to its potential. Then as we eat it, we can focus on how nourishing, healing, and strengthening it is for our body, mind, and spirit. This is so much room to be creative in this.

Stressful times are an opportunity to go looking and to find, healthy recipes to make for ourselves and our families. There are so many amazing, healing recipes out there. I'm a huge fan of anti-inflammatory, auto-immune, and cancer-fighting recipes as a base. Generally, the more earth grown the better. It's much more medicinal that way. Choosing as conscious of foods as possible is important.

So much has to do with the energy we put into things. Blessing our food and giving thanks can change the dynamic of the food (water molecules like we already talked about). We just need to have some intention when creating and eating our meals.

Another fear chaser and healing modality is frequency. I will get deeper into frequencies in a few chapters, but I want to mention it here because it is an absolute game changer when it comes to our immune health, and our mental and emotional health. Frequencies powerfully impact every aspect of our being, and very much so, our health. They can work to bring our nervous system back into balance, amongst many other beautiful potentials.

Recordings and videos can be found online that have been created with serene, beautiful background music. Some are created with a specific purpose in mind such as to release anxiety, fear, or pain, some are made to help with indigestion, high blood pressure, and so on. Sometimes I listen to a few before I settle down on which one, I'm feeling the most. They can create an almost instant shift in our mood, and bring in a calm, serene, peaceful feeling. You almost don't even notice your mood shifted from not good to great until you assess where you've been for the few minutes you were listening. Frequency music can be used to uplift our spirits and give us more energy, it can help balance and harmonize our cells, our DNA, and can even help us get in some truly peaceful sleep. It has a powerful effect on our nervous system hands down.

Many of you have heard about the *Om* sound, usually we've heard it chanted by monks somewhere along the way. This can go along with the humming aspect we just spoke about. This chant and practice, has been around for thousands of years. Listening to the 'Om' sound is powerful beyond measure, and doing it along with the music or on your own, is also quite powerful. It is known as the primordial sound of the Universe, the sound of creation, preservation, harmony, and healing. It's known to decrease stress and regulate emotions as well as connecting us to the infinite realm of all that exists. It can also be found on videos with beautiful music in the background.

It's generally super easy to find music that naturally uplifts us, most of us have some of our own favorite types. Many of us know music can totally change our emotions and uplift our spirit. We can use music to serve us in a time of despair and sadness, or in this case, to strengthening our system. It's important to choose that which uplifts us and makes us feel good and elevated.

Let's chat a bit about how we speak to ourselves, and how we speak about things, as we've talked about in other areas already. When we're in the face of adversity or some kind of crisis, this is one of the most important times for us to speak positively to ourselves. To focus on and speak more about the *good* things that are going on. We really only have the time and energy to lend to this kind of stuff these days, because we're needing to strengthen ourselves more and more it seems. We don't want to waste time and energy thinking about or speaking the negative into our world when it's already there.

Affirmations can create a space for where we want to be. Stating what we want with intention and as though it is already happening. Speaking in the present tense as though we already have it. What we speak about, we bring about.

Over and over again throughout history, it's been proven that what we think, feel, and focus on, manifests. It's even logical if you think about it, something happening because we are so fixated on it. So, let's work on thoughts and sentiments we can purposefully think about to move into a stronger, healthier, more elevated place for ourselves. Here are a few to boost our strength both physically and mentally.

- I am safe and protected.
- My body is healthy and strong.
- I breathe love into every cell of my body.
- My body is powerful and can heal itself.
- I am so grateful for my body's healing.
- My immune system is strong and supported.
- I love and take care of my body.
- My body is built perfectly to overcome challenges.
- My body is a gift, and I am blessed because of it.
- I am so grateful for my body, this life, and all the beauty that surrounds me.

I encourage you to create your own. Focus on what you want, rather than what you don't want. If we stay dwelling in the negative, like the

I'm going to catch it mode, we are just weakening our immune system further, as well as opening ourselves up to it. We depress the potential, processes, and hormones we need to keep our bodies strong and healthy. Stating something as simple as *I love myself* or, *thank you for my healing,* will attract a healthier mindset, which keeps us above the chaos and fear that's constantly being thrown at us.

There's truth to just about everything, it's just what we decide to give our energy to, and what we want to invite into our life. I personally don't give energy to certain things, and truth be told, they don't affect me in the ways that they seem to affect others. I just don't give them power. Of course, I am always working on where my focus and energy goes, but you can catch yourself at any point, and redirect it. We're constantly deciphering what is true for us and what isn't.

We all get to decide on what resonates with us and what doesn't, just like these concepts I'm presenting around healing and strengthening ourselves. So, if any of this isn't for you, you can just pass it by. There is an affirmation section later in the book that might be more helpful for those that are interested.

Another part of helping ourself stay strong and protected is through the acknowledgement of our energetic field. You know, the one that we have surrounding us that I mentioned briefly, earlier. There isn't enough being said about the body's energetic field, not enough focus on it, nor much, if any energy put into knowing about it, however, it was once acknowledged, and it is quite fascinating.

Our energetic field is affected by external frequencies and energy such as microwaves and cell phones, which also affect the electrical system in our body. Quantum or biofield science explains more around our energetic field and it helps for us to recognize it and realize that even our thoughts affect our energetic field. Thoughts emit a certain frequency, as well as does visualization, which can help us realign the energy within our fields.

As per the research and studies I've read, it is possible to create a shield or protective forcefield around us. It can be done in many ways; one way is by visualizing a blue protective shield around ourselves. This serves as a field of energetic protection which even includes external threats including the recent fear and biological organisms going around. This also embraces the ability to protect ourselves from people or environmental stressors. I apply this in moments that I feel unsafe, when someone is sick around me, or I can feel negative energy from the people or situations around me. I just envision the shield like a bubble of protection around me.

If someone's energy feels heavy, negative, or off to us, we can shield ourselves. We kind of have to be mindful of all aspects of life, these days especially. Personally, I refuse to be around draining, negative energy that's being put out by others. When we encounter a draining person, we might notice our energy feels off, or affected by it. There are so many ways people can be draining. We might even begin to feel sick, tired, irritable, or just super uncomfortable around them. It affects our fight and flight response, our immune system, and our nervous system. We need to be regulating and enhancing these systems when we're trying to work on strengthening ourselves, so it's important to avoid draining people or situations when we can.

Whenever we feel a need to protect ourselves, this can always help. We can create our own version of how we want your protective shield or forcefield to look, if this resonates for you.

We might then find ourselves wanting to do some deep cleaning in our life and start releasing the energy-draining people or things from our life. It's not always easy to let go of people, especially those who we've known for decades, people who we've had in our lives, family and friends we couldn't imagine letting go of. And sometimes we can't altogether detach from people, but we can choose how much of our time and energy we choose to lend to them. Through this process, we end up finding we want more positive people around us instead, ones who love us, care for us, and support us. People who are healthy minded and who add to the world in a positive, beautiful way. It starts happening naturally once we decide we won't allow fear-struck, negative people and things to continue taking up space and time in our life. It's very refreshing, to say the least.

It's also a good time to clear the clutter and overwhelm out of our environment. Having too much stuff around us, garbage, excess junk, and keeping things just because we paid for it, adds to our stress. It's always a good time to clean up our environment and create more free space in the place that we live. We don't realize just how heavy and sickening clutter and keeping stuff can be. Take some time to give things away and get rid of things you no longer need or use, and watch your life feel more open, elevated, and free.

Now, onto some of the physical things we can do for ourselves. We spoke of breathwork, some food stuff, and thought processes, but let's get into a little more depth around the things we can do to direct help our physical body and how they help.

Again, I am not a doctor, I am not advising, prescribing, nor telling you what to do, what to take, and so on. But we need to know and want to know about other forms of things that we can do so that we can keep our bodies strong.

No matter how it went in the past, maybe we fed into the fear and got ourselves wrapped up in misery the last time, but it doesn't have to be that way next time around. We can always do stuff to help ourselves whenever we feel like our bodies (or minds) need a boost in the face of anything that may be *going around.*

The two most common vitamins that do a ton to boost our immunity are Vitamin C and Vitamin D. First of all, I am a proponent of and do strongly believe in obtaining these vitamins as naturally as you can, like getting Vitamin C from fresh fruits and vegetables and Vitamin D from the life-giving, glorious sunshine that exists for us. Sunshine as you know, helps our body to produce this vital and necessary hormone/vitamin.

Vitamin D is an absolutely essential component that bolsters immune function, promotes calcium absorption, helps greatly in reducing inflammation, assists with cell growth, is *absolutely necessary* for bone growth, neuromuscular function, and glucose metabolism. Ideally, a good sun soaking of a minimum of 15-20 minutes a day (with some sungazing on the very edge of the sunrise and sunset) is absolutely necessary for healing and rejuvenation. I know not all of us have sunshine 365 days a year, but it even shines through the clouds, so being outside is important.

Our bodies *produce* Vitamin D via the sunlight entering our retina or through the skin, then processed in the liver and kidneys. Taking a synthetic supplement form is not utilized by the body in the same way, though that goes with almost everything synthetic. However, if someone's Vitamin D levels are terribly low, or the sun isn't happening in our day, a supplement is necessary.

It's difficult to get Vitamin D from food, although it is said to be found in salmon, tuna, mackerel, beef liver and egg yolks. The flesh of fatty fish and cod liver oil contains the most. Lack of Vitamin D not only decreases your immune system's strength, it also causes depression and decreased hormone production in the body. People with low Vitamin D tend to have opioid/drug addictions and tend to be more depressed, requiring drugs to keep them going.

Vitamin C is an easy one and well known by most. Vitamin C fights free-radicals. Free radicals move our bodies towards more diseased states and accelerate the aging process. Vitamin C is quite lovely as it can be taken in large amounts, especially when a person is under the weather and feels sickness coming on. Vitamin C is relatively safe to take in high doses, even up to 8000 mg can be taken in a day. Now that's on the high end, so don't just head into maxing out. Research has shown with an onset of cold symptoms, anywhere from 1000 - 2000 mg or up to 6000 - 8000 mg per day is effective. The side effect of taking higher amounts of vitamin C is generally loose bowel movements.

As a side note, I would like to state that in an alternative treatment protocol such as for illness and cancer, Vitamin C is given in high doses via IV infusions. Vitamin C is a game changer and easy to come by. There are *tons* of studies out there on this.

There are also wonderful naturopaths and IV infusion clinics with a licensed doctor where you can get IV vitamin and mineral infusions that have been proven over and over again to have amazing results. There are several formulas used specifically in strengthening the body. One that has become popular and is noted for its powerful properties is Glutathione, a powerful anti-oxidant. You can find information about it online, *if only* western medicine used these vitamin and mineral formulas to help people heal at a greater capacity.

When it comes to Vitamin C, citrus fruits are one of the most powerful sources for it and happen to also contain anti-oxidants. Lemons are one of the most powerful citrus fruits with its astringent, cleansing, and tonifying properties that have a wonderful impact on the liver, kidneys, and the bowels. Drinking room temperature water in the morning with freshly squeezed lemon and a pinch of Celtic or Himalayan salt, is a phenomenal way to flush our system in the morning, as well as giving us a good dose of Vitamin C and charging our electrolytes.

It's also wise to take a B Vitamin Complex. B vitamins are essential for our overall health and well-being, helping our cells do their jobs. They are essential for our heart and gut health, brain and nerve function, cellular health and growth, as well as assisting our hormone production and energy levels. B vitamins can be found in dark leafy greens, nuts and seeds, blackstrap molasses, nutritional yeast, wheat germ, root vegetables, avocados, bananas, citrus fruits, watermelon, beans, whole grains, eggs, liver, red meat, soy, poultry, cheese, and some shellfish like oysters and clams.

There are other supplements that we can invest in to support our health like other vitamins and minerals, as well as herbal and other natural supplements. Today's pharmaceutical medicine after all, came from plant medicine. Being that our diets are unfortunately highly deficient in the vital nutrients that we need (at least here in the US, due to farming, pesticides, poor soil conditions, and GMOs) it's a good idea to have a few things on hand in case we fall into a place where we need to boost our nutrient profile.

The ones I will mention here are some I've personally taken and are known to be effective by science and health experts. They have been mentioned by endless health gurus and doctors throughout this recent pandemic situation, though gained little attention on the mainstream media. I'll give you a small briefing on what they are good for, but again, do some research, and look beyond the usual websites.

*** OF COURSE, check with your doctor on any of these if you take medications. I am not prescribing, nor suggesting, I am just sharing some popular supplements and powerful superfoods out there that are safe when taken appropriately.

Zinc: is a mineral found throughout the body. It's an abundant mineral found in the earth's crust and in the soil where it infuses into our food. It assists with immune function, nervous system function, cell growth and division, DNA recognition, wound healing, as well as being essential for bone and eye health.

Zinc activates enzymes that *break down proteins in viruses and bacteria*, destroying them. Zinc helps to activate immune cells helping to destroy microbes. Zinc also helps reduce inflammation in the body. It can be found in nuts, beans, pumpkin seeds, watermelon seeds, spinach, asparagus, cacao – dark chocolate, brewer's yeast, grass-fed organic beef, lamb, pork, chicken, crab, lobster, and oysters. When taking the supplement look for chelated zinc which means it's more easily absorbed.

Quercetin: is a potent anti-oxidant that helps your immune system. It is a flavonoid with anti-inflammatory and anti-viral properties that also acts to protect your cells and tissues from being damaged. It helps to restore the tissues of the lungs and reduces inflammation. It has a protective effect on the cells of the gut blocking damage to the lining of the gut. Quercetin can be found in grapes, berries, cherries, broccoli, onion, citrus, apples, tomatoes, kale, capers, leaves, and seeds, as well as an over-the-counter supplement. Best taken alongside Zinc.

L-Glutamine: is an amino acid found in abundance in our blood stream. It is the foundation of protein. It is used in large amounts by the body to maintain the immune system and intestinal function. The body uses it to boost white blood cells and regulate immune response, so it is beneficial for those suffering from immune system disorders and diseases such as cancer.

It assists on repairing ulcers and leaky gut, it nourishes the cells in the small intestine, helps to eliminate viruses and bad bacteria in the gut, as well as helps normalize bowel function. It is used to improve brain function such as memory and concentration. It helps reduce fatigue. It also assists with recovery and repair of muscles, tendons, and ligaments, as well as in the healing of surgical wounds (apparently sometimes prescribed). Best when taken in combination with B-12.

<u>Elderberry:</u> The father of modern medicine, Hippocrates, called Elder trees his "medicine chest". This dark purple berry is one of the top antiviral plants on the planet and it happens to contain quercetin! It boosts our immunity supplying us with tons of antioxidants which fight viruses and bacteria. It has a lot of Vitamin A & C. Its rich in potassium, and has compounds that are highly beneficial to heart health, regulating cholesterol levels, and promoting better circulation.

Elderberries decrease mucus production. They assist with glucose metabolism and are currently being studied for their effects on lowering blood sugar levels. Studies have also shown their powerful impact when it comes to fighting cancer. They are indeed *superberries* that also assist with many other things such as brain function and are beneficial to the skin.

<u>Green powders:</u> These are a wonderful and easy way to get your greens, chlorophyll, and oxygen content into your diet. Green powder is generally made up of green grasses and leafy greens, such as wheatgrass, alfalfa, barley grass, kale, spinach, as well as chlorella, spirulina, root & fruit powders, enzymes, and sometimes even probiotics. These green powders offer dense, concentrated nutrition, create alkalinity (which viruses and opportunist organisms do not like), and help with oxygenation.

These powders are a wonderful boost for the immune system or pretty much all the systems in the body. They are a wonderful addition to one's daily intake. Of course, if you are on certain blood thinners, you may not be able to take this because of the interactions with the medication you are taking, best to check with your doctor if you are on blood thinners or copious amounts of medications.

<u>Adaptogens:</u> These are plants and mushrooms that help your body adapt to stress. They assist your body in being resilient during times of physical, emotional, or environmental stress. They are greatly supportive and healing for the adrenal glands and the entirety of the endocrine system. They have been used for centuries in two of the most powerful medicinal cultures, Chinese medicine and Indian Ayurvedic medicine.

The adaptogenic herbs most widely known and safely used are: Ashwagandha, Panax Ginseng, Rhodiola, Maca, Holy Basil, Turmeric, and Schisandra Berry. The *mushrooms* that are adaptogenic are:

Cordyceps, Chaga, Reishi, Shitake, Lions Mane, and Turkey Tail. All can be taken in capsule form, you can make teas with them, eat some of them, and of course there are powders available with different combinations of adaptogens you can add to your smoothies or food. You can even grow some of your own mushrooms, there's tons on information online and wonderful companies who can supply you with all that you need to do so.

Colloidal Silver: A powerful pathogen killer. Safe when taken as directed. Silver is used in the medical profession for wound healing, burns, and eye treatments. It's also been proven to kill MRSA as well as many other organisms like strep, influenza, respiratory infections, fungal infections, *viruses*, and even cancer. It's helpful for teeth and gums, digestion, skin rashes, and the list goes on. It has not gained momentum because it cannot be produced or patented by pharmaceutical companies.

Echinacea and Goldenseal: these two herbs when combined are immensely good for boosting the immunity and supporting the liver. Echinacea on its own is very beneficial as it acts to stimulate the cells responsible for immune function as well as that it has anti-viral qualities. Goldenseal is an immune stimulant. It is an anti-bacterial, anti-microbial, and anti-fungal. It is used in the treatment of inflammation of the mucous membranes in the respiratory, digestive, and urinary tracts.

CBD: This wonderful plant has recently gained popularity for many reasons. It's made from hemp, or can also be made by the marijuana cannabis plant. The hemp version is legal in the United States. In regards to the immune and nervous systems, CBD is a golden remedy to ease and support both (I will talk more in depth about CBD later) I do want to express that it's best to get it from a trusted brand or source, not just at some gas station situation. I will list a few good companies in the back.

Mineral supplements: Minerals are essential for functions of the body. They help run the heart and cardiovascular system, the brain and nervous system, are vital for bone and muscle growth, as well as help with the production of necessary hormones and enzymes. Many of us are depleted in minerals, as our soil and food lack the essential minerals due to the farming practices and pesticide and insecticide usage. There are several sources of mineral supplementation.

My favorite two are Sea Moss and Shilajit. Sea Moss contains over 102 essential minerals that we need and is easy to prepare and add to our food such as smoothies and soups. Or there are capsules available. Shilajit is a thick resin that contains over 84 necessary minerals. It is a strong anti-oxidant and anti-inflammatory, protecting against cellular damage. Science has shown it to be protective even for Alzheimer's, has anti-aging properties, and energizes the kidneys.

There is also other plant sourced or trace mineral supplements that can be found in your local health food store. Of course, if you are already on mineral supplements like potassium check with your doctor before taking these, although chances are they will not have good information on these. Adding sea moss to your diet, in my opinion, is really only good for you.

Celtic Sea Salt: has 82 minerals and contains 3 types of magnesium, which help our cell membranes to pull water inside of the cell. It is unprocessed so does not contain chemicals, preservatives, or additives. Refined, table salt (iodized) can *cause* high blood pressure and contains harmful ingredients, but natural salt with adequate water intake can help stabilize both the heart rate and blood pressure, whether low or high.

It helps to eliminate mucus buildup, alkalizes the body, balances blood sugar, improves brain function, increases energy, builds immunity, helps with muscle cramps, a restful sleep, and helps to balance electrolytes. When it comes to getting in enough hydration with you water intake, make sure to drink half your body's weight in ounces, as that's the general knowledge.

The next best thing for your physical body in keeping it strong is through exercise and movement! I know, it's one of those obvious ones and not exactly everyone's favorite, but I feel it's important to impress upon the fact that it's essential in keeping our bodies moving and our stress levels down.

While everyone was sitting at home during lockdowns and the pandemic, people were less active than ever. Unfortunately, being inactive is actually weakening to our immune systems and bodies on the whole. Inactivity weakens our connective tissue, muscles, bones, and can reduce cellular activity (which is vital). So, it's time to get moving! Watch an exercise video, sign up at your local gym, get a trainer, go for a daily walk, and work your way up. Go for a run, get off the couch and do something, even if it's just some jumping jacks, squats, push-ups, or a couple sets of sit ups. Whatever motivates you, do it. We will get into moving more in the next section.

A great way to detoxify, boost your immune system, and recharge your electrical system is by taking an Epsom salt and sodium bicarbonate bath (which is baking soda). 1 cup of each in a warm/hot bath will help relieve tension, move toxins out, and recharge your energetic-electrical field. It boosts your immune system and also helps to settle and recharge the nervous system. This is also wonderful as a foot soak, relaxing and detoxifying.

There are plenty of natural, even free ways to get ourselves stronger, healthier, and ready for whatever comes our way. The biggest part of it all, is your belief in yourself. If you seriously believe that your body is weak and you'll never be able to combat something you foresee as bigger than you, then you likely won't.

On the other hand, if you truly believe in and work to support your body and yourself, you will indeed be able to overcome so much more than you thought. We need to work towards bettering ourselves and gaining our health and strength, no matter what age we are or what condition we are in. There is *always* room for change and improvement. Remember, you got this.

HOMEWORK:

1. Name 3 things you can do for yourself when fear creeps in to bring you back to calm and balance.
2. What if any, immune boosting supplements do you have on hand? What comes to mind when you think about doing a few things to give your immune system some extra love?
3. What kind of new activity are you wanting to try to release your fears, depression, or anxiety? Is there something you love that helps with this?

MOVE

You are only as old as your spine is flexible. "That which is used, develops. That is which not used, wastes away."
- Hippocrates

eing flexible and limber throughout our life, even into our elder years, is vitally important. Once we slow down and stop moving, stretching, and keeping ourselves in somewhat of good shape for our age, we begin to lose function and essentially, our health.

Like Hippocrates said, *use it or lose it.* When it comes to our physical body, lack of use creates a loss of the muscle's abilities and strength, which means less agility and flexibility. It also means less oxygen pumping through. Exercise not only helps our actual muscles, it helps the internal ones as well as our organs and systems, as we are pumping more blood and oxygen through our bodies when we're active. The brain is another one of those muscles and if we don't exercise it, we end up losing knowledge, memory, and cognition. Without movement, muscles will end up weakened, breaking down, and eventually wasting away.

When we're active and moving our bodies whether it be through running, dancing, swimming, walking, lifting weights, or whatever it is, we create contraction of the muscles. When we contract our muscles, they secrete chemicals and proteins that scientists call *hope molecules* which act like anti-depressants. This is big.

These hope molecules go from your muscles into your bloodstream and reduce stress, depression, bringing a sense of peace, happiness, and serenity. That's why we are told to get outside and get some exercise when we're feeling down and depressed. Movement always helps the body and mind on one level or another.

Exercise and movement increase our brain's functioning and capacity, as when we have oxygen pumping through our bloodstream it is only good for the tissues of the brain and nervous system. People who are active and exercise well into their elder years, have a stronger memory and overall healthier functioning of the brain.

We can also help our brain with other exercises, activities, and mind building practices as they work to help to form new synapses, again, enhancing memory and learning capacity. Many of us know about keeping our brains active which we can do through reading, studying something, or in learning things. People also like to do crossword puzzles, sudoku, and other brain games to help this.

Physical exercise improves the cellular health in the body, especially that of our cardiovascular system, immune system, and digestive system. Exercise is also vital for our bone strength and to help our body get rid of toxins and waste products. The list of benefits to exercise is honestly endless, every part of our body benefits from movement and exercise, as well as our mental and emotional health, without a doubt. We also tend to stay younger and more flexible keeping us freer and happier during our days.

It's often that we hear people state how hard it is for them to fit in an exercise routine or take time out of their day to do it. Sometimes it's just too hard to get motivated, especially having not been used to it, or when there's so much already on their plate. Many feel as though they cannot find the time.

I myself, have come up with many reasons in the past as to why I couldn't, and have had some truly unmotivated moments in my life. Especially, when I was really going through something depressing or emotional. It felt easier to *not do* something that required effort, than it felt to just sit around and dwell on my problems.

Sometimes when we hit a vulnerable or rough patch in our lives, we can go one of two ways. We either throw ourselves into exercise and use it for our benefit, or we neglect it altogether. We might even know that it would *be good* for us to do and would essentially help us feel better, but the motivation isn't there. Sometimes we need someone or something there to help motivate us and give us a good push.

We all know in the end the reward is great. When we, in the least, accept that we need someone or something to help motivate us, it allows us to begin with some confidence and encouragement. We also give ourselves permission to go forward with things and they start to happen. New neural pathways are created and a new formula to strengthen our health, is carved out. It helps us move into things much easier.

Of course, there is no *one way* for everyone to exercise and move their bodies. People get trapped thinking it has to be that they go running or go to the gym. That limitation in itself will cause almost anyone to close the door to it, especially people who don't like either of those. No two people are the same. It's important that we do things that resonate with us so that we're happy with our activities and so that we want to continue moving forward with things.

To start off simply, we can start by doing the extra *little things* that will make us move more than we are. Like parking farther away from the store entrance, or taking a 15-minute walk every day after lunch. We can dance around our house for 15 minutes. We can do some stretching or yoga at the beginning and ending of each day. We can even include others like our neighbor when we take a walk, or our kids as we stretch or dance around.

It's always best that we pick a few things that don't seem so overwhelming to us, especially in the beginning if we're just getting started. Even better, something we wouldn't mind and actually feel good about doing. Things we feel happy about doing. Having a few options is always ideal so that we can have choices to choose from, and so that we don't end up getting bored too quickly.

We are reworking and rewiring our brain and body and setting ourselves up for a more expansive outlook on movement and staying active. Doing things that resonate with who we are and what we like, is so important.

We can tailor to our specific likes with everything that we do in our life, which includes our movement and exercise. Following our own ideas, desires, and being able to fill up our toolbox with specific activities and movements that we enjoy, helps build our confidence and brings on a natural motivation. Including fun into the mix tops it off and creates greater gains both in success of our moving and in feeling so much better about ourselves. It helps to feel like a little kid sometimes, let's be honest, adulthood can sometimes be too serious for our own good. Personally, I think adding fun or happiness to our movement even adds to our youthfulness, physically.

When we take a good look at where we're at to begin with, it's important not to be too judgmental and hard on ourselves for what we *haven't* done. So, starting with realistic and easy going efforts will always bring more progress in.

If we're too out of shape to go to a gym or do aerobics, ride a bike, or weight lift, we can start by making everyday things like cleaning the house, a workout. Engaging our muscles in our movements of wiping, sweeping, or bending down for things, is also just as conscious of a movement for our body. If you are thinking about the muscles you are using, put focus on keeping them in good alignment, and most always, contracting and using your abdominals while doing everything, you'd be surprised the workout you might get from vacuuming the house. Alternate using different sides and arms, and be conscious of your breathing.

Of course, be smart and don't bust a move and break a hip, but putting on some of your favorite music will help you feel more motivated while doing chores to your benefit on now more levels than as to why you're there in the first place! You can wiggle and shake in between rooms.

Fifteen minutes of your everyday is not hard to allow for. We can throw ourselves a 15-minute dance party in the middle of the day just to get our blood pumping. We can jog in place, do some jumping jacks, or some squats while standing up at our desk. We can include movement into random moments of our day. We can do some push-ups or sit -ups during commercial breaks. I like to do squats while food is cooking or while I'm waiting for water to boil. I do toe raises while waiting on line at the store or stretch my quads and hamstrings. Moving is important, but it's important to remember so is stretching. Stretching is so essential.

There's always a way to keep ourselves moving even if we're pent up at home. Of course, if you're pent up, getting outside is pretty important. Taking a walk around the block or through the field, depending on where you live, is one of the easiest things for those who are less active. To boot, you're getting fresh air and hopefully some sunshine. Walking daily, will over time, turn short distances into longer distances with the ability to withstand activity for longer periods of time. In no time, you'll go from from half a block to six. The more active we are, the more endurance and strength we gain.

This is certainly not meant to tell anyone what to do, what you *should* do, and how to do it. If you are content with being immobile and have the absolute belief that you can't do anything, everyone is their own person with free-will and unique mindsets and I am not here to upset you or cause any stress. I honor everyone's choices they make Please do not overdo *anything*! We all need to be honest with ourselves and be smart. Our health and wellbeing are of utmost importance, first and foremost.

If you are completely inactive and get out of breath easily, I *do not recommend* that you park a mile away from the store. These are all just loving, gentle suggestions and ideas to get yourself moving more. Maybe, park 5 spots further out, it doesn't have to be on the other side of the parking lot. To do the little things is what's important, when you're just starting out. Things that are just one small step up from what you're already doing, and building from there.

The key is to always listen to your body. If you feel or sense some part of you is on overload or overwhelm, stop. Reassess the situation, did you go too far or push too hard? What's your body trying to tell you? Which part needs your loving attention?

Sometimes we too go hard and fast into it, coming from nothing and I would say that's never the best idea. Easy to burn that bridge right off the bat. Unless you're moderately in good shape already, someone who's been super inactive for a long period of time likely shouldn't try to walk a mile, after not having walked at all for the last seven years. In this case we need to be rational as well as gentle with ourselves. We can approach it and go at it to a lesser degree than that.

I think it's also useful to have a guide or fitness coach to work with if it's feasible. Having someone build realistic and clear expectations and a game plan with you, is great. The support and even accountability it gives are great to have when you really want so much so, to turn your life around.

Some people have had physical therapists for one reason or another, and they can be quite helpful if you happen to have one, otherwise getting a personal trainer who works with your age, abilities, and desires, is awesome. There are many out there, even ones online. You don't even have to leave your house, or you can use the gym at your complex all while video calling your trainer on the phone. It gives us the ability to still have the support and training if we don't have people close by or leaving home is an issue. Coaches and trainers bring in more motivation.

Right now, you can probably ask your doctor for a referral to see a physical therapist to get your muscles stronger. Generally, they agree to this type of thing, and it gives you a connection through your care team as well as is something beneficial your insurance will pay for. It's nice to have someone who is able to assess where your body is at on a muscular, structural level and help us to work from where we're realistically at. It's an excellent and realistic assessment of where you should begin. You're given homework, like exercises and stretches to do at home, sometimes even give you tools to use. And best part is that they see your progression and help you to see that you are getting get better and stronger in just a short period of time.

Of course, there are always people who have a super difficult time working out or getting exercise in, as with the elderly, handicapped, and highly disabled. Disabled is a word that we could write a chapter on, hence my saying *highly* disabled.

In these cases, they need someone to *actively* help them get in their exercise. Paraplegics as an example, need someone else to move their leg for them to keep the muscles moving. And they need this even twice a day. It's actually vital for them, for blood flow and oxygenation.

There have been quite a few stories I've heard over the years about people who had been in accidents, severely injured, even paralyzed, who were told that they would never walk again, actually walking again. Against all odds, they did what was scientifically considered impossible.

These beautiful people had experienced a life-altering, damaging event but had a miraculous, unexplainable recovery. But it's not all unexplainable. Some of them were actually able to explain what they did to get themselves to that point. To be able to walk again. And their truth was, that it came from their mind and belief.

They held on in their mind that no matter what, their body was going to heal and they were going to walk again. They told themselves that like they knew it was true. They had nothing more to do with their day than to envision themselves walking and telling themselves that they would. Or at least they choose for these to be their thoughts and take up their time, others may drown in the negative of everything. You can imagine where they end up in contrast.

People don't want to believe this kind of thing is how it goes, afterall we've been told this type of mind creating literal physical is just ridiculous, nonsense, or just some airy-fairy crazy talk, but let me tell you. This whole mind, feeling, and belief combination, has got some serious goodness, strength, and power to it. It's funny, because you'll have people who push away this type of thinking yet they'll state something was a miracle. Or, they may just think that it was the body being stronger than the doctors thought, which may indeed be true, but the other truth to how these people healed themselves and walked again was because of their mind, emotions they chose to focus on, and their beliefs. This truly applies to most everything in life.

Many of these amazing people have written books about their experience and what they went through. It's very worth reading some of them because if they can do it and get themselves moving, what's stopping us?

Their stories also show us that we can rewire our brains to accomplish things others say is impossible, or that we may have never thought was possible for us, before. This is also not to give some false claim or false hope for those who are paralyzed, maimed, or suffering. I *do* very well understand that some people are rendered to never being able to walk again.

This is presented in here to give light to the fact that some people do find their way through their determination and desire to be able to something, instead of living hopelessly. They use their inner vision to see themselves where they *want* to be, which triggers synapses in their brain that activate that pathway, even helping to fire off the muscle fibers as if they were doing it. The brain doesn't know the difference between what we're thinking we're doing and what we're actively doing.

As we know, exercise and movement improve our mood because it pumps endorphins like dopamine, as well as oxygen through our body. This is a reason why exercise and movement are suggested, and known to be greatly beneficial for people who suffer from depression, anxiety, or other mental health issues. Having oxygen and endorphins pumping through the body will definitely get people to feeling better, and then add to it those hope molecules created by the muscles, there's nothing better!

For those out there that suffer from sleep issues, movement and exercise is key and widely known to help to improve the depth and soundness of our sleep.

I'm sure you already have a few ideas in your head and some things in mind that you can personally do to get yourself moving more. Maybe there are some things that you *haven't* done yet, but want to try. I find it's always helpful to write things down, make a list, or even journal about your ideas and feelings around things, so you can check back in with yourself or just get out some things you needed to. It's good brain exercise to write. Then you can follow your progress and feel accomplished or see areas you need to work harder on, as it all will keep you moving forward.

Finding, maybe even searching for things on line to find a variety of ways to move, can be a good idea. I'm sure Pinterest and YouTube have loads of ideas people have come up with that aren't so traditional, on keeping themselves active and moving. We can always modify things even to work with us. Being creative with things is a blessing especially if we're not able to follow such a solid place and time, we can find something to do no matter where we are, whatever the weather, or time of day it is. It's always good to have options.

There are even ways to get tiny workouts in while we're sitting, like when working a desk job. We can do isometric exercises, which are basically tensing up our muscles and releasing them. We can work our abdominal muscles, glutes/buttocks, calves, thighs, even our arms. We can take 5-minute breaks to stand up and stretch, do some squats at our desk, or go for a 5-minute walk around the office. At lunchtime, we can use 10 minutes of it to take a walk around outside and also get some sunshine into our day.

Even if we are someone who is only going for walks as our form of exercise, we can jazz it up a bit by finding new places to get in our walks. We can add in some nature trails or new spots into our routine, maybe some music or intentionally listening to the sounds around us. We can add variety and even a meditative aspect to our activity and exercise.

When we do something we enjoy, we're more likely to keep doing it because it elevates our mood and uplifts us! Even if it does make us breathe heavier and sweat! Which we need. Moving also boosts our metabolism. Our metabolism is a vital function of our body that works in sync with our *immune system*. Our metabolism carries the energy around the body so things like breathing and digestion can take place.

DO WHAT'S GOOD FOR YOU.

When we're doing something good for ourselves, we benefit in more ways than one. The obvious being that our body has a better chance to thrive and maintain its healthiest state. But let's also remember, we're impacting our body energetically by uplifting our vibration, resonance, and frequency. We are literally activating our atoms and molecules who carry sound and light.

Exercise and movement literally raises our vibration. Jump and dance around for 5 minutes and then stop completely. Do you feel the buzzing in every part from your head down to your toes? An uplifted feeling and the energy flowing? Moving creates a positive charge in our energy field as well as working to invigorate our energy potential in our bodily systems.

Finding something that invigorates us is pretty essential. It creates a new form of self-love and care that we may have not focused on before. The love we receive from ourselves without realizing is reason enough. And to reap the benefits physically, mentally, and emotionally is top notch stuff.

So, what can you do to get yourself moving more? What inspires you to take action? Your health issues? Your weight? Your mental health? What have you always wanted to try or learn to do? Have you wanted to try that Zumba class or self-defense place? How about going to that rock-climbing gym or seeing what a spin class is like? Or even to do a hike you always wanted to, building up to completing a trail little by little.

It's good to know that most exercise classes or centers, generally offer a free first class or entry in, so you can see if it's something you actually like or enjoy doing. There is such a variety of classes out there. If you can think it up, it exists. Especially if you live near a city, the chances are that you will find a ton of different options around you. If you live in a small town and there isn't much happening (which chances are there's something), you can explore the endless online resources of just about every type of workout imaginable.

You can always start something yourself, too! Why not get a few friends together a certain day of the week and go for a long walk, or do an hour workout of some kind together. Friends or groups tend to keep things motivated and going. Perhaps as a group you love to go for hikes, walks, a run, bike ride, or maybe you even like going to the gym together. There are also groups like on the app MeetUp that are basically people meeting up to go for hikes and activities they like doing. And you never know, you become so passionate about an activity that you, yourself starts a program, class, or group in your community. You never know the inspiration that may come.

I've had a few elder patients who wanted to be active but had no interest in going the gym, understandably so. Some of them discovered a workout that they loved by joining their local pool. Many pools and community centers have water exercise classes which are generally designed for adults and elders, as a great option for a workout that isn't hard on the body. The buoyancy of the water takes all the pressure off the joints, keeps you weightless, flowing, and making it easy to move around, all the while giving you movement and muscle activity.

For those who cannot do big workout classes, there are chair and sitting exercises available at most community and senior centers across the country, at places like the YMCA, and of course, you can find many of them online. I'm a fan of the gentleman Justin Agustin who has streamlined workouts for people who haven't touched an exercise in 25 years. His website is www.justinagustin.com. He offers gentle, well formulated workouts that are easy to do, underwhelming, and get one's body into motion. There are tons of wonderful experts and people out there with these kinds of videos, who offer gentle movement exercises for people with all abilities.

I'd love to share a beautiful story about a US Army Veteran named Arthur Boorman who became disabled after serving his time in the military and then moved on living a very unhealthy lifestyle. He was depressed, just shy of being wheelchair bound, overweight, and didn't have the help within the healthcare system that he needed to rebuild his life.

He lost control and began to give up, was heavily medicated, and was given very little hope for getting any better than he was. In a last attempt to save himself, he came across a yoga instructor who felt driven to do all he could to help Arthur get out of his situation. This instructor became the one person who believed in him when all of the others said there's was nothing that could be done.

His transformation was magical. He went from being unable to walk, bend, over, or move without pain, to walking, leaping, and dancing through life, despite all of the odds that were once against him. He broke through the barriers and limitations others had placed on him and he was finally given permission to believe in himself and his recovery. His desire and motivation grew as he built the healthy and fulfilling life that he wanted, and most importantly, he put in the work for it.

Deep down, he really didn't want to give up on himself and his life. This is a truth for many people who are burdened with mobility and health issues. His story proves that having someone to believe in us, especially ourselves, bears powerful results. I highly recommend looking for his video on YouTube and finding his story on the internet, as I do not do it justice. He is now lean and fit with a new lease on life. It's truly inspiring.

Yoga is a life changing practice. Not only is it beneficial for our physical body and our flexibility, but it's also therapeutic for the mind and spirit. There is an ever-growing number of yoga teachers and instructors being born daily, because once you start doing yoga and realize the amazing benefits and peace that comes with it, it's hard not to want to share it with the world.

You don't have to leave home to join in on a yoga session, again, there are a ton of online sessions and plenty of classes on video. I will say though that my experience in starting with the in-person version is top level. It's really a great way to get started if you're just beginning. Another reason to take a look around in your community to see if there are any classes. There are even classes for different age and experience levels.

I've seen people of all statures move themselves and get stronger. Some even blew my mind. There were people who are bedbound doing workouts and physical therapy in bed. Some elderly people could bend and squat better than people way younger than them. These people all decided to do this for themselves. They knew there were only going to benefits. They let go of other's limitations and the fear associated to it. They were more afraid *not* to move!

Of course, it's wise to listen to ourselves if we're in an activity and fear does come up. Although it may be our limiting thoughts talking, it's always wise to check in with ourselves and ensure we're not doing ourselves more or unintentional harm.

As we mentioned earlier with people who broke through limiting barriers, visualization played a big role in their ability. The last thing I want to include here is just that. Visualization.

I like to use NASA here as an example because they've literally done the studies, along with other high profile government agencies, where they had test subjects hooked up to equipment that monitored their brain and nervous system activity, heartrate, breathing, muscle firing, and even their eye movement. In the study, the test subjects visualized themselves doing whatever activity they were told to visualize, whether it was running, fighting, driving, and so on, in order to see how the brain and body responded.

What they found was that during the visualization, the person's brain acknowledged the activity as though it was *actually* happening. Their heart rate increased, breathing increased, neurons were firing. The visualization activated their autonomic nervous system (*which controls breathing, heart rate, blood flow, digestion*) creating the same effects as if they were actually doing the activity. The brain did not know the difference between the actual physical motion or the visualized version.

Visualization in itself, is powerful. It might take some effort and the concept may be foreign to our brain, as we think about it more so as an imagination little children have, but it's good to realize, it's not just for children. There are wonderful benefits that come with visualization. It works in all aspects of our life.

It also doesn't hurt to tell ourselves things that are a little more supportive while we're trying to get our bodies to move more because let's face it, motivation isn't always thriving, when the struggle is real. I like to say things like, "I got this!" or "I can do this!" or even "You got this, Trish!" Why not be your own cheerleader?

Silly or not, it really does shift our mindset, it's even proven to boost our confidence, so why not? If it actually enables us to do more and go farther, it's only a good thing. So go out there and give yourself some kudos and support. It's good to have your own back.

HOMEWORK:

1. What does your exercise and movement situation look like? What about it do you want to change or transform?
2. What is the first form of movement/exercise that motivates you?
3. Think about a kind of exercise or activity you haven't done that sounds like something you would be willing to try. What have you always wanted to do but never pushed yourself to do it?
4. Do you have any negative self-talk about being active or when you're about to work out? Do some of your limiting beliefs or self-talk come from other people? What are some new things you can say to support and motivate yourself?
5. Try out the visualization of something active, see how long you can stay in it. Just an interesting concept, and can be used in just about every area of your life.

HEALTH TOOLS TO HAVE AT HOME

et's talk about a few lovely tools that we can have at home to help our body on one level or another. This is not a promotion or suggestion for people to go out and buy these, nor are these going to be for everyone, but I find it helpful to mention them and explain the benefits and the advantages of using them. In my personal opinion, they are easy to use and their impact is life-changing.

A few of them can be used for flexibility and strength and a few serve in helping the body move things around, or out. These tools help to improve our muscles, movement, immunity, nervous system, digestive system, *all* of the systems and organs honestly. They help us to achieve a greater state of health.

Along with other modalities and avenues to keep ourselves active, fit, and healthy, these tools will compliment anyone's daily health practices.

YOGA MAT

Yoga mats are so great to have. They are a personal sized exercise mat that have a fantastic gripping ability and are great for so many types of physical activities, not just yoga. They're usually made out of a rubbery, often times recycled material, although you can get rubber-free versions. The gripping nature of these mats when barefoot, is perfect for yoga, stretching, and balancing exercises. It keeps your feet planted and free from slipping. It's amazing for any floor work whatever that may be whether it's sit-ups, push-ups, isometrics, and so on.

My yoga mat stays in the same place, at the foot of my bed where I cannot ignore it. It speaks to me every morning, night, and on occasion sometimes randomly during the day. It's where I do my morning and nighttime stretch sessions as well as my meditations. The morning stretch really sets me up for the day (though I believe everyone should do a few stretches in bed before getting out of it). It keeps my body more flexible and honestly prevents a lot of pain I might otherwise have without the stretching I do.

Before I began doing this daily practice, I was having a lot of difficulty with my back, hips, and overall spinal comfort. It has genuinely changed all of that for me, and my flexibility has improved immensely without my realizing. Having a yoga mat somewhere you will see it often, can serve as a reminder which may trigger you to want to do a quick stretch, or sit and meditate. It's a wonderful tool that you can use as part of your routine, or perhaps you will be more motivated to create one that you don't already have.

Here in the US, you can buy one for $10-30 in stores or online. They are very transportable, so even when you take a road trip, there's no reason *not* to bring it. If you decide to take a yoga class, you will happily have your own to bring instead of borrowing a mat. There are even bags to carry it!

REBOUNDER – *THE SMALL TRAMPOLINE*

Here's another great way to get moving more, especially if you're a less active person. A rebounder is basically a mini trampoline. They say rebounding is equal to jogging, so 15 minutes on the rebounder is like 15 minutes of jogging. It requires some energy and movement on one's part, but you don't have to be masterful or be super coordinated to use one. A rebounder is a wonderful tool to get in some movement, as well as that it is super helpful for the lymphatic system.

A lot of rebounders come with a handlebar which is a great thing to have, as it can help keep you stable allowing you to hold on to it while doing your bouncing. The handlebar can help prevent falls, as it's a great stability feature that is especially good for older folks or more nervous people, lending more security and ability to be more cautious.

We really only need to bounce lightly, unless you are very active and you use this for more intensive exercises, because you can get in a really good a workout on a rebounder. If you're into it, definitely check out some videos online.

Using a small trampoline or rebounder is *obviously* not a go to if you're injured, have serious spine, hip, knee, ankle, neck, joint, or back problems. Although rebounding is quite gentle on the body when done therapeutically. Of course, if you are fearful of incurring injury with it, skip over this one, you can get exercise and lymph movement in another way.

But if you are down to try it, the rebounder is loads of fun! It honestly makes you feel like a kid again, which in my mind is only ever good. When you're on the rebounder, **your feet don't have to leave the rebounder** to get the bounce going. You simply raise up onto the balls of your feet almost like standing on your tippy toes, lifting your heels up, and lowering back down. If any balance stuff arises, this is where the handlebar comes in.

We can engage other muscles while on the rebounder when we feel confident and strong enough to do so. It can build up our ab strength if we work on contracting our abdominal muscles during the bouncing, we can do air punches, arm movements, or use arm weights to work on our biceps a bit. Do whatever feels comfortable and you can always switch it up and get creative. Of course, always be wise and careful, using any device or equipment as a general rule. Know yourself well enough so that you can prevent any unnecessary injuries. Having body awareness is key no matter what we're doing.

Generally, I love the rebounder because it is an excellent tool for the lymphatic system. Rebounding will help move the lymphatic fluids. If being used for aerobic exercises, there are tons of videos out there that will give you an actual workout to do. Some rebounders come with their own programs. Depending on where you live, there are rebounding classes out there, too. If you're lucky, you can sometimes find these gems at a garage sale, at a sporting goods store, or online for $40-50. The exercise rebounders with a handlebar range from about $80-400 online.

FOAM ROLLER

This large, cylindrical piece of foam is a wonderful tool for breaking up tension and rolling out areas that need some massage. When rolling a body part over this foam piece, it uses your body weight to add a firm, yet gentle pressure to the area, which helps to unlock and release tension, stimulates blood flow to the area, and gives the muscles and tendons some much needed massage. The foam roll also helps in stretching and lengthening the spine when rolled over slowly. Personally, I find that it gives me a bit of an adjustment, cracking a few of my unaligned vertebrae which helps me out and keeps me from having to visit the chiropractor as often.

It can be used both directions, horizontally and vertically. I will warn though, that the vertical position can be a bit trickier to get onto. Once you're on it though, it's easy to work with. The horizontal position tends to be easier to utilize and helps release compression in tight areas from the neck down to the tailbone.

When using this device, it's important to go *slowly* so that you have better control if something doesn't feel right. It's important to relax as much as possible, but to know your limitations. It's quite easy to stiffen up when you fear relaxing on it, which can cause injury, so always be wise.

Either you know your body is capable of being down on the floor using it, or you know it isn't, so be a good judge of this. As just stated, you have to get down onto the floor for this tool to be utilized, so if getting onto and off of the floor is not ideal for you, I might suggest avoiding it. You can always see a physical therapist who do work with these and can assess your ability as well as show you how to use it.

This tool should not be used by frail individuals, people with compression or other known fractures, serious disc issues, delicate spinal situations, or after having back or spine surgery. Please ask your doctor if you have any doubts.

DRY BODY BRUSH

A dry body brush is also known as a lymph brush. It's an excellent movement tool for the lymphatic system and is also helpful for many other reasons. This soft bristled brush is easy on the skin when applied. It's used to stimulate the lymphatic circulation which happens to be closer to the skin surface than we realize, so this soft brushing stimulates the movement of it. The brush is also excellent for exfoliation, removing toxins, increasing circulation, energizing the meridians, and reducing cellulite. This is wonderful to do before you get in the shower.

When using a lymph brush to stimulate the lymph system, ideally you want to start by doing circular motions over the center of your body, the mid torso area over the stomach or so, essentially close to where the spleen is. Then begin on one side of the neck, close up to the ear and on the side of the face, brushing downwards towards and over the chest, towards your center. For the ladies, brush in a clockwise circular motion around the breast and in towards the center. Move into the armpit and down your side brushing in towards the center. Work your way up the inner arm, up to the wrist and brush down the arm towards the center. Then move to the other side starting on your neck again.

After that second arm is complete, do a couple of circular brush motions at your center again and then start working on the lower extremities. Begin on one side of the lower abdomen and upper groin area, brushing upward towards the center. Brush the inner groin and like with the arm, work your way down the inner leg, brushing upwards, getting all the way to the ankle and back up to center. Repeat on the other side. You can then use the brush on your head and scalp, buttocks, back of the thighs, and your back if you have a brush with a longer handle. The whole practice should take about 2-4 minutes.

You want to open up the channels for things to move and flow easier. As we mentioned earlier, the lymph system doesn't have a pump so it needs some help and it flows in the direction towards your center, so try not to brush in the opposite direction, away from your center.

It's never too late to get things moving and help your body, so get yourself a lymph brush and start today! You can start at any time. It's so important to put in the effort of loving and supporting our body's overall function and well-being. This practice connects you to your body and is a wonderful way to support your body as part of your daily routine. Doing this before taking your morning shower is the best time to do this however, doing it morning *and* evening is even more effective.

TONGUE SCRAPER

This simple, genius device is a wonderful tool for removing bacteria and pulling out mucus and stagnancy from our lungs and digestive tract. It can be used however many times of the day we choose, essentially after we brush our teeth, especially in the morning, as people find they have the most mucus build up upon rising.

It's fairly self-explanatory and easy to use. It's a U-shaped metal device, where the U is perfectly designed to scrape along and down the tongue. You hold it by both ends, starting at the back of the tongue and scraping down and out. Rinse the scraper and repeat. This will remove a layer of gunk and the film covering our tongue that contains bacteria and undesired mucus. Each session requires at least 5-10 times.

Many people have a white or yellow film on their tongue which is indicative of their intestinal and respiratory situation. It helps to remove that undesirable layer (with time). It brings mucus up and out believe it or not, creates a pulling of sorts to help the body remove the excess buildup. You'll be surprised at the amount of mucus that you get out. It's wonderful for gut and lung health, just be careful not to set off your gag reflex too much, you don't want to cause yourself to vomit.

Tongue scraping has been practiced for centuries, dating back to ancient India in their medical teachings known as Ayurveda. The tongue is a direct connection to the vital organs in the body: the kidneys, heart, lungs, spleen, liver, and stomach. Inspecting the tongue is proven to be a gauge of one's overall health. The dynamics that Chinese and Ayurvedic medicine use are undoubtedly genius, revealing, and can actually guide us towards discovering weaknesses and stagnancy in our body. Please do look into the tongue and the organs aligned to it online if you're interested. There are other body parts like the face and the iris of the eye that are also powerful diagnostic tools.

The white or yellow coating on the tongue along with bad breath is highly indicative of poor digestive and bowel function, poor liver function, and stagnation. Other symptoms that often times go along with this are brain fog, confusion, and fatigue.

Benefits of tongue scraping are:

- Clearing toxins, bacteria, and dead cells
- Promotes good dental and oral health
- Gently stimulates your internal organs
- Helps pull out and remove mucus

The best tongue scraper one can buy is a copper one. Stainless steel ones are second best, and getting the ones that are U shaped are ideal. There are some other kinds out there, just find what works for you. They are very transportable so when traveling they are easy to bring along. Tongue scraping is *only* beneficial and an absolute wonderful addition to your oral hygiene routine.

ENEMA KIT

Enemas are extremely useful and can be a life-saver when you're sick. It's an old practice that's been used for thousands of years, and not even forty years ago, most households and families had an enema bag on hand for when someone fell ill. It's still a powerful first defense when someone is getting sick. A large percentage of the present-day population would greatly benefit from these, considering all of the toxins we're exposed to every day.

Enemas can help to move stagnancy out, get rid of some of the poisons in the system, and lingering leftover waste. They hydrate the colon and give the body what was once called by the medical profession, *internal washing.* It's overall helpful for the system that is overwhelmed by all the types of foods and products we ingest.

You can find one at your local pharmacy or drug store usually, but a lot of choices online. Mikacare makes a great one. Some hot water bottles come with the attachment for an enema. Remember to lie on your left side when doing an enema, and you might have to get some help, as it can be cumbersome to maneuver for the elderly or those with disabilities. Use distilled or purified water whenever possible, and you can heat it up beforehand to body temperature of around 98-100 degrees or so (check temp like you would check the baby milk on your wrist). Warmer water feels better going in and is also more effective on loosening up old debris.

Many people have heard about coffee enemas. There's a lot of power behind doing these. You really don't want to just use your everyday regular coffee considering what they contain nowadays, it's best to grab some that is more medicinal in this way.

There is special coffee that is best used for this method that is pure, clean, and mold free. This coffee is roasted in a way that helps to retain all of the nutrients and elements maintaining a golden color. I love S.A. Wilson's coffee for this.

Coffee enemas are different than ones done with only water. A smaller amount of this coffee is instilled into the lower colon and held for about 12 minutes. You don't want the coffee to fill up the entire colon, just the lower portion. A coffee enema helps to stimulate and remove toxins from the liver and the blood, as well as increases the production of glutathione s-transferase which is a powerful detoxifying enzyme.

It's important to choose to eat enzyme and probiotic rich foods or supplements to maintain balance in the system when utilizing enemas or colonics. This therapy is key for removing any leftover matter, giving the body a greater chance to reestablish and maintain a healthy gut bacteria balance. It assists the body when things have slowed down, have gotten stagnant, and the system is constipated. Helping the body to release and eliminate leftover poisons is so vital in keeping the body healthy and strong.

CASTOR OIL PACK

Castor oil has been used for thousands of years to treat a large variety of health issues. It was a big thing when illness hit to give someone a spoonful of castor oil. Castor oil has been known to boost the immune system and is most commonly used to help improve liver function.

However, I am not here to promote oral consumption of castor oil, instead share with you an ancient practice known as a Castor oil pack. This castor oil-soaked cloth helps to relieve pain, break up congestion, relieve constipation, increase circulation, reduce inflammation, heal the skin, and moisturize. Here's what a castor oil pack is good for:

- Improves blood flow, breaking up stagnancy
- Intestinal disorders, constipation
- Headaches, migraines
- Cysts in the breast tissue
- Skin issues
- Arthritis
- Muscle aches
- Backaches
- Lung infections
- Improves lymphatic flow, helps lymphatic drainage
- Inflamed joints, rheumatism
- Parasitic infections
- Ovarian cysts and fibroids, menstrual issues
- Liver or gallbladder pain, stagnancy, or stones

Castor oil softens hardened matter and deposits in the body (where it is applied) by stimulating circulation to the area and adding a softening agent through the skin. It's also used as an aide for hair growth. When placed on the central abdomen, the action of the castor oil pack helps to boost the digestive system, spleen and lymphatic system helping to increase lymphocyte production (disease fighting cells). Lymphocyte production increases when the skin absorbs castor oil speeding up the removal of toxins from the tissues.

It increases immunological function overall. Castor oil packs can also be used for thyroid issues as they help to nourish the thyroid, stimulate blood flow to the area, and calms inflammation. They are wonderful for female issues and menstrual difficulties as they help break up blockages and increase blood flow to the area. Castor oil packs are proved to help to shrink uterine fibroids, ovarian cysts, and even help to reduce symptoms of PCOS.

Of course, if you've never used castor oil before, I would do a spot test and make sure you don't have a reaction to the oil. Let's cover what is needed for this, as many people have it all of these items already at home.

- Good quality castor oil (organic, cold-pressed is best)
- A piece of flannel cloth (size may vary depending on the area you want to cover)
- A container or mason jar (to pour the oil over and soak the cloth)
- A piece of plastic wrap or a small towel
- Hot water bottle or heating pad
- One hour of free, undisturbed time with somewhere to relax and rest during the treatment.

My favorite thing to use is a <u>castor oil pack wrap</u> which is available online, because it comes with the cloth to soak and a covering that you can actually Velcro around you to keep everything in place. It's also great to not have to deal with plastic wrap which as we all know, can be difficult at times, as well as that your clothing is protected.

Directions:

1. Soak the piece of flannel, making sure its saturated. You do not want it dripping off the cloth so not to overdo.
2. Place the cloth over the area you wish to treat and cover it with plastic wrap or the small towel to prevent soiling other materials.
3. Place the heating pad or hot water bottle over the area. If using a hot water bottle, get the temp of the water as high as the bottle allows for. With electric heating pads, always use with caution.
4. Now try to relax for the next 30-60 minutes. If you can, focus on the healing of the area, visualization is great. When you finish the session, use a towel to clean off the area to remove excess oil. You can then store the soaked cloth in a mason jar or container in the refrigerator for your next use.

Always consult with a doctor if you have questions or health issues that are severe. Note that most doctors do not have the training or understanding around castor oil packs unless they've been around a few decades.

* If you start feeling nauseated, have abdominal cramping, vomiting, or diarrhea **stop** using the castor oil pack and reassess. It can stir some things up and depending on your condition, cause your body to move too much, too quick. Shorter time frames like 15-20 minutes may be best to try in the beginning working your way up to 40-60 minutes to allow your body to get used to it. **This is not a *daily practice*.** This can be done 3-4 times a week, spaced out.

* DO NOT USE IF BREASTFEEDING, PREGNANT or on the lower abdomen if you have an IUD. Castor oil can induce labor.

SAUNA

If you can access one of these, what a blessing it can be! Many of us have been in a sauna at some point in time, but perhaps you never have. They've been around for thousands of years, used by so many of our ancestors. There are different types of saunas such as dry and wet saunas, infrared saunas, Finnish or Turkish saunas, steam rooms, or sweat lodges.

We can find saunas at a lot of health centered places such as gyms and exercise centers, pools, spas, holistic and alternative health clinics, hotels and resorts, and even there are some apartment complexes that have them. If you're one of the lucky ones, you have one of your very own either inside your home or somewhere outside.

A sauna is an enclosed structure, like a small room or building designed to entrap either wet or dry heat. Saunas consist of a heating element, such as an electric heater or stove. Rocks, wood, and tile are elements used inside as a conduit for the heat. Water can be splashed onto the hot rocks to produce steam.

The temperature ranges from 90 degrees to over 200 degrees, with a usual temp usually around 165 degrees (Fahrenheit). The degree of heat and amount of time you can spend in a sauna depends greatly on your health status and current disposition. The recommended length of time is usually around fifteen to twenty minutes, however when just getting started, start at five to ten minutes to judge how your body handles the heat. Short stints are better than wanting to pass out. And always get up slowly from sitting when inside.

It's serious and vital that you are hydrated well and continue to hydrate yourself after using a sauna. Eat light avoiding heavy meals before using a sauna. Sitting on a towel prevents skin irritation and keeps the area clean. Most people go totally without clothing, although people sometimes wear towels wrapped around them.

Saunas have amazing health benefits, however, _ALWAYS CHECK WITH YOUR DOCTOR BEFORE USING A SAUNA!_ People who suffer from cardiovascular disease or blood pressure issues are people who should not use a sauna (unless their doctor says yes to it.) An unrestricted and balanced blood flow is _essential_ for a hot therapy like this. Those with high heart rate, atrial fibrillation, blood pressure issues, or who have a pacemaker, should stay away from saunas, as well as hot tubs.

It's also important to avoid the sauna if you're pregnant. Not to go in if you have a hangover or have drunk alcohol, take narcotics, diuretics, beta-blockers, sedatives, or have street drugs in your system. People who are obese should check with their doctor. Endocrine, especially thyroid disorders should check with their doctor (remember Thyroid is the main temperature regulator). People with neurological disorders, brain traumas, tumors, or who have spells of dizziness should all avoid saunas, check with your doctor. Lastly, if you have any metal implants, it's best to avoid using an infrared sauna.

Saunas help to open up our pores, especially a moist or wet heat. The intense heat causes us to perspire, or sweat, which helps in releasing, expelling, and in carrying toxins and impurities out of the body. Saunas help the body to detoxify. They're great for the skin by removing dirt and dead skin cells from the pores.

They're also wonderful to improve immune function, as they stimulate the production of white blood cells. Saunas help to slow down the aging process by helping the cells to release free radicals and toxins from within the cells. They stimulate the cellular response on so many levels, even improving insulin sensitivity.

Saunas heat the body up, helping to fight off unwanted organisms.

They assist in improving cardiovascular health. The heat opens up and dilates blood vessels, increasing the blood flow. They can help relieve pain through the heat and moisture, which penetrates more deeply, reducing muscle tension and stress, and by bringing blood to areas that need more oxygen. Being in a sauna promotes an overall relaxation of the body. When you get out of a session, you feel lighter.

Science has proven many benefits to saunas, even decreasing one's chance of dementia or cognitive disorders. The list in seemingly endless.

Just always know your limits. Work your way up from five minutes, especially if you aren't in perfect health, take your time getting used to using a sauna. Your body needs time to adjust to the heat and work its way up slowly. Especially if we are highly toxic, we don't want to dump toxins out too quickly. ALWAYS BE CAUTIOUS. It's never going to be to our benefit to push ourselves. Nothing happens overnight so take your time with this one.

There are all kinds of saunas available for purchase or you can build your own if you're feeling the pull. There are ebooks on Amazon that are free as well as tons of information and science online.

PH TEST STRIPS

These are a great at-home, simple tool to measure your body's pH level through your urine or saliva. When you are highly acidic and working on becoming more alkaline, this is a good gauge to get an idea of where you're at. When you start changing your diet and eating higher alkaline foods to give your body a break from all the acids, you will be delighted to see the pH level on the strip more on alkaline side, which is a step towards your healing success!

The last thing to say about using all of these tools and truly any modality or therapy, is that it's important to acknowledge our body during the time that we're using them. *And,* that we should speak words of love and gratitude to our body while using them, (even to the tool, too!) as a part of it.

As an example, when you're using the lymph brush, it's actually beneficial to watch yourself use it as you brush it along your body.

Your eyes are hitting all of the parts of you, and the visual of seeing the brush moving along, helps move the energy. Also, it's important to can acknowledge each part (leg, armpit, breast, etc.) as you pass over it and tell it *"Thank you"* and *"I love you."*

It's great to say it out loud, but we don't have to, we can just think in our heads. We can even look in the mirror and say it to ourselves in the mirror. I even do it differently each time. Sometimes I just say *"Thank you! I love you!"* over and over again, or sometimes I take the time to acknowledge each and every part. Lastly, smile while you're doing it, it stirs in the emotion of happiness and joy. You can't not feel good when you smile.

Being conscious like this is a superior way to be, especially when it comes to taking care of ourselves, our health, our body. We can do this at any time, and in just about everything that we do. There's no limit as to when we can do and speak these things.

Gratitude and smiling create such a high vibe, and it's good for healing.

HOMEWORK:

1. What tools sound like something your body could benefit from?
2. If you try a new one or two of these tools, write about some of your process as you begin using it. Include the practice of adding words of love and gratitude while using them. Journal about anything you notice, new feelings and any changes you may experience.

MEDICINE CAME FROM NATURE

"The plants have enough spirit to transform our limited vision."
– Rosemary Gladstar

We are made from the same cellular concept as all other living beings on the planet. We are a part of the animal and plant kingdoms connected through our biology, chemistry, and energy. We are a part of the Earth. The wise intelligence in our body is directly connected with nature. All living beings have a unique and divine intelligence of their own, especially the plants and animals.

Plants closely resonate and harmonize with our biological and cellular structure, which is why we get the best nourishment and nutrition from them. Almost all of the vitamins and minerals that our bodies need, are found in these colorful, beautiful foods that are grown out of the Earth. The Earth provides us with the nourishment and food that we need. It also supports our healing on powerful levels.

Every plant that grows from the ground, has chemical compounds within it, many that are helpful towards our wellbeing in one form or another. For thousands of years, these plants have been known to affect specific ailments and body parts. It's the wisdom of the past that has been carried down for generations.

Plant medicine has been around since the beginning of time. It's been used by every single one of our ancestors, no matter from where we've come. It's a part of all of our bloodlines; it's a part of our DNA.

The beautiful thing about plant medicine, is that it works so powerfully, yet so simply. Plants interact with our body so harmonically and perfectly. They not only bring in physical assistance and healing, but also emotional and energetic remedy as well.

Our bodies can assimilate the molecular and biological structure of plant compounds, most perfectly. This means our body can easily break down and use the components that are contained in the plant or herb, that we are ingesting or utilizing. Our bodies can interact with the ingredients more effectively, as they resonate on a much greater level compared to synthetic compounds. They are closer to our genetic and molecular makeup, as well as our vibrational frequency.

Synthetic chemicals do not possess the same potential as plant chemicals, and there's a disconnect that occurs, especially on the energetic level. They don't resonate in the same way on a cellular level as plants do.

When taken in safe and effective ways, plants will work gently to find the pulse of what's going on in the person's body. They have an intelligence.

Plant medicine knows how to work with the body's vibration and is there to help uplift it. Plants nurture the energy within the body, and bring balance back into it. Plants assist the body with its healing process.

Plant medicine, herbs in particular, have powerful qualities that help the cells in all of the regions in the body, assisting them with cleansing, tonifying, strengthening, protecting, and the actual healing of the cells and systems. Herbs help the cells get their health back, so they are able to work properly and efficiently.

Each herb has different properties or actions that assist on different levels. Some herbs can help calm the nervous system, moving the body out of stress mode; others can assist in cleaning out toxins, triggering waste release. Some herbs support the regrowth and renewal of various body parts, while others help regulate glands and fight off organisms. Each herb possesses numerous amazing qualities.

Herbs can work quickly and effectively, or they can be used slowly over a long period of time for a more gentle approach. They are especially helpful with chronic health problems, the ones that take time to reverse or heal from. Plant medicine is a wonderful guide and healer that can help our bodies work their way back towards a more balanced state of health.

As a nurse, I never learned how the drug and chemical formulas were actually thought up or created, nor from where actual chemicals that are used, originate from. Less than one-hundred years ago, plants were an integral part of the medical, health, and healing profession. All of the medicinal formulas, were originally made with plant materials that were found to have specific action and purpose within the human body.

Today's modern medicine and its science have sadly cut off the connection to plants and their medicine, even going as far as to ridiculing them and claiming them harmful, inadequate, or useless. Understandable on the level knowing that they do interact with the chemical medicine that is out there.

Since the beginning of time, plants were used to heal. There's tons of documented research and studies that have been done between the 1600's to the early 1900's that's somewhat available for us to see.

Plant medicine and herbal remedies were also used for spiritual, emotional, and mental imbalances and disruptions. Healing of the body wasn't only about working on the physical symptoms and issues, it included acknowledging and working on the spiritual, emotional, and mental aspects of the person, as well.

Science once acknowledged plant medicine as a crucial element for healing, but as we know, chemical medicine eventually took over. With it becoming the primary component of healthcare, the inclination to rely on nature diminished. Why bother when fast-acting chemical compounds seemed capable of providing instant relief for a while?

However, this era didn't endure for long. We soon came to realize that there is a place for everything, and no single remedy, especially synthetic chemicals, can address all of our needs. The demand for more natural medicine and healing has returned, so much so, that even the chemical companies are now working to produce more herbal based formulas and products.

Lavender, tea tree, peppermint, cinnamon, and ginger are some of the more commonly known plants that we see infused into formulas and products that are on the shelf today. Whether it be skin care products, cleaning products, or medicine for symptom relief, these herbs are gaining recognition by the majority of folks.

Plant based medicine or ingredients are now being appreciated and seen to be much safer, than synthetic, chemically based ones. People are taking notice. Most parents would rather give their children something natural, over something chemically based. So, many children's medicine formulas are now being produced with herbal ingredients, such as elderberries, lavender, and other flowers and plants that are highly effective, gentle, and safer for our children.

Although the new found demand for natural has been working its way into things, there's still some distrust occurring, and understandably so after a century of conditioning and pushing it out of the picture.

However, many cultures never stopped using plant medicine or old remedies and continue to use them as a first line of defense for themselves and their families. They have learned to turn to modern day doctors only when things weren't improving.

Of course, we don't always know what our ancestors did to help heal themselves, as much of that information has been lost or is hard to find. However, with each passing day, more of our connection to it seems to be revealed. Many of us feel more drawn to it than the current and usual suspects, i.e., the chemical formulas.

Once you realize how powerful plant medicine is, the chemical, synthetic versions don't seem as appealing. Of course, chemical pharmaceutical medications have their place and use, but there are natural, herbal ways to assist the body in helping to heal itself. Now instead of trying to shush a cold, we are able to give our body nourishing and supportive herbs to help it get through the process.

When you look back at the old school medicinal formulas, it's pretty cool. They *only* contain herbal and natural ingredients, and there were generally only about 2-7 ingredients found in each. All made very simply, no fillers, chemicals, or preservatives added, just the herbal or natural components in it for the reason indicated. Generally herbal formulas used alcohol to pull the medicinal constituents out of the herbs, which also acted to preserve the formulas.

Some of the drug companies that exist today have been around for a few hundred years, some for over *three hundred and fifty years*. These old school, popular companies used to make these herbal formulas. Some even continue to make a few of them today, but for whatever reason they generally aren't being prescribed or used here in the US. Back in the day, not even ninety years ago, they even had cannabis as a *major* ingredient in over two hundred medicinal formulas, before it was pushed out of the picture.

Whatever the situations have been in the past, the important thing is that plant medicine is making a comeback. People are now more accepting of it, feeling less fearful of, or threatened by it. Many people have come to realize that nature does indeed have powerful medicinal qualities and that it was put here on the planet *for* us.

What I love about plants is that they can be used in so many different ways, through different therapeutic methods, depending on the reason that we need them. Incorporating them into a health plan is easy, because we can often use whatever form we prefer. For example, we may prefer tea and tinctures, over pills and capsules. Herbs are easy to work with, and are even beneficial to our senses. We gain benefit from their smell, colors, and their beauty. Herbs are excellent for their variability. Here are some of the methods in which they can be taken or used:

- Tea, infusion
- Capsule
- Tincture (liquid herbal solution that is alcohol or glycerin based)
- Skin cream, ointment, salve
- Enema, suppository, douche
- Eye wash
- Compress (a soft, cloth pad held in place used to supply moisture, cold, heat, or medication, or apply pressure)
- Poultice (herbs moistened, spread on a cloth and applied to part of the body; used to warm, moisten or stimulate an aching or inflamed part of the body)
- Soak, bath

As with anything medicinal, herbs and plants must be respected and used wisely, just like with the use of chemical, pharmaceutical medications, we need to be well informed of their effects and precautions. There are many plant formulas out there on the market that are safe, tested, and come with instructions and precautions that are sold at your everyday drug store or grocery store.

Of course, the biggest rule of thumb is if you are someone who is on several medications, **you must talk to your doctor.** Better safe than sorry. Do your research. Take it upon yourself to also learn what it is that you're taking. There is a lot of information out there for us both online and of course through some truly amazing books and textbooks, but don't ever go it alone if you have a lot going on and are just starting out. Remember there are naturopaths who know both pharmaceutical and herbal medicine, they are great resources.

Let's take a look at a few commonly known plants and herbs, and some of the wonderful healing qualities they possess. These are generally easy to access. Of course, use caution and be smart. If I were to forage and pick any of these growing in the wild, I would make sure they weren't contaminated, growing next to a busy road or sprayed with herbicides and the like. And for the umpteenth time, please be cautious if you're on medications.

Dandelion, is known as a common weed, yet holds high medicinal and nutritional value. The leaves and roots are the most commonly used parts, and the leaves can be eaten raw or cooked. Dandelion is rich in potassium, which is critically necessary for every cell of our body to function. It has **detoxifying** properties (removing and destroying toxins and poisons) because it contains nutritive salts that the body uses to purify the blood. Properties of dandelion are:

- Liver detoxifier- dandelions stimulate the flow of bile
- Helps to dissolve uric acid, relieving stiffness in the joints (anti-rheumatic)
- Its high in organic sodium and potassium which combined, is the balancer of electrolytes in the blood
- Acts as a **diuretic** used for water retention related to kidney or heart problems, increases the flow of urine. Decreases edema
- Acts as a **tonic** (restorative, invigorating, and refreshing agent) especially for the liver and urinary system
- Acts as a gentle laxative
- Used for calcium deficiencies
- Nourishing and good for anemia, **high in iron**, builds blood nutrients

- High in Vitamin A
- Invigorates and strengthens the body
- Restores gastric balance after severe vomiting
- Great survival food
- Contains inulin, which is a soluble plant fiber that helps stabilize blood sugar levels- helpful with diabetes and pancreatic issues

Calendula, is also known as Golden Marigold. The leaves, flowers, and petals are all used for medicinal purpose. Works as an antiseptic, helps to heal infections and wounds, is known as the *best tissue healer*, and is soothing to all parts of the body. Calendula works to heal internal membranes of the body, it's an anti-inflammatory, astringent (drawing and constricting, stops blood flow) and hemostatic (an agent which stops bleeding and hemorrhage).

- Antiseptic properties similar to witch hazel because of its high iodine content
- The ointment is used to help heal cuts, wounds, burns, injuries, bruises, and varicose veins when applied
- Using a poultice is good to help heal wounds and cuts
- Constant applications can help and even prevent gangrene and tetanus
- Is an anti-fungal, can combat internal and external fungal infections
- Great for insect stings- bee stings, scorpion stings, wasp stings, etc.
- Used as a nasal wash or as a gargle, to soothe and heal mucous membranes. Helpful with gum diseases
- Taken internally for inflammatory conditions of the colon, stomach, liver, and healing after operations
- Used for gastric and duodenal ulcers
- Helps relieve gallbladder problems
- Known to help normalize menstrual cycle
- Works to help stop external bleeding
- Strengthens physical body tissue

Chamomile, also known as Ground Apple, is a commonly known for its relaxing qualities. It was highly revered by the Egyptians, Greeks, and Romans in ancient medical texts. Although chamomile is known to be relaxing, it's actually labeled as a stimulant. However, it works as a nervine (calming on the nerves & nervous system) and soothing tonic, so it is best known for its calming and sedative qualities:

- It is beneficial for a good night's sleep
- Relaxing and good for anxiety
- Used to help children with nightmares
- Relaxes nerves in the gut- soothes bowel complaints, nausea, vomiting
- Stimulates blood flow for poor circulation
- Effective relieving menstrual cramps and stomach cramps

Chickweed, otherwise known as Starweed and Stitchwort. It can grow year-round even under the snow. The flowers, leaves, and stems are used medicinally. Helpful for the skin, respiratory system, circulatory system, and digestive system with its anti-inflammatory properties. It can break apart and dissipate fat and diseased tissue. Chickweed has cooling and soothing properties. It is good for:

- Rashes, dry itchy skin, diaper rash, abscesses, boils, sores, eruptions, ulcers, burns, acne, skin infections
- Gout, rheumatism
- Pink eye (as an eyewash)
- Asthma, bronchitis, coughing
- Allergies, hay fever
- Breast inflammation, lactation
- Stomach ulcers, inflamed bowels, colitis, hemorrhoids
- Swollen testicles

Works to **break down fat** and absorbs and **dissolves diseased tissue,** helping:

- Cellulite
- Circulatory system- plaque in blood vessels and arteries
- Blood poisoning
- Fatty tumors, cancerous tissue

190

Parsley, well known for its culinary use, has spectacular healing properties. The leaves, stems, and roots are all used for health purposes, the roots being the most potent. It has a high content of chlorophyll and three times more Vitamin C than citrus fruits. It also has a high content of iron and potassium. Parsley is easy to ingest whether eating it raw, juicing it into a juice, or as a tea, making it easily accessible. It works as a tonic, diuretic, and helps break down hardened matter. Parsley:

- Is an ancient remedy for kidney stones, used to dissolve and pass them
- Works for gallstones as well
- Greatly beneficial to the urinary tract system, increases diuretic activity, especially in case of an enlarged prostate
- Good tonic for blood vessels and capillaries
- Highly nutritive, high iron level, potassium
- High chlorophyll content which has cancer-fighting properties, oxygenates the body, and boosts the immune system
- Due to the blood cleansing and blood building properties, it's very helpful for the liver and the spleen
- Provides kidneys with nutrients needed to detoxify and clean out
- Stimulating during the menstrual process
- Helps to ease flatulence and accompanying colic pains.
- Works to assist with low blood sugar if there is adrenal malfunction.
- Acts as a gentle laxative and lowers blood pressure.

It's true that doctors **do** need to worry about the herbs you take, and yes, they can be dangerous because *they can have an interaction with your medications.* Remember, pharmaceutical drugs are rooted from the chemical properties of plants. Both the herbs and the pills work biologically and chemically when in your body, meaning, they can indeed interact with one another, and not always in a positive way. If you are on medications, please find a practitioner or doctor who understands all of them who can further guide you, instead of just braving it on your own. Naturopaths are wonderful with this as their schooling incorporates plant and pharmaceutical, chemical medicine.

The herbs I've listed here are relatively safe, but be sure to check with a doctor.

CANNABIS AND HEMP

Cannabis has surely gotten a poor rap over the last century, or so, but don't be fooled. The fact of the matter is that this plant has some amazingly, powerful medicinal properties, and it can be very safe for use.

The version of cannabis that is most popularly known is marijuana, which can indeed have a psychoactive effect, altering one's state of mind and perception. However, this is not true for all species of the cannabis plant, as there are two that are most utilized, one being the marijuana plant and the other being the hemp plant. Both of these have medicinal properties with amazing healing effects, as well as that there are certain plant chemicals within these plants that do not cause the psychoactive effect.

Hemp and marijuana are two versions of the same plant species. Hemp, however, has very low levels of THC and is usually referred to as industrial hemp. The hemp plant is able to be transformed into cloth, building materials, and fuel.

When you look back at medical history, cannabis was last found in over two hundred formulas only a hundred years ago, and was well-known for its healing capabilities and prescribed by doctors often. Unfortunately, in the 1930's it became an illegal substance and was taken out of medicinal remedies because of certain industries and the takeover of synthetic, chemical medication. It was proclaimed to be dangerous and propagandized to be harmful and make people unstable.

Cannabis dates back to Ancient China, documented as far back as 2737 BC. Emperor Shen Neng known as "The Father of Chinese Medicine" used cannabis quite frequently. The roots were used to remove blood clots, the juice of the leaves to combat tapeworm, and the powdered seeds were used for constipation and hair loss.

The Chinese at this time, discovered that when the plant's leaves were ground and consumed as tea, or were smoked, they brought pain relief caused by illness. They believed cannabis numbed the body of pain and it was used during surgery, as it was also noted to increase chances of recovery, thereafter. The Chinese listed cannabis as one of the 50 fundamental herbs to be used for illness.

The Egyptians used cannabis suppositories for hemorrhoids. In India cannabis' psychoactive properties were used for insomnia, headaches, digestive disorders, and pain. They used cannabis to cure dysentery, sunstroke, and to bring alertness to the body and mind. Ancient Greeks used it to dress wounds and sores on horses, used the dried leaves for nose bleeds, and the seeds to expel tapeworm.

In 1545, the Spanish fleet brought marijuana to North America. This was then followed by the British, who brought more in 1611. By this time, cannabis was used for the production of industrial strength rope and was considered to be as important as wheat. In 1890, Sir John Russell Reynolds, the president of the British Medical Association and physician to the royal household, wrote a paper reviewing thirty years of personal experience in prescribing cannabis tincture and to advocate for its legitimate medicinal uses, which at the time was for a wide variety of ailments such as agitation and insomnia in dementia, migraines, neuralgia, seizures, and menstrual cramps, to name a few.

It was once prescribed as an anti-spasmodic, sedative, and narcotic. By the twentieth century, over a hundred papers were published in Western medical journals and cannabis was found available at most pharmacies.

In the 1980's a new system in the human body was discovered called the Endocannabinoid system. This system is a network found in the human body that works as a neuromodulator in our body, which means it helps to control motor function, cognition (perception), emotional response, regulation, and motivation. It works to specifically help modify *pain signaling* through the nervous system, releasing the body's natural endocannabinoids, reducing sensitivity to pain. Our endocannabinoid system works on one end with our brain and nervous system and on the other, with our immune system.

In 1988 Judge Francis Young ruled that cannabis had medicinal value, and so began the road towards the *rediscovery* of cannabis and gaining deeper insight into the plant. Studies since, note that cannabinoids can block the mechanisms that promote the pain in headaches, fibromyalgia, irritable bowel syndrome, and muscle spasms. Also, science has confirmed that underlying *deficiencies* of these compounds that *should be* in the body, can actually contribute to these conditions.

On October 7, 2003 the United States government obtained a patent on the anti-oxidant and neuroprotective properties of cannabis, patent no. US 6,630,507 B1. If that's not evidence in itself, I don't know what is. There are now thirty-eight states that have legalized marijuana on some level (medical or medical/recreational) and forty-seven countries who have legalized it for medical use, with a handful legalizing recreational use as well.

Today, cannabis has been identified as medicinally appropriate for cancer, glaucoma, severe pain, severe nausea, muscle spasms, PTSD, autism spectrum disorders, Crohn's disease, epilepsy/seizures, depression, panic and anxiety, HIV/AIDS, Parkinson's, Sickle Cell, spasticity related to ALS and MS, spinal cord injuries, and terminal illnesses, with more being presented as time goes on.

Cannabis, once used all around the world by practically every culture for pain and other maladies, is why it wasn't going to stay away for very long. It came back on the scene with a positive vibe and showcasing its medicinal value. Cannabis has become popular in its use as an end-of-life medicine for pain, anxiety, neurological symptoms, GI issues, and to ease the person's fear of transitioning out of their physical reality.

The opioid epidemic has also brought cannabis back into the light because opiates have caused more problems and deaths than cocaine and heroin combined. People wanted non-toxic solutions for their pain and began pursuing other methods of pain relief that didn't have such addictive or harmful side effects. Regardless of the narcotic/opiate's pain relief, people grew tired of the effects these substances have on their body. Narcotics taken in large doses or with chronic use can suppress breathing, disempower the digestive system, largely causing severe constipation, and essentially work towards shutting down the nervous system. Some doctors and anesthesiologists I know used to state that opiates turned one's brain into mush, for lack of a better term.

The main medicinal components of Cannabis are known as *cannabinoids*. These compounds interact with our central nervous system and immune system through our endocannabinoid system. Cannabinoids imitate compounds our bodies naturally produce. Two of the most popular cannabinoids are THC and CBD. The others worth mentioning that are being studied as we speak are CBG, CBN, THC-A, and CBC. THC, or Tetrahydrocannabinol, regardless of the negative stigma put upon it, has significant, positive medicinal effects on the body. THC offers these healing properties:

- Pain relief- blocks pain signals from being sent to the brain, especially useful for nerve related pain.
- Antiemetic- Manages nausea and vomiting
- Stimulates appetite
- Improves sleep
- Helpful for Glaucoma by helping to lower eye pressure
- Anti-inflammatory
- Suppresses muscle spasms
- Neuromodulator- Helpful with autism, ADD, ADHD, OCD, and Tourette's
- Reduces tremors- Useful for Parkinson's, seizures, MS

CBD, otherwise known as Cannabidiol, is the second most popular cannabinoid found in the cannabis/marijuana and hemp plant. Unlike its counterpart THC, it does *not* create the psychoactive effect. CBD can actually *cancel out the psychoactive effects of THC.*

CBD regulates the cannabinoids you already have in your body and prevents them from breaking down. CBD displays a broad range of potential medical applications. Cardiologists working with mice at Hebrew University have found that a dosage of CBD immediately following a heart attack can reduce damage by about 66%. More studies are being done with each passing day. Here are *some* of ways CBD has known to be helpful:

- **Reduces Inflammation**- CBD engages with receptors that help in modulating inflammation. It shifts the immune response from inflammatory to anti-inflammatory. CBD reduces inflammation when applied topically to an area of injury or trauma reducing damage done. CBD enhances physical performance and recovery from exercise. It reduces central nervous system inflammation. Useful for neurological diseases such as Epilepsy, Parkinson's, MS, encephalomyelitis, Alzheimer's, Degenerative Disc Disease.

- **Epilepsy/Seizures**- Works as an anti-convulsant. Reduces and eliminates seizures. Seizures, by definition, are any uncontrolled electrical activity in the brain, which may produce a physical convulsion, uncontrolled shaking, thought disturbances, loss of consciousness, or a combination of symptoms. THC-A is also known to be effective.

- **Antioxidant**- A potent antioxidant. CBD protects brain cells from damage. The body's natural process of breaking down from oxidative stress, is slowed down by CBD according to studies done. Also, studies world-wide are showing CBD affects cancer cells and contributes to their possible death, meaning CBD has some anti-cancer properties.

- **Pain Reliever**- CBD has analgesic properties, aka, it alleviates pain. CBD helps to break down and boost the effects of a chemical in our body known as Anandamide, which helps functions in the body like pain sensation, memory, sleep, ovulation, and appetite. CBD has been shown to have amazing results with *neuropathic pain.* It stimulates the capsaicin receptor, known for its impact on pain and inflammation, helpful for those who suffer from arthritis.

- **Relieves anxiety & depression**- CBD has calming properties. It can relax and promote calmness, promoting resilience to stress. Studies show it causes the over activity of the limbic/paralimbic system of the brain to *slow down.* The limbic system supports a variety of functions including emotion, behavior, motivation, long-term memory, and smell. Our emotional life is largely housed in our limbic system. It also has a great deal to do with the formation of memories. CBD stimulates serotonin receptors, which is helpful for depression. CBD improves mood and relieves irritability.

- **Relieves Nausea**- Cannabis has been proven to relieve nausea in chemotherapy patients, primarily with THC, however, CBD appears to halt the *psychological sensation of nausea*, by binding to receptors in the brain that tell the brain to "turn off" the signals that cause a person to feel sick.
- **Strengthens Bones**- A study that was first published in the Journal of Bone and Mineral Research strongly suggests that the active ingredient in Cannabidiol (CBD) stimulates enzymes and osteoblasts (*bone cells*) that are involved in the strengthening and healing processes of bones. It assists in bone healing with a break or fracture. It also helps to increase bone mass and minimize the likelihood of fractures in the future.
- **Diabetes**- Cannabinoid receptors have been identified in the pancreas, heart, blood vessels, nervous system and several other organs – all of which suggests a potential role for cannabinoids in treating diabetes. CBD has been shown to be beneficial for the pancreas and sugar metabolism. Unlike insulin and other existing medications for diabetes, CBD may actually reverse and perhaps even resolve the disease itself while working on other levels such as its anti-inflammatory and regenerative properties.
- **Neuroprotectant**- CBD has neuroprotective qualities and *regenerates nerves*. CBD protects the nervous system from degeneration, and it has been studied and shown to have protective qualities when there is reduced oxygen in the brain (strokes, brain injuries). CBD reduces Central Nervous System inflammation. A team from Neuroscience Research Australia has published the first evidence suggesting that CBD may reverse some of the cognitive impairments of Alzheimer's disease. Alzheimer's causes neuron loss and cognitive decline such as memory loss, CBD helps with regeneration.

Another cannabinoid found in hemp is **CBG**, referred to as the *stem cell cannabinoid*. It's been noted to have pain killing properties, continuing to be researched. So far, CBG is being proven to reduce inflammation and pain, enhance appetite, increase energy and productivity, helpful with sleeplessness, nervousness, and anxiety. It's also helpful for eye health such as with glaucoma, helps with bladder dysfunction, skin issues, even is beneficial for bone health. More studies are being done, as I'm sure this list will grow with time.

Cannabinoids have been shown to target cancer cells, shown to kill cancer cells and slow tumor growth. This was mainly studied with THC. Studies have shown that the THC connects to the cannabinoid receptors on the cancer cells causing a process to occur that causes cell death, all while leaving the healthy cells alone. It targets the cancer cells.

While most of the studies around curing cancer with herbs and other natural methods are done outside of the US, it's finally showing up more in our country. The National Cancer Institute has done research of its own showing that cannabis does in fact, kill cancer cells. In various types of cancers, cannabinoids have been shown to stop tumor growth, block cancer cell growth, trigger cell death, and block the blood vessels that feed the tumor. They inhibit the spreading of cancer from one part of the body to another.

While we are still very early in our understanding of how to best use cannabis to fight different types of cancer, this information is now becoming more well-established. It is presently permitted by the medical profession to be used to assist with symptoms of cancer treatments such as the side effects of chemotherapy. Western medicine does have a synthetic version of THC available as a pharmaceutical drug called Marinol.

The studies done on cannabinoids is quite extensive, I was very surprised to see so many studies within my own government and health agencies proving how powerful cannabis is, each cannabinoid. I don't have to look crazy anymore, it's all online for anyone to see if they want to look. Now to apply all of their research to start getting people healed.

Another beautiful component to cannabis is its other naturally occurring compounds that make up the aroma, taste, and colors of the plant. These compounds are called terpenes. The terpenes have their own therapeutic properties who interact with the cannabinoids in the plant, causing medicinal, therapeutic effects. Each plant strain has its own terpene profile.

One of the most well-known terpenes is Myrcene. It's found in some cannabis strains, and is also found in basil, bay leaves, lemongrass, thyme, parsley, mango, and hops. Myrcene has anti-inflammatory properties, is a muscle relaxant, and can act as a sedative. Myrcene-rich hops are used in Germany as a sleep-aid.

Others commonly found terpenes worth looking into are Beta-caryophyllene, Limonene, Pinene, and Linalool to name a few. All carry different aspects that help on a therapeutic level.

Cannabis can be used and taken in a variety of ways. The most familiar or well-known way of using cannabis medicinally, is through smoking it. When it is smoked, 10-15% of the cannabinoids and medicine are absorbed. When it's eaten through food, tea, or a tincture form, 25-30% of the cannabinoids are accessed and used. If it's inserted rectally via a suppository, 75% of the medicine is absorbed into the system.

There are advantages and disadvantages to each method depending on what you need the medicine for. Ingesting it as a tea is a quick reliever for stomach issues and nausea, whereas ingesting an infused food item may not work well for stomach issues as well as that it takes about forty-five minutes to take effect. The condition of the digestive system and how much food is on board both effect the absorption.

Smoking has an immediate effect, within two to five minutes, as it gets absorbed quickly into the bloodstream through the lungs. However, with smoking you are taking smoke into your lungs, as well as inhaling some residue. As there is burning occurring, smoking may not be best suited for everyone. If someone needs a more immediate effect and cannot smoke, taking a sublingual or under the tongue cannabis remedy would be within that range of time. There are sublingual forms available or can be achieved with tincture form held under the tongue for 10-20 seconds, then swallowed.

There are also ways in which you can take THC without any of the psychoactive effects or the "high". The first way is by juicing the raw cannabis leaves. Raw cannabis has more powerful medicinal properties, as most plants do in their raw state, with high chlorophyll content, minerals, as well as anti-inflammatory and anti-cancer properties. This is super good for digestive troubles and cancers. You can juice it and freeze it in ice cube trays, adding it to smoothies, or of course, you can drink it like a glass of juice.

The other method to not getting the "high" and psychoactive effect, is by taking it in suppository form. This is a good way for people who need to take large doses for medicinal purpose, such as cancer treatment. By administering through the rectum, you bypass the liver, where THC converts and metabolizes, leading to the creation of psychoactive or "high" effects.

Bypassing the digestive tract allows it to be absorbed efficiently with very little loss of the cannabinoids. The only side effect with rectal administration is some drowsiness. Cannabis suppositories are also very helpful with menstrual cramping and pain, either distributed rectally or vaginally. The medicine is absorbed and maximizes muscle relaxation and pain relief.

Of course, cannabis and hemp as medicine should be treated respectfully and taken responsibly, especially when THC is involved, as it can cause impairment. "Dosage is everything" -Paracelsus. You must take care of yourself when using any kind of medicine, and that of course includes any form of plant medicine such as cannabis.

Being aware of your surroundings and being in a safe environment and situation, is important when ingesting or smoking marijuana. It's also vital to stay well-hydrated and have food on board. It's wise to know the side effects of whatever medicine it is you're using, including cannabis, and how to reduce or get rid of any unwanted effects, if experienced.

CBD will *counter* the psychoactive effects of THC. It is also said that orange juice, lemons, and black pepper can also bring down psychoactivity and paranoia. The known side effects cannabis can bring forth are: rapid heartbeat, lowered blood pressure, dizziness, hallucinations, anxiety, and paranoia. If a person is taking certain narcotic pain medications or benzodiazepines, such as Valium, Ativan, and Xanax, caution is strongly indicated as the combination can suppress respirations and breathing.

The paranoia factor that everyone worries about, comes about for several reasons. Firstly, the foundation we have around what cannabis is and what it does, sets us up mentally. If we were taught it was evil and that we would become a drug addict if we touched it, that energy around it will likely cause fear, paranoia, and guilt if consumed. If we go into it knowing that it is indeed plant medicine, we can find it in ourselves to at least have more respect for it, and see and treat it as the medicine it is.

However, the main reason people have the paranoia effect is because of the actual cannabinoids themselves and their effect on the nervous system. Some people cannot tolerate cannabis in any form or dose, whatsoever. This is why it should be tested in the smallest increments upon initial exposure, like 0.5 mg – 1 mg for an adult.

THC's psychoactive and perception altering property can have positive effects on those who use it medicinally. It can bring one's awareness into a more focused state. It can deepen our senses, can affect sensation, enhance creativity, and even enhance sexual drive. When taken in smaller amounts, THC can induce relaxation, and with larger amounts, it can be more sedating.

If someone takes too much, they might pass out into a deep sleep, or with those who are more sensitive, full panic mode can set in. The sativa version of the cannabis plant has a tendency to be the version that brings on this paranoia, panicky and nervous energy, because it acts more like a stimulant. As mentioned earlier, CBD, orange juice, lemons, and black pepper, can all bring the heightened activity down. There are terpenes in the foods that help calm things down.

There are now medicinal tinctures, patches, salves, food items, and, concentrates made available for use. There are two main types or species of the marijuana plant. There's one that is more activating known as Sativa, and one that is more sedating known as Indica. Let's look at their properties.

SATIVA:

- Mind-dominant
- Activating, increases alertness
- Energizing, uplifting
- Enhances creativity, boosts motivation
- Anti-anxiety
- Anti-depressant

INDICA:

- Body-dominant
- Sedating, relaxing
- Muscle relaxant
- Treats acute pain
- Reduces nausea
- Increases appetite
- Increases dopamine

Many doctors are slowly moving towards suggesting CBD as well as being open to marijuana, mainly THC, as healing treatments for their patients. A doctor named Dr. Justin Sulak has dedicated his life and purpose to understanding and teaching others about cannabis. He brings the information forward in all aspects of cannabis, the medicinal uses for THC, CBD, and all of the other cannabinoids. Dr. Sulak recommends exploring THC and CBD usage under the guidance of a medical professional especially when being used for certain ailments or diseases.

Wonderfully so, there are more and more doctors gaining awareness and exploring the mechanisms of cannabis as the science gains momentum and legalization continues.

I am not licensed to be able to speak more in depth about dosing, but what I will tell you is that *less is more* when you begin. Especially when it comes to THC. Having *too much* THC can cause the opposite effect of what you desire. Over usage and overly high dosing can **increase** pain and suffering associated to your problem. Beginners should always begin with small amounts, even when it comes to CBD, to make sure all is well.

One of my family members had a traumatic brain injury where he suffered from a concussion and bleeding to the brain. He was released from the hospital with Tylenol and a seizure medication for a few days. These medications did not help the pain, confusion, or healing process.

This is where CBD came in, thankfully I brought it knowing what had happened. For nine days, I gave him a healthy dose of CBD, two to three times a day. He so beautifully began to recover. Besides the CBD, he had adequate rest, hydration, and nutrition, and that was it.

He was able to do more for himself little by little as the days went by, slowly working his way back, and eventually into a full recovery. After several weeks of taking CBD, his CT scan showed that there was no more bleeding, swelling, or even signs of trauma. The healing aspects of CBD helped his brain tissue and nervous system relax, heal, and rejuvenate. Something I had never witnessed before.

In my eyes, there are no drugs quite like that. Steroids are used to bring down swelling so that the body can do its healing, however, they come with a list of side effects and are highly stressful on the body, especially the kidneys. CBD on the other hand, has no side effects, is not stressful on our body, and works to bring down inflammation and regenerate nerve cells. Along with many other healing properties.

It's important to always use caution when taking any kind of medicine, whether it be pharmaceutical or plant based. As for cannabis, never drive or operate machinery while medicated. Please be aligned with what you're doing in your life at the time you are using it, as well as any form of medicine. You absolutely know what's best, just tune in with yourself.

Cannabis is a plant that is grown here on the planet to serve us, just as most all of the other plants are that are grown here. Cannabis has amazing medicinal and healing potential, as well as that it is a wonderful resource for fuel, building materials, rope, and clothing (hemp). Hemp bricks are even pest proof and fireproof.

Please do your research or find an educated health professional. Know that if you choose to make it a part of your health care regimen, it's absolutely vital to *pay attention* to your body's signs and signals. Make sure to utilize other health promoting practices and interventions, as well as to tell your doctor, if you are someone who is closely watched and on several medications. These plants were grown on this planet to help us heal and thrive, but respect and caution is always necessary.

HOMEWORK:

1. What plant, herbal, botanical medicine, if any, do you already use?

2. How can you incorporate more herbs into your diet? Adding more fresh herbs to salads, juicing them, what feels easy to bring more in? What do you want them help you with or feel they could help you with?

3. Do some research on your own to explore what plant medicine can do for your health concerns. Look beyond the monopolizing websites, although they sometimes have decent information. Books are gold. Find a naturopath or herbalist if you would like to consult with someone to help you along your herbal, plant medicine journey.

AMAZING HOLISTIC THERAPIES

There are many wonderful and powerful methods and therapies out in the world that can help us get ourselves into a better state of health. Methods and therapies can include food, plant medicine different cultural healing practices, ancient methods and practices, as well as newer technologies and rediscovered techniques.

Alternative, complementary, and natural therapies are gaining momentum and popularity for good reason. People are feeling more comfortable with old remedies and are starting to look back in history to learn more. With each passing day, the number of people going back to more natural methods is growing.

Personally, I've had experience with many different alternative therapies through my own health journey, and would not know where I would be without them. They have provided a safe and effective base for many of my health and wellness needs throughout the second half of my life.

As with anything, it's always so vital and important to listen to ourselves, tune in, and be discerning with the people and therapies that we choose and use to help us. It's always a good idea to learn about these methods, therapies, and techniques before we make a choice to use them. And, it's just as important to find people who are knowledgeable and trained, even looking for people around us who have had care with them.

As with any choice we make, it's important to listen to our gut instincts as we take in the information. Nothing is for everyone, but as you get to know and trust yourself, you will end up following the best path and choosing the best therapies that resonate with what it is you need.

After having witnessed hundreds of thousands of lives change for the worse throughout my career, I felt so driven to want more for people. If it were up to me, nature would be brought back into medicine and be utilized and respected just as much as the medications are. People would have more options around their care, more nature-based treatment plans, or the choice of a more pharmaceutical one. However, their care plan looked, it would be designed specifically for whatever their ailments and illnesses were, as well as their preferences.

How wonderful to have access to *all* of the healing modalities that are out there. To have the knowledge around food, herbs, plant medicine, and of course, how to renew and rebuild our bodies, as well as our spiritual, mental, and emotional health. This would get our health back on track on a more expansive and lasting level, where we could actually *heal* from diseases.

The truth is, we already have the power to do this and to achieve a greater state of health, we just need better access to more of the healing mechanisms and modalities that are out there.

Finding new methods and therapies to help us take better care of ourselves means, we need to have and understanding around our body and about what each of them do. As we develop an understanding and see the bigger picture around what it is our body needs, we can find the ones that will help us reach our healing goals. These therapies can work harmoniously with the body to help cleanse, release, rebuild, regenerate, or realign things from within.

Herbs work in the same kind of way, hence being labeled as *complementary* medicine. Besides the great benefit we receive when receiving these therapies for our specific purpose, we soon find that other areas of our lives begin to improve indirectly, as well, bringing positive changes we didn't necessarily expect. Healing some parts of our health and wellbeing will sometimes trigger something else to respond and connect into something that we also, and unknowingly needed to happen.

There have been tons of questions in my mind over the years while in the profession wondering why certain things weren't being included, especially when they're so beneficial. Of course, I do understand things better now, it's been such a shame that everyday people who don't necessarily know about these therapies, have missed out greatly. I could only imagine the lives that would've been changed had they had these therapies included in the health plans with their doctors.

I want to share with you a few of the more well-known therapies. There are so very many therapies out there available all around the world. Many countries use a lot of these in their medical clinics and centers in this present moment, as they are trained in and allowed to utilize different therapies, not just the ones of the western medical model.

As with anything, one must be cautious and wise with any therapy, method, medication, herb, etc. Always consult a professional and an expert in the area of therapy you are wanting to explore, and of course, speak to your doctor if that's appropriate.

First and foremost, never overdo anything in excess, or in an attempt to speed up the healing process, or to get out of a situation quickly. Nothing in excess is ever the answer, nor are things always going to heal quickly. Listen to yourself first and foremost and if it feels wrong, then don't do it. Your body knows. Don't just do something hoping it will save you or to get a quicker result. Although, combining treatments and modalities can accelerate our body's ability to heal itself.

These are a few of my favorites and ones that are pretty well-known. You can find out more about any of them in books or online, as well as research other therapies. This expansive side to health and healing can indeed bring us a renewed sense of hope and bring motivation into our life when we gain a deeper understanding, as well as a genuine connection with ourselves, our body, and these wonderfully healing, holistic therapies.

- **Hyperbaric Chamber and Oxygen Therapy**

I briefly mentioned this one earlier, and as we know, oxygen is *vital* for optimal cell and body function, and for our overall physical existence. We take for granted that we automatically take in oxygen with our breathing. The air we breathe is approximately 21% oxygen on average. However, with all of the pollution outside and the toxins inside of where we work and live, it's been thought that we need more oxygen to help our bodies thrive just as well. We need oxygen to help filter out toxins, helping our cells to detoxify. Oxygen is an alkalizer and detoxifier.

In 1662, a device was created to provide a high level of oxygenation to people with health issues. Almost 400 years ago, scientists and doctors were aware of the fact that oxygen was involved in illness and disease, rather the lack *of* it and the need *for* it.

This device that was created was a chamber that created a pressurized atmosphere, where in because of the pressure, the oxygen content increased. These pressurized chambers were once called 'air baths' and in the 1830's France created chambers that help as many as 12 people at once. It spread throughout other countries in Europe, and eventually made its way to the United States in 1861.

This pressurized, highly oxygenated chamber was found to resolve nervous system disorders, as well as lung and kidney disease in the 1920's, but then ten years later, the American Medical Association deemed it as to having *no scientific justification for its treatments* and shut it down in 1930.

In the 1950's it was studied by heart surgeons in Australia, who noted that it treated a variety of congenital or acquired coronary diseases. It has continued to be utilized around the world for its benefits. Here in the US, it now used for burn and wound healing even though hyperbaric treatments are greatly known to treat *many* conditions, even used for cancer in the alternative and naturopathic medicine world. There have been so many studies done, providing tons of evidence that is just left out of mainstream information.

A hyperbaric oxygen chamber is usually one of two things. There's a hospital grade one that is a clear, spacious, large chamber where a patient can relax on their hospital bed during their treatment. There's also a smaller version that looks like a capsule that is able to hold one person laying down. Some are slightly bigger and you are able to sit up in them, however, they aren't great for those who become claustrophobic easily. They can be found in alternative doctor's offices such as naturopaths and chiropractors, as well as are found in other alternative clinics, spas, and practices.

This airtight, sealed chamber becomes pressurized slowly providing

100% pure oxygen. The pressure is built gradually, to give the body the optimal opportunity to absorb the oxygen. Increased pressure allows the oxygen to absorb into the blood stream, tissues, and the *stem cells*. The oxygen in the chamber increases the amount of oxygen delivered to the tissues by up to 600%. It stimulates the body's production of oxygen-rich blood cells.

Hyperbaric chambers are presently used for diving accidents, in cases where someone gets compression sickness. They are excellent for wound healing, as it helps regenerate the tissue. Hyperbaric oxygen helps with poor circulation because it improves blood oxygenation and circulation. It also promotes relaxation and decreases stress levels. The oxygen absorbs into the bloodstream, which reaches cancer cells, and as we know, cancer does not like oxygen no matter what modern science may claim.

This is the list from the FDA here in the US of the *approved* reasons for use of the hyperbaric oxygen chamber. Personally, I would add a lot more to this list, cancer being the first. And it's strange that there aren't any nervous system disorders, lung, or kidney problems listed here, which is what they found it to be helpful for, over 150 years ago.

These are the present-day approved reasons here in the US:

- Air and gas bubbles in blood vessels
- Anemia (severe anemia when blood transfusions cannot be used)
- Burns (severe and large burns treated at a specialized burn center)
- Carbon monoxide poisoning
- Crush injury
- Decompression sickness (diving risk)
- Gangrene
- Hearing loss (complete hearing loss that occurs suddenly and without any known cause)
- Infection of the skin and bone (severe)
- Radiation injury
- Skin graft flap at risk of tissue death

- Vision loss (when sudden and painless in one eye due to blockage of blood flow)
- Wounds (non-healing, diabetic foot ulcers)

Hyperbaric oxygen treatment is presently being studied in regards to the recent virus here in the United States, proving how absolutely helpful and beneficial oxygen treatment is for those that have gotten the virus. It's extremely assistive for the lungs, themselves. You can find the continuous studies on clinicaltrials.gov. It's very exciting to see that this being studied more, although it should be widely accepted and actively utilized right now, for the information and evidence has already been shown. It should be widely available in every hospital and doctor's office across the globe. I will intend for this to be the case.

Worth mentioning, is another form of oxygen therapy called *exercise with oxygen therapy*, discovered by Dr. Otto Warburg, a two-time Nobel peace prize winner. In 1931, he discovered that cancer cells were unlike other cells and organisms, as they did not use oxygen, they produced their energy *without* oxygen.

If our cells do not get enough oxygen, they become disabled and eventually die. They can't then keep us alive if they do not survive. Oxygen is vitally essential.

Exercise using oxygen therapy is a very simple technique with very empowering effects. The person wears an oxygen mask while they walk on a treadmill or cycle on a stationary bicycle for 10 minutes. Doing one of these mild activities raises the heartrate, increasing the absorption of oxygen which then gets pushed into all of the cells, including any cancer cells. The oxygen floods in and uplifts the cells and organ systems that need it the most.

He may not have been the first to discover this therapeutic use for oxygen, but he brought it out into the world for one glorious moment before it was taken out of the equation. With the research Dr. Otto Warburg performed with oxygen therapy, he was able to cure the top 200 diseases in the early 1900's.

- **Colon Hydrotherapy**

Colon hydrotherapy, otherwise known as colon cleansing, or colon hygiene, is an old school method used to help flush old, leftover waste, out of the colon. It's truly a great way to get rid of waste that's been laying around for too long (sometimes even decades). The instillation of water, otherwise known as a colonic, loosens and breaks down the leftover waste, hydrates the colon, and helps move it out. Removing excess debris and freeing up the areas and walls of the colon helps it to breathe easier and work more efficiently.

Doctors once called it 'internal washing' and believe it or not, colonics were found in emergency rooms and medical centers across the nation, as well as in other parts of the world prior to the 1930's. Internal washing has been around for centuries, if not thousands of years, and was once used by western medicine. It was once prescribed, and performed by both doctors and nurses.

Built-up waste is more common that you think. Think about every bowel movement you've had in your life. Have all of your meals fully been let go of? Leftover waste causes a host of health issues, we spoke about this earlier. Waste creates strain on the bowel walls and affects its muscle tone, which weakens the colon muscle affecting its ability to evacuate food. A backed-up bowel is one of the major causes of auto-intoxication, or creating a toxic environment where the leftover material rots. The rotting releases toxins and poisons which end up being absorbed into the bloodstream, then circulating around the body.

Waste can build up for many, many years. Some people start having elimination issues in their childhood. And, although you would think all of that's probably dissolved by now, there has been plenty of research showing waste can hide in small crevices, covered over by newer waste and hold on for decades.

Certainly, a thorough cleansing requires more than a few laxatives. It involves adopting new habits, adjusting diets, incorporating occasional fasting, and embracing cleansing practices or methods. Sometimes, a bit of extra assistance is needed, and water proves to be extremely beneficial in the cleansing process.

A colonic introduces warm, gentle streams of purified water into the colon, which fills and releases throughout the session. The waste in the colon absorbs the water, softens and loosens up, allowing it pass out of the body. Colonics stimulate peristalsis and the hydrate the colon walls.

There are several colonic techniques and systems and a few of them involve or allow you to do it on your own. For myself personally, I find it more effective and therapeutic when there's a practitioner present to do the colonic for me. This way you can relax and work through the process in whatever way that's needed. The practitioner will do tummy massages aligned to the waste removal, use some acupressure points to help the release, and help relax you throughout the process. You can always massage your own tummy, and it's good to remember to do some good deep breathing during the session.

The method I am trained in and prefer is called the Woods Gravity method. This where the purified water enters into the bowel via gravity. The water container is higher up than the body allowing the water to flow down, naturally into the colon. There are other systems that use a motorized mechanism that propels the water into the colon, kind of like a gentle pressure washer. It is known to offer the great benefit of breaking down old matter, but for those with more delicate or fragile colon walls, the gravity method may prove to be a much safer approach.

If colonics are unavailable or unaffordable, you can get always an enema kit for at home enemas. With enemas, the use of purified, warm water is preferred, and holding the infusion in for 5-20 minutes is recommended. You can always split the enema into two parts if it's difficult to hold a lot in. Always follow the general rule of never overdoing things, no matter what it is. Be wise and really tune into your body when administering any kind of therapy to yourself.

Both colonics and enemas act to hydrate the colon and its contents. Important factors when doing any type of colon cleansing:

- Limit meat, grain, breads, dairy, and sugars both **prior** to and **after** the colon therapy.
- Have abundant hydration; drink plenty of fluids such as water, coconut water, vegetable juices, fruit smoothies, and clean soups.
- Eat lots of fresh foods like watermelon, berries, and seasonal fruits and veggies.

- Avoid alcohol.
- Get plenty of rest, and take notice (relax) when your body asks for it.
- Keep your plans to stress free activities, meditation, and always practice gratitude after a treatment.

Throughout my time as a colon hygienist, I was excited to witness elderly people who couldn't use the bathroom for weeks, get some results. And I'll tell you, the waste that left them was *old*. Cleaning out the colon has been shown to clear one's mind, mental state, energy levels, relieves the excess weight, takes stress off of the digestive and detoxifying organs, and has even proven to helpful in cases of dementia and Alzheimer's. It is effective for people with mental health disorders, autism, liver and intestinal issues, as well as to help one's overall health and wellbeing. Because, as we know, the gut directly affects our nervous and immune systems.

There is great power and benefit behind getting waste out of the body through this method. It's not as scary as it sounds.

- **Hydrotherapy**

Hydrotherapy is a general term for any kind of water therapy. There are several types of hydrotherapy, more than just in regards to the colon. Water therapy has been around since as early as 4500 B.C. It is known to promote wellness with its powerful ability to relieve pain and break up congestion. It can be used cold, iced, hot, or steamed, depending on the issue being treated.

Back in the early 19th century, hydrotherapy ice cold baths or walking in the snow was popular. A well-known method was going from a hot sauna to an iced cold bath. Today, people have reignited this movement, especially for ice baths because of their powerful impact on one's immunity. Even if you don't have a bathtub, you can rinse off with very cold water at the end of your shower for 10+ seconds, or you can even dunk your face in a bowl of ice water for 5+ seconds at a time.

Hot water opens up or dilates the blood vessels, causing the blood flow at a greater capacity. Cold constricts or tightens up the vessels, which makes the circulatory system work more efficiently by helping the blood move through the body more quickly. Hydrotherapy is known to be helpful for people with poor circulation, high blood pressure, and diabetes. Also, cold water therapy stimulates leukocytes, which help your body to fight off infection, and in a study, showed to help the body be more resistant to cancer. If you have very low blood pressure, hot to cold hydrotherapy is **not** recommended.

- **Acupuncture**

Acupuncture has gained momentum and popularity all around the world. It's been around for thousands of years, birthed and originating in China. It was discovered to be a subtle but powerful healing tool used to bring the body back into balance when illness or disruption began to occur.

According to the Chinese, illness is caused by disruptions in the energy pathways of the body, these pathways are known as the meridians in the body. Acupuncture uses these meridians of energy to attune and balance out the energy flow of the body, which is known as the Qi (sounds like chee). When Qi is blocked or weak, the blood flow becomes stagnant or sluggish and can cause pain and proneness to illness. Small, hair-thin needles are inserted into the skin on certain meridian points to unblock and open up the channels and flow of energy. Acupuncture works to balance the flow of Qi to the organs, glands, and tissues of the body.

Chinese medicine focuses on the channels in the body, the meridians, fluids, and energy flow. The Qi, blood, and body fluids are vital substances that are essential to sustain the body. They keep the organs, tissues, and channels in good working order. There's been tons of research done on acupuncture and how it activates the pathways between the nervous system and the endocrine system. It's basically turning the circuits and pathways back on in the body.

There are variations in acupuncture practices today. Some versions have taken the traditional Chinese or Japanese acupuncture and added elements to the practice, such as in Five Elements Acupuncture or Shamanic Acupuncture. There are many reasons to receive acupuncture, the list is endless, as everyone unwell or bogged down could likely use some energy shifting and balancing of their Qi.

- **Chiropractic care**

Chiropractic care relates to the musculoskeletal system, mainly the spine and the joints, and its connection to the nervous system. The word chiropractic means, to be done by hand. Chiropractors do adjustments to restore joint function and to support the central nervous system. The Central Nervous System is the connection between the spine and the brain. It regulates communication and the coordination of the body, and affects *every* organ, tissue, and cell.

The goal for chiropractic work is to correct misalignment of the joints and vertebrae by helping to reset and realign things. This is done to support the body's natural ability to regain its balance and fluid movement, as well as to keep the nervous system flowing and running smoothly, as it runs through the spine and connects inward to the organs of the body. Essentially, this supports the body's ability to heal itself.

Often times our vertebrae are misaligned or out of place (subluxated), which causes inflammation, swelling, irritation or the cutting off of a nerve or nerves, muscle tightening, and most often, pain. Misalignment also breaks down the communication and response system of the central nervous system. Scientific research has been done proving that chiropractic care has a positive effect on the respiratory system, digestion, immune system, and assists the other organ systems to function optimally.

Our spine has also been proven to hold memory, being directly linked to the brain and neurological network in the body. Our spine contains part of the nervous system, and part of our subconscious which is where traumas and memories are held. Science has proven that when the brain and nervous system get stuck in trauma, they rewire themselves in a way that makes healing a challenge. This stuck energy is held in the body, often times in the spine itself.

Network Chiropractic, or Network Spinal Analysis is an expanded version of chiropractic work created by Dr. Donald Epstein in the 1980's.

Unlike regular chiropractic care, network spinal care does not require drastic manipulations, cracking, or sudden, swift motion. Rather, it is a non-invasive technique that works gently with the nervous system (which is again, infused through the spine) where tension and traumas are held, working therapeutically on *emotional* release.

This technique was developed specifically to involve the nervous system in helping to reestablish the connection back to the body's self-healing capability. It's a very empowering therapy that helps the body reach new levels of nervous and endocrine system regulation. Once the body tunes in more soundly with itself, it will be better able to move around the energies and emotions within it, helping to release and integrate them easier.

I have seen the usual negative banter around this care online, about it being a scam or some other nonsense, but I myself, as well as my son since he was a baby, have used network chiropractic care and in my eyes, it's by far the best chiropractic technique out there. Gentle, but powerful beyond measure. It does more than force vertebrae into place by working with the spine and nervous system's intelligence.

- **Craniosacral therapy**

Craniosacral therapy is another hands-on technique working with the membranes and movement of the fluids in and around the central nervous system through gentle touch on the joints of the cranium (head). Children often respond to this therapy instantaneously. It has been proven to be effective for children with learning disabilities in helping them to come back to a more balanced state.

The practitioner works with the bones of the skull and the pelvis. These are the beginning and end points to the spine, incorporating the spinal cord and cerebrospinal fluid, which is essential for circulation and balance. This spinal system also carries information and a consciousness. The practitioner is able to sense what the body needs. It has both physiologic and intuitive healing aspects and is practiced as a holistic, shamanic, or meditative practice.

Craniosacral therapy is performed by chiropractors, osteopaths, physical therapists, and massage therapists. It's used to treat migraines, chronic neck and back pain, stress, tension, emotional problems, depression, neurovascular or immune disorders, anxiety, asthma, autism, fibromyalgia, PTSD, scoliosis, difficulty with walking or movement, chronic fatigue, concussion, traumatic brain injuries, and spinal injuries. Not to be done with skull fractures, injuries causing brain bleeds, or with a diagnosed aneurysm.

There is sometimes an emotional release known as the Somato-Emotional Release which varies for each individual, and may show up in the form of crying, laughter, anger, or fear as the body is releasing the trauma and emotional stress that have been bound up. Craniosacral therapy works to clear the emotions in conjunction with adjusting the bones of the cranium.

- **Rolfing**

Rolfing was founded by Dr. Ida P Rolf, is a hands-on therapy that relieves tension in the connective tissues that helps to improve posture and flexibility. Dr. Rolf recognized the network of connective tissue (fascia) that supports all of the muscles, bones, nerves, and organs, strongly affects one's overall health and well-being.

Our fascia connects just about everything in our body, even the brain is covered in fascia. The nervous system sends signals and messages to the fascia, giving it the thumbs up to keep functioning properly. The fascia helps keep the body and its parts in alignment, which means it does a lot of adjusting and compensating. The compensation can create problems down the line.

Rolfing enables the body to regain the natural integrity of its form, using deep manipulation of the fascia tissue working to reorganize it. It relieves tension that is caused by tight and misaligned fascia, helping to improve posture, relieve chronic pain, and in turn it enhances neurological function. Rolfing breaks up restrictive patterns in nerves and muscles in the chest to maximize full chest expansion in people with asthma. Rolfing helps to restore flexibility and re-energizes the body.

It's very helpful for lumbar lordosis, low back pain, scoliosis, plantar fasciitis, frozen shoulder, and chronic neck and shoulder tension. It's great for athletes, especially those who get repetitive stress injuries. A Rolfing treatment generally consists of ten sessions that work to balance and optimize the body with a purposeful succession. Each session focuses on different regions to optimize the progression of the work. You can learn more about this fascinating and greatly underused therapy at www.rolf.org.

- **Naturopathy**

Naturopathy emerged from thousands of years of natural methods of healing. It was brought together by the wisdom of a combination of many different cultural healing practices: Indian (Ayurveda), Chinese (Taoist), Greek (Hippocratic), Arabian, Egyptian, and European (monastic). A German Catholic priest Sebastian Kneipp came up with the idea and helped people with 5 things: Hydrotherapy, Phytotherapy, Exercise, Nutrition, and Balance. A group of Kneipp practitioners formed a committee and decided to incorporate all-natural methods of healing into **one** medical practice, later known as Naturopathic Medicine.

Naturopathic medicine incorporates botanical medicine (herbal/plant), nutritional therapy, physiotherapy, psychology, mind-body connection, homeopathy, and manipulative therapies. The first school of Naturopathy in the United States was opened in New York City 1901 by Dr. Lust. It gained some popularity in the 1920's, but with the rise of pharmaceutical drugs and the medical industry changing hands in the 1930's, came the decline of the nature-based medicine world. By the 1970's the desire for natural medicine began to build back up and more colleges began to up. Now Naturopathic medicine is becoming more widely accepted and is gaining popularity, some insurance plans even cover a portion of the care.

- **Homeopathy**

Homeopathy is a section of naturopathic medicine that was first discovered and invented by Dr. Samuel Hahnemann in the 1700's in Germany, with the first homeopathic school birthing in the US in 1835.

Homeopathy came before germ theory and antibiotics were discovered. The principal of homeopathy is "like cures like". In other words, drugs which cause specific symptoms can be used to cure diseases which cause the same symptoms.

The law of infinitesimal (tiny, nanoscopic) doses became the primary characteristic of homeopathy, which was a dilution of the medicinal component of a plant, mineral, or animal such as crushed up bees, to 1:100. It is then taken in repeated doses between 6-30 times.

The goal of a treating one with homeopathic remedies was to combine all of the physical, mental and spiritual problems, the person's body constitution, and prescribe a remedy to treat the "totality" of the patient. Homeopathy gets a bit more complex, and if you're interested in learning more about it, there's tons of info online and many Naturopathic practitioners who still work with it.

- **Reiki**

Reiki is a Japanese energetic healing technique that's been around for thousands of years, and it's been said to be the healing work that Jesus used. Reiki came from the words Rei which stands for "God's Wisdom or Higher Power" and Ki meaning "life force energy". Reiki works on the energetic biofield of the body incorporating body, mind, and spirit.

It works in alignment with the cellular function and the nervous system of the body. Reiki works to clear blockages, releasing stuck energy to bring back balance so that illness, old wounds, and patterns can be accessed, transformed, and released. It's proven to relieve pain both physical and emotional, as well as relieve overwhelm and stress.

Reiki helps people become calmer and more clearheaded as blockages are removed. Security, peacefulness, a sense of wellness, relaxation, and anxiety reduction are all benefits of Reiki. This healing technique is performed by practitioners with the laying on of hands, although it can be done from at a distance. The practitioners who perform Reiki become a channel for Universal healing energy and unconditional love, opening the energy flow wherever the body or spirit needs it most.

Medical reiki is being used in hospitals, becoming more popular with time because of the amazing effects and undeniable results. Medical Reiki is documented in use for nausea reduction, pain reduction, muscle tension reduction, sleep improvement, and in the *acceleration of healing*. It stimulates the immune system as well as the healing of tissues and bones after surgery or an acute injury. It's used in operating rooms, as well as before and after surgery, in cancer treatment areas, cardiology, orthopedics, internal medicine, and of course in hospice care as a *complementary* healing practice in conjunction with other medical treatments.

More people are becoming aware of the benefits of Reiki and seeking treatment. It is absolutely life changing. I will list a medical Reiki website that notes studies and research done at medical centers, as well as several trusted Reiki practitioners whom I trust and adore, in the back section.

There are so many other forms of natural and alternative therapies and practices, I couldn't possibly cover all of them here. Here are some other ones I have worked with, or have confidence and faith in, in regards to their benefits.

- Aromatherapy
- Ayurveda
- Biofeedback
- Body Code
- Emotional Freedom Technique (EFT)
- Emotion Code
- Flower Essence Therapy
- Hypnotherapy
- Neurofeedback
- Neurolinguistic Programming
- Quantum Healing
- Shamanic Journeying
- Somatic Therapy
- Zero Balancing

HOMEWORK:

1. What natural therapies have you heard of? Which ones have you tried?

2. What holistic therapies and practices resonate with you? Which ones do you feel that may be of benefit to you, and that you are willing to look into further?

3. Find holistic practitioners in your area just to see what's available around you.

OUR DIVINE MIND &
BEAUTIFUL SOUL

"if only our eyes saw souls instead of bodies,
how different our ideals of beauty would be."
            -Lauren Jauregui

YOUR CHILDHOOD AFFECTS YOUR MIND & HEALTH

We all have stories about where we've come from and what we've been through. The story of where we grew up, how we were raised, all of the happenings good and bad, the victories, battles, scars and all. Regardless of who we are, we all have a unique story that made us into the person that we are today.

Some parts of our story we can remember vividly, and others as though they never even happened. Some of us don't realize just how powerful those early years in our childhood were and the impact they had on our life going forward.

We can say, that much of what we've been through has helped us learn how to survive, live, and make it by in life. Maybe it even brought us to a point where we created a really good life for ourselves because of it.

Of course, there's the other side to how some of our stories went, some weren't great and helped to create some not so good experiences and setbacks in our life. Maybe our stories even put us in an eternal state of fear and survival mode.

Our childhood has a strong influence on how we receive life and how we respond to it. There's a part in all of us that still works through some of these things unconsciously (or consciously), as the years go by. We're usually not fully aware that our stories are having an effect on what's happening in our lives presently, including our health.

Some of us use our childhood stories as fuel or a means to get by, or maybe to keep us motivated towards our betterment. It's all dependent on what our stories are, how we tell them, and how we use them. Letting go of the stories of the past that no longer serve us, is something that can reinstate a part of our personal power that we might have lost. To live in the sad moments of when we were five, while we're forty-eight years old, is very likely keeping us held back in some area of our life.

Deep down we know that it's time to let go of some of our stories so we can move forward, but for some of us, the hard part is actually letting go.

From birth until the age of five is when they say a child's concept of the world is built. The brain is developed most rapidly during these years. Whatever we go through, feel, and experience, will mold and shape our view of life and the world going forward.

As children we don't rely much on verbal language, instead we largely operate through our senses and inner knowing. We pick up vibes from everything and everyone. We all know that children are the most honest and purely intended little people. They're the most inspired and creative. They are in tune with the world on a level that we as adults have forgotten, because as we move through the years getting older, our outlook changes drastically. We are formed by familial, institutional, and societal thinking, rules, and limitations.

Children take on *everything*. They take on what's going on in their surroundings, the energy, emotion, and mentality of whoever and whatever they're around, especially of those they are raised by. They are highly sensitive on every level, starting life off pure in spirit, until the world around them affects how they feel about themselves, others, and how they see the world.

Children are such innocent, pure little loves that they so easily absorb other people's stuff, even often times feeling responsible for things that happen around them. Children internalize so much of what they encounter and what's said to them. Most of the traumas that are experienced by children are due to the actions of others. Most often these events and experiences are never properly dealt with or worked through. Children don't altogether have the tools or capability to work things out for themselves logically or rationally, nor are they always able to explain what is going on with them and how they're feeling because of something.

As we all know and have been there, children are very often

misunderstood or not believed because of their age and their ability to fully verbalize and express themselves. Even if they are able to, and are believed, often times adults don't know how to work through and manage things, nor have the tools to help. An incident that creates stress or trauma, can often be difficult to work through with a small child. It's not like working with an adult, and because of this, things might then remain unresolved, the child misunderstood, and this is where the buildup begins.

It may affect their self-confidence, how they trust themselves or others, or can cause an overwhelm to their nervous system which connects to a host of other problems for them. This is unfortunately where the dimming of their pureness begins and the disconnection is created.

A lot of children experience something that's unfortunate early on, whether it be losing a pet or loved one, issues with peers or at school, encountering some form of abuse at home, neglect, or even being witness to something that is less than desirable on one level or another. Of course, there are some children who never have these experiences, which is a big blessing for them, and in a perfect world, how I wish it were for all children.

However, this is not the case. Most of us experience something, but some of us undergo serious traumas, or continuous trauma and abuse which is absolutely damaging beyond measure. Children are known to be quite resilient, but it's mostly because they have no choice but to learn to move on, with or without healing. It's also because they have the most receptive and brave little souls. They continue on their journey taking everything with them.

Generally, the most painful events that happen to us as children get shoved down into a place where we can't access them easily, so that the events or occurrences don't affect our everyday lives so deeply. Our brain and body do this on purpose to protect us and to help us survive. The experiences don't fully go away, the emotions and feelings linger, and our nervous system builds up protective mechanisms that we can function from.

The residual memories and effects, get embedded into our subconscious mind and cellular memory, remaining there to serve us at a later time, as a form of protection when something similar happens. Of course, these embedded memories and events can cause a variety of other issues in other areas of our lives as we get older, impacting our behavior, our responses, our physical health, our relationships, how we view the world, the decisions that we make, and most of all, how we see and feel about ourselves.

When we experience trauma or a negative event at a really young age, sometimes the adults around us truly aren't equipped with what is needed to help us get through it, so no matter how much they want to help, it gets left on the sidelines with the hopes that it will heal on its own. Some children don't even have someone to help them, so much of what they've been through gets brushed under the rug.

These unresolved childhood wounds usually cause some type of damage. They have a powerful effect on our mental, emotional, and physical health going forward. When a traumatic event occurs, it activates our brain and nervous system, first and foremost. After the event takes place, the memory gets stored into a part of the brain and body where it becomes harder to access, and as mentioned, as a way to protect us further.

When future triggers arise, the response or emotion around the old trauma may come up. The trigger causes the nervous system to recognize the scenario as being similar, but the mind works hard to try to keep the original memory from resurfacing. We do know that regardless of this attempt, the original trauma can indirectly cause us to respond in the same way and maybe even relive the original experience.

For some, however, the memory never shows back up and gets pushed further and further away, being completely forgotten about eventually. The reason why we end up responding the way we do moves further away from being realized, causing us to forget why we even react this way anymore. Many of us claim *"that's just how I am"*, or *" this is who I am"* claiming it as though it's what we are and who we are.

Some children may even have an out of body experience when experiencing trauma. We've all heard about a child who was traumatized saying they would leave their body, even able to see what was happening from above. As though they were floating up above the scene and watching what was happening. This trauma is usually severe enough that the child develops an amnesia of sorts, so they can continue to live their life without staying locked in the trauma. This amnesia stops the fear and emotional pain from controlling their every move, thought, and feeling. However, this is usually nearly impossible, as the trauma is held and felt deeply throughout that person's life in one form or another.

Even if the memory or trauma is suppressed, it will show up in how they see the world, how they receive it, and how they behave in the world, well into and throughout adulthood. They might even attract similar situations, or have the unfortunate occurrence of having flashbacks, especially when it's physical, sexual, or harsh mental and emotional abuse and trauma.

Most of us as adults don't identify our triggers and responses as to being based on, or connected to a childhood trauma or experience that we had. Or our childhood, in general. We might have nightmares, attract similar experiences, isolate ourselves due to lack of trust, or just end up plagued by feelings of fear in different areas of our life. We might live our life with feelings of unworthiness, guilt, shame, anger, sadness, detachment, numbness, denial, or the overall feeling of not being loveable. These become a part of our everyday existence, sabotaging aspects of our well-being, health, and growth.

Trauma causes the brain and body's stress response system to activate, signaling the fight or flight response. The activation of this stress response over and over again, which can occur daily for those who are chronically abused, keeps them in an endless state of stress and weakens their body and its systems. The immune system is affected and weakened, the nervous system including brain function is decreased, and the body's ability to live outside of survival mode, becomes foreign. There is an increase in oxidative stress which further causes break down and weakness physically.

When it comes to these traumas and experiences showing up in physical form, as an example, when a child has had sexual trauma, they can end up having sexual organ issues, growth issues, kidney and urinary issues including bedwetting, and may even develop asthma or some other type of childhood illness.

It also has a hugely negative effect on their emotional and mental health, obviously, as they experience problems with their intimate relationships, self-esteem, self-worth, a lack of trust in themselves and others, as well as problems in school, with their peers, and their overall academic performance.

There is a TED talk from a few years back by Dr. Nadine Burke Harris who speaks on childhood trauma and how it affects a child's physical health. Dr. Burke Harris is a licensed pediatrician who covers the medical science and has documented scientific research on how childhood abuse, trauma, and toxic stress in a child's environment can cause literal physical health problems. She calls these traumas Adverse Childhood Experiences (ACE).

Many of these children during childhood, especially during the time of the trauma occurring, may be diagnosed with a disorder or an illness such as diabetes, asthma, and ADD, as well as many others. These children may have difficulty in school or have behavioral issues. As they grow older, some of them can continue developing health problems, even being diagnosed with life threatening diseases such as cancer or heart disease in their early adult years. Some end up having a shorter life expectancy because of the trauma.

People who suffer from any form of abuse may find themselves in deep states of depression, with heavy anxiety, bipolarism, schizophrenia, poor boundaries, OCD, ADD, as well as being highly likely to abuse substances to alter the pain that they feel. The engage in self-harming activities, risky behaviors, and some even become suicidal. Many may even continue the cycle becoming abusive towards others, and generally destructive to much in their life.

Those who have suffered and carry unhealed trauma, do their best to function in society and keep themselves going, however, often times they suffer from self-sabotaging actions and thoughts, experiencing relationship problems, health difficulties, and a constant flow of unfortunate events that keep them in survival or stress mode. The constant flow of negative events have them feeling like the world is always against them and they have no one in their corner who cares or understands them.

All that we ignore or suppress, eventually rears its head and shows up in one form or another down the line. We end up attracting a lot of the same case scenarios that we went through or similar types, because it's as though we're programmed for it, almost expecting it.

Many of us may live our life stuck in victim mode, which is understandable, but as we get older and are no longer captive to that time or experience in our life, it does become our responsibility to make the necessary changes and let it go, so that we can move into living a peaceful, healthy life. Victim mode has us living in a less than desirable state, unable to take responsibility or action towards bettering ourselves or lives.

It's understandable that things can trigger us if we don't work through our traumas and heal the past hurts and pains that have occurred in our life. Of course, it's not what anyone really *wants* to do, trust me I would know. No one wants to hash up the past and bring back painful events, but if we don't work on forgiving ourselves and others, and letting go of these events and timelines that greatly affect us, the road we continue heading down isn't going to be a fun nor healthy one.

It's important to know that we don't have to relive the details moment by moment, and doing this doesn't mean what was done is okay, but it will serve us without a doubt. Revisiting the reasons for our emotions and our emotional setbacks is necessary so that we can work on moving out of the trauma state we're stuck in.

Some people do end up taking all their hurt, anger, sadness, resentment, and pain with them to their grave. They leave their life still feeling angry, hurt, betrayed, victimized, or feeling unloved and unseen. Science has proven there is truth in the creation of disease that comes from unhealed psychological, physical, emotional, and mental circumstances and trauma.

In my years of doing Hospice nursing, I got to know a lot of my patients on a deeper level. People can open up the flood gates at the end of things. Listening to some of their stories and things that happened to them growing up and throughout their lives, was utterly heartbreaking. You could palpably feel the emotion and pain still present all these years later.

I could then see the connection to how some of these things they held onto played out in their life, how they ended up where they were now, and just how broken they still were. In the end, some of them did ask for forgiveness, forgave, and let go of the past. Those people seemed to pass more peacefully and were able to let go more easily, having finally let go of the pain they were holding onto. Those who held onto their pain, unforgiveness, and resentments seemed to suffer more agonizing deaths and had a more difficult passing.

We know that memories, traumas, and emotions can be held in our cells and that our DNA holds programs and memories, so it's easy to see that whatever it is we hold onto whether it be trauma, unforgiveness, or unfortunate childhood experiences, all get programmed into our nervous system, our gut, our heart cells, even our immune system affecting our overall wellbeing. If we don't heal from it, it will remain with us and translate into our future in one form or another.

I might guess that we've all heard about people who get organ transplants such as a heart transplant having strange experiences, dreams, and thoughts. There was a little girl who received another little girl's heart. She began to have nightmares and memories of the things that happened to the little girl who was her donor. She was able to recall some of the trauma that the deceased girl had gone through, which was very traumatic for her to experience considering she did not encounter those events personally.

Another woman who received a heart transplant from a young adult male said she began craving beer and hamburgers, something she'd never liked prior. It turned out that her donor loved and enjoyed those two things often. Both of these people who received the organs were able to confirm the experiences as being related to their donor.

Through research, science has found the amazing evidence around how the heart contains certain specialized cells that are like brain cells, but are only found in the heart. They store certain memories that are independent from the brain. These specialized cells are called sensory neurites. They think, feel, and remember things independent of the brain. This gives us more viable proof that we hold memories and events in our body, specifically in the heart especially when what happened is based around love or a lack thereof. We also hold these experiences and emotions in our energetic fields.

When we reflect on a positive memory, it can bring about good feelings such as joy and happiness. When thinking about something funny that happened, we can find ourselves laughing about it all over again. These types of memories can work to enhance our wellbeing because of the positive emotions and feelings they bring forth. It goes without saying that the same happens when a negative experience or memory comes up for us.

When we hold onto a negative event that causes us to relive the stress, anger, victim consciousness, or unforgiveness, it will absolutely cause issues in our lives in how we handle things, relate to others, and experience the world around us. It may eventually cause physical issues and find somewhere to fester in our body.

If we hold onto it and it's causing more strife as we move forward, it will affect the life that we create for ourselves. What we hold in our memory and in our cells, 100% affects the way our life turns out for better or for worse. We can also use our pain and anger to create drive and motivation to change our lives for the better but at some point, we still have to let it go.

So, when you have heard of someone who's been through some of the worst experiences through their childhood and see them thriving in their life today, this is not by chance. That person had to do the work and likely went through some very uncomfortable things to get to that point. They may have come to a breaking point in their life where they realized they could keep living in the pain, or they could break themselves out of it, ending the cycle, and changing things for the better. There is often a need for help in many of these cases, having others to help get through the rougher, seemingly impossible patches, is most often essential. We don't have to go through these things alone.

It's also so important to reconnect to the child we once were, or our child-like self. To find a way to nurture and help that little version of us, no matter how disconnected we are. The reconnection to this part of us is vital. From here, we can let go of the past moments that were so hard on us and that became the story of who we are. We can be there, so to speak, for our little selves and help them to realize it wasn't about them or who they are. Reconnecting with our child selves will also bring in much more joy and ease in how we handle our lives.

Try and imagine that little version of yourself, seeing him or her in your mind. Look them in the eyes and send them your deepest love and compassion, tell them how much you love them. You can acknowledge how much they (you) struggled and felt so deeply unloved, and the pain that they felt, by telling them that they *are* truly loved, that's it's all okay now, and that we will always be there for them.

We can assure them that someone is going to help them heal through everything… that being us. We are who are the ones who need to be there for that little version of us who's still holding onto so much. Although it may sound silly to many people, you'll be amazed at how life changing this is and begin to feel more love for yourself than you may have ever felt before.

Often times, I'll be honest, there's a lot of crying that happens, but this is washing away and releasing so much that we've held onto from childhood. The letting go becomes easier as we practice this, because we're able to receive the love now as an adult, our own love for ourselves, which helps us to let go and move through the issues that need healing.

We truly need to be there for ourselves in all of the versions of who we are on all past and present timelines. We can move past the limitations that were handed to us, realizing that we *can* rebuild ourselves and our lives in a way that we know we deserve. We become a more loving and fearless version of ourselves. We gain a renewed connection to that little, pure and beautiful child inside of us, realizing how perfect we are at our core, and that we are love in its deepest form.

Reconnecting with our little self, even our teenage self, will transmute the energy in a way that we would never expect it to. We even find that we can reconnect to a more spiritual aspect of ourselves because we've expanded into a deeper connection, as we become more aligned and in tune with ourselves on a whole new level.

With each passing day, there are more resources and tools available and more being created that can help us heal through our past, and walk into our futures feeling liberated and free. We can take back our life and heal our bodies from all kinds of things we've carried for years on end. We just need to decide that we are tired of feeling this way and that we deserve more out of life.

This decision and the desire to move out of our past, and out of the places in which we feel stuck, is everything. The minute we decide this, things begin to align for us as if almost spontaneously, uplifting us towards what it is that we need and towards a better place.

Stuff begins to show up for us, that therapist just stumbles across our path, we might read something that is exactly what we needed to hear, we begin to take better care of ourselves without even trying, we may even decide to release toxic people or walk away from unhealthy situations in our life. We feel more strongly about releasing ourselves from being stuck in things that aren't good for us and bravely decide what we will allow into our lives going forward, and that which what we won't.

Having someone to talk to, whether it be a therapist, counselor, coach, or close friend or family member, is beyond valuable. Having someone to be vulnerable around, someone who we can feel comfortable crying in front of and releasing our angst to, and who essentially holds a safe and sacred space for us with compassion, is a gift.

There are beautiful people out there who we can trust that will treat us with great care. We can stop masking our traumas and emotions with chemicals or in ruining our lives, and start living a healthier, more abundant life that we deserve.

Our childhood is a gold mine of information. Our health issues, personal relationships, wealth and abundance issues, our work and life goals, are all affected by where we've come from and how we moved through things that happened in our life.

Our childhood does need some revisiting but the good news is, sometimes we end up remembering those truly wonderful memories and past people who touched our lives for the better. I have gone back and remembered countless good things that brought me so much joy that I could literally connect back into that feeling again and almost relive the moment. Those good moments that we remember, are the ones that feed our heart and can even help us to heal.

It's without a doubt fully possible to move through and heal our traumas so we can become the greatest version of ourselves. We deserve it. We deserve to release and be done with the past pain, everything that holds us back, and keeps us sick and unhappy in our life. When we move through it, we can recreate what it is that we want in our lives, what we will allow going forward and that, my friends, changes everything.

We end up on a new, refreshed journey that takes us down a better path towards a more beautiful, fulfilling, healthy, peaceful, and love filled life with a new appreciation for ourselves. The reward is greater than we ever knew it could be.

HOMEWORK:

1. What parts of your childhood do you feel most affected by?
2. What pattern or response do you feel like you're stuck in? Is there a time in your life that feels connected to this?
3. What avenues can you take to help yourself in processing and letting go of these issues and past traumas?
4. What fears come up for you as you think to work through these?
5. Who can you trust or turn to with any of this? If you have no one, how can you find support?
6. There are guided meditations and videos you can watch on healing these areas of your life. If you feel inclined, do some searching on YouTube to see what comes up for you. Never know, something might appear and be exactly what you needed.

AFFIRMATIONS

I f a person wants to heal themselves, they need to talk to themselves. Science has proven that our self-talk has everything to do with the circumstances that come into our life. It's been studied that by saying positive statements about what we want to change, three times a day for twenty-one days, it begins the process of rewriting our mind, our DNA, and the script within our body.

To **affirm** is to *state or assert positively; to confirm or ratify; to assert solemnly; to express agreement with, or commitment to; to support giving approval, recognition, or encouragement.* An affirmation is a statement or sign that something is true. They can be phrases we say out loud or in our mind, repeatedly and often, to interrupt negative thought patterns and create more positive ones.

It's literally like rewiring and reprogramming our brain to think more empowering thoughts. More of what we want. Of course, this can work on the opposite level and we can create quite negative affirmations.

Not only is affirming like rewiring, it's helping to program (or reprogram) the subconscious mind. The subconscious mind is there to help us produce results of that which we focus on, think, and speak the most. It cannot make a distinction between the thoughts that we think and the things that are actually going on in our physical reality. In other words, it cannot tell the difference between our imagination and our reality. If we visualize, think, or believe something, it's just as good as the real thing to our subconscious mind.

Our subconscious mind will offer us experiences to match the thoughts that we put forth, so knowing this, why not design our thoughts or the statements that we make in a way that supports the outcome we want?

Our subconscious mind will give us that which we focus on and think about most, so giving it positive thoughts and feelings towards what it is that we want most, brings on more of that. It also helps our subconscious let go of the negative stuff that no longer serves us that it's been holding onto from our old programming.

If we repeat the phrase, *"I am healthy"* over and over again, it begins to translate into our internal programming. Even if we aren't perfectly well, and someone may think, *"well, it's not true!"*, it's by far always going to be better than saying *"I'm so sick"* over and over again. How do you think your mind and body will respond to one over the other?

Our mind and body will respond to our words and thoughts, so creating positive phrases for where we *want to* be, is going to have a profound effect. As proven time and time again, our mind creates literal physical experiences. Speaking statements in the present tense is especially more powerful and helpful because we are confirming the statement as if it is already the case.

It's important to acknowledge the statements and words that we speak both out loud and internally. Words have great power, and can either destroy or create. Knowing this is golden.

We can use this powerful knowledge to assess our words and thoughts more closely. We can even connect the dots as to how and why some of our life might be going a certain way, observing how we have had a hand in creating certain things to be the way they are with our negative, worrisome thoughts and statements. This gives us the power to change it.

Historically, this has been used by the ancients, our ancestors, masterful leaders and conquerors. Those who have created the impossible, or thought their dreams into realities, like Henry Ford as an example, used this principle for that which they wanted most. They focused on their intentions.

Intention is having something in our mind and planning for it. We intend to do certain things because we desire a certain outcome. Historically, those leaders and masters had intention behind what they strove for. Intention brings *attention* to what it is we desire. Speaking, thinking, believing, and intending bring results forward. These leaders created an intention for what they wanted and made the plans as they went along.

Beautifully enough, intention also brings about inspiration!

Our thoughts can create an emotional state within us. If we're thinking a lot about something bad happening to us, and we think it over and over again, fear and worry creep in. We're actually stating things out of fear, and we accentuate these emotions within ourselves. We're then digging a deeper hole for ourselves into a place where we might even feel like we've lost control.

Our physical body will also respond to our thoughts, and if we're immersed in fearful thinking, our body is going to respond by going into stress mode to prepare for the fearful event it believes will come. And as we know, this stress mode will then slow other things down in our body such as our immune system and digestion, weakening us, just through our thoughts alone.

We all experience trauma, loss, emotional hurts, and pain in our own way. How we process these things and the mindset we have around them, comes from the culmination of our life experiences. We're all raised differently with different trains of thoughts and beliefs, and this is where we, as adults, need to take a good look into those old thought patterns and statements we're so used to and when they came into our lives. We don't have to hold onto the negative thoughts and statements that others around us have practically ingrained in us.

This way we can begin to clear the old out of our subconscious mind by actively working on new thoughts and statements to replace them. We want to create thoughts that work *for* us, instead of against us.

Luckily, we are not limited to how we once thought and spoke, as we can change it at any moment we choose to. The reason why I love this time in history so much is that we're finally back to realizing all of the power that we actually hold. That we can redesign and recreate the kind of life we want to live through our words, thoughts, feelings, and actions.

Even if the conditioning and mindset from our childhood is negative, we can create new thought patterns and inspired intentions for ourselves going forward. Again, the new cancels out the old. Affirmations will help to transform our old mindset into something more productive and positive for our lives going forward.

I discovered affirmations through my first yoga teacher who read a page of Louise Hay's book '*Heart Thoughts*' at the end of every class.

I was completely in love with how those affirmations felt as I laid on the mat. After a few classes, I went out and bought the book so I could read the affirmations on my own time. As I looked through the book, I realized how many aspects of my life I needed to work on. I picked it up every day, and to this day I still love that book so much. Louise Hay is one of the first self-transformational teachers I studied under when I was twenty-one. I came to realize how powerful affirmations and intention setting really was.

If we say something enough, eventually we start to believe it to be true, whether it is or isn't. Modern day psychology speaks greatly on this. We can literally speak a total fabrication out of nowhere and render it as true if we speak it and believe it enough. We've seen and heard of people who do this. It's the amazing power of the human mind and emotion in combination.

Affirmations can be used to create new thought pathways around the desires that we have. They are used as a tool to rewire our mind to guide us towards certain things, events, or situations that we're wanting to create. High functioning parts of society along with the military, NASA, and several agencies here in the US have done tons of research on all of this and are quite familiar with this technique, using it along with other intentional, creationary techniques that the public hasn't been taught or made aware of.

It's not been taught to us in school like it should be. Regardless of the lack of education we've received around it, we're here now to understand it, so we can use it from this moment forward and pass it onto our children who would be quite honestly, the most powerful ones to use it.

Saying affirmations to ourselves while looking in the mirror is a powerful method. It's a bit uncomfortable to be quite honest, and even somewhat strange. We don't realize even with the abundance of times we look in the mirror at ourselves, we don't actually *look into* our eyes when we're checking things out.

When we try and look directly into our eyes and speak to ourselves, it's going to feel foreign to most of us. Louise Hay was a big advocate for looking right into your eyes and telling yourself, "*I love you. I really, really love you.*" This statement truly hits you in all kinds of ways when you first try it out, because it actually proves to be difficult, believe it or not.

To say it, look at yourself, and actually mean it, can feel uncomfortable and even untrue.

However, doing this over and over again is beyond transformative. Part of why we're in the situations that we're in has a lot to do with our lack of self-love and our self-talk. This *"I love you"* affirmation alone can move mountains if practiced daily.

Building our own affirmations is rather easy, as long as we have a few positive words in our vocabulary. I'm all about grabbing a journal or notebook and writing some down. It's one of the best ways to begin. This way we can actively write them or read them aloud on a daily basis.

Of course, it's important to remember to always speak in the positive and present moment. Using words like *don't* or *not,* should be left out of our affirmations. As I once heard, our subconscious doesn't hear the words don't or not, instead it hears the main words. For example, *"I don't want mean people in my life."* What's protruding from that statement is *mean people* and *my life.* So, a different way to put that is, *"I attract loving, positive people into my life."* or *"I have good people in my life."* Or, *"I am so happy to have wonderful, thoughtful, and supportive people in my life."*

Also, when it comes to things we don't want, the same applies to stating things like, *"I am free from disease"* or *"I am free from debt".* Although these are positive statements and are more productive than stating something like *"I don't want to be in debt"*, our subconscious will still hear the word disease and debt, so we have to switch it up. It's better to use words like health and financial abundance than disease or debt. We can try using something that states the positive, like, *"My body and cells are healthy and strong"* or, *"Money flows abundantly into my life, and supports me with everything I need and desire."* These statements work more in favor towards what it is that we want.

We can apply affirmations to every area of our life. Health, wealth, relationships, spirituality, career, adventures, experiences, you name it. Now we just have to create a way to affirm these new, beautiful phrases into our days and make it a daily practice. We can do it at any time of the day, as many times as we can think to do it, there's no limit as to how often we can say these statements. Writing them down every day makes it even more powerful.

You can say anything to yourself out loud or in your mind, and besides having a notebook full of them, we can also create simple reminders for ourselves in other ways that we can see throughout the day to inspire us to take action. I like to write a few affirmations down on a piece of paper and stick it on the bathroom mirror. You can stick them on your computer monitor, somewhere on your desk, on the wall next to or across from the toilet, the car dashboard, wherever you might be looking a few times a day. There are endless places to put them.

You can also practice saying the same one over and over again. I do this when I've woken up and can't get back to sleep, or when I'm needing a boost of confidence, feeling a little fearful perhaps. They truly do soothe the mind and spirit, and can move us out of fear and worry quickly.

I've had several nights lying awake feeling awful about or hung up on something, and just spent a few minutes repeating one or more empowering statements, essentially falling back asleep. My two favorites are "*I am safe and protected*", and "*I am the light, I am the love, I am the truth, I am*". Without fail, these bring me back into a sense of security, strength, and calmness.

These spoken repeatedly literally change how I feel within 15-30 seconds. Another beautiful way to affirm goodness in the moment is by saying how grateful we are about our life and anything we are using, experiencing, or enjoying. Gratitude is a huge affirmation in itself! Saying *thank you* for everything we have, the people in our lives, what we receive, eat, or enjoy is so powerful.

It's also vital for us to connect the affirmations that we're saying with the *feeling and emotion* of what it would *feel like* to have or receive them. We can visualize ourselves in these affirmations seeing how impactful they are on how happy and grateful we feel because of them.

The emotions and feelings we have around our desires is so important in bringing them into fruition. The more we can tune into what it would *feel like* to have that which we seek, the easier it will be for it to find its way into our reality. We will attract things at a greater level and faster pace when we connect them to a feeling and emotional state.

When things aren't in a good place for us, the more love, good vibes, words, thoughts, and actions we throw in to the mix, the better the outcome. It's time for us to be inspired in finding new ways to heal ourselves mind, body, and soul.

Over the years, I've collected certain affirmations that always spoke true for me. There are beautiful books and websites out there that have affirmations listed that anyone can use. Eventually, you will find yourself creating your own. Just remember, when speaking them, make sure to invoke some emotion of excitement or goodness, as well as a sense of knowing it to be true, as though it's already happening. Speaking our affirmations out loud is generally more powerful, but stating them in your mind is just as effective. Here's a few of my favorites...

- All is well in my world.
- I am safe and protected.
- I love life and life loves me back.
- It is safe to look within.
- I love and approve of myself.
- I am healthy, whole, and complete.
- My body is powerful and healed.
- I am oxygenated and alkalized.
- My income is constantly increasing.
- I am greeted by love wherever I go.
- I am changing for the better.
- I deserve all that is good.
- I am in charge and I am powerful.
- It is safe for me to speak up for myself.
- Life is the ultimate gift.
- I am more empowered with each passing day.
- I forgive myself for all my past mistakes.
- This glorious body of mine is strong and healthy.
- I am a sovereign, free being.
- Abundance flows through all areas of my life.
- I am successful and aligned to my life's work.
- I attract positive opportunities into my life.
- Love comes easily to me.
- I am a magnet for all that is good in the Universe.
- I forgive and release all that is no longer needed.

- I attract abundance in all forms.
- My nervous system is balanced and at ease.
- My heart is strong, and I am so grateful for it.
- Thank you for my healing.
- I lose weight easily and effortlessly.
- All the cells in my body are returning to their perfect, original, and healthy form.
- My cells are vibrant and healthy.

There's an author named Napoleon Hill who brought into light the path to self-induced success through patterns of speaking and thinking. His book *Think and Grow Rich* is a timeless classic that explains the realm as to how producing and expecting positive results and success takes form.

He mentions the term *auto-suggestion* which is the absolute power our words and thoughts have on our body and mind's objectives and actions. You are *suggesting* what it is you focus on and speak about. Self-suggestion is when one comes to believe what one states to themselves, whether it is truth or false, just like affirmations.

Conducting ourselves as though we are already in possession of the non-material or material thing that we are demanding is an action performed by the subconscious mind. The way the subconscious mind works as mentioned earlier, is that it will figure out a way to make something happen. The mind takes on the nature of that which dominates it. A mind dominated by positive emotions, thoughts, and words will express those in action. This is all science.

Faith is also a state of mind that is induced by auto-suggestion. Faith is the external elixir to give power to one's thoughts. The subconscious mind will translate this into its physical equivalent. A thought impulse of a negative or destructive nature is just as easily translated as one of a positive nature. Thoughts mixed with any positive emotion will affect the subconscious mind more powerfully.

Faith or the expectancy and belief that what we desire will actually take place, is huge. I know it's a bit repetitive, but just want to get the point across. It's time to pass onto our subconscious mind that which we desire most. We can absolutely transform our life by working with our words, thoughts, and emotions, so why wouldn't we?

HOMEWORK:

1. What areas in your life do you find you struggle with the most? What thoughts, words, or statements do you find yourself speaking around these areas?
2. What aspects or areas of your life do you want begin to create positive affirmations around?
3. Write down some affirmations you feel comfortable with and excited to start using. Start and affirmation and gratitude journal. Then grab a piece of paper that you can post somewhere with a few affirmations and find a place to put it. Start a practice of speaking them in the morning and at night before bed.

FREQUENCY & SOUND

F requencies exist in everything. We carry frequencies. They exist in the trees outside, our indoor plants, our cell phones, viruses, the ocean, the thoughts we have, even our emotions emit certain frequencies. The list is long, as everything alive, even inanimate objects, hold frequencies.

Everything is made up of vibrations and frequencies, including us. We are made up of atoms and molecules, unseen to the eye, that vibrate and create these frequencies. There is endless science and instruments that can prove this, measure it, and confirm it. Each organ in the body also has its *own* vibration and frequency. Organisms carry their own vibration and frequency including bacteria, parasites, viruses, cancer cells, and so on. This is very important to acknowledge.

A frequency is the rate of an electric, magnetic, acoustic, or mechanical vibration, measured in Hertz (Hz). Our body has a specific frequency when in a healthy state that's somewhere around 62-78 Hz. We each have a specific harmonic song so to speak. When the frequency of our body drops, which can be caused by a number of reasons, our immune system becomes compromised, and disease and illness can start taking place if held there for prolonged periods of time.

The frequency to each specific organ of the body can be used to realign the organ back to its optimal state of being, especially after overcoming illness. If the body's frequency drops to 58 Hz, cold and flu symptoms appear, and at 42 Hz, cancer can show up. The lower the frequency, the more sick and weak our physical state will be in.

Emotions also have frequencies. We don't even have to know the science around it to have all experienced feeling differently when we're around certain emotions. For example, when there is a person angry with us and yelling, we feel that harsh, negative energy. It makes us feel smaller or fearful, or something. The emotion and expression of anger emits a very low frequency. The feeling and state we absorb is one of a low vibration and frequency.

This is why when we hang out with certain people who carry negative or heavy stuff around, we feel heavy or anxious. If we're around people who are joyful and laughing, we take that vibe on. Joy and laughter resonate at a much higher vibration and frequency than anger.

There's scale showing the frequency of emotions from high vibrational to low that was designed by Dr. David Hawkins. These emotions have been measured with scientific instruments that show the level of the frequency being emitted while the emotions are transpiring. It's not difficult to understand why enlightenment would be the highest number, and shame would be the lowest.

This is the chart of the Emotional frequencies in order, which is otherwise known as the Map of Consciousness by Dr. Hawkins.

700 Hz	Enlightenment
600 Hz	Peace
540 Hz	Joy
500 Hz	Love
400 Hz	Reason
350 Hz	Acceptance
310 Hz	Willingness
250 Hz	Neutrality
200 Hz	Courage
175 Hz	Pride
150 Hz	Anger
125 Hz	Desire
100 Hz	Fear
75 Hz	Grief
50 Hz	Apathy
30 Hz	Guilt
20 Hz	Shame

Everything can change our frequency. What we think about, eat, consume, do, say, and emote. The more positive and loving of these things that we do, the greater we increase our vibration. Whereas, choosing the negative, unhealthy versions of these things helps to lower our vibration. Obviously, the vibration and frequency in which we hold, will attract more of the same, as like attracts like. So, if we're in a more positive vibration or more of a negative one, we will attract the same type of resonant experiences or physical circumstances into our world.

Toxins, poisons, pollutants, and synthetic chemicals all have low frequencies, causing our body's frequencies to lower. Processed foods have a frequency of 0 Hz which lowers healthy frequencies within the body bringing us towards disruption and illness. Fresh produce has up to 15 Hz, dry herbs from 12 to 22 Hz, and fresh herbs from 20 to 27 Hz. Essential oil frequencies start at 52 Hz and go as high as 320 Hz which is the frequency of Rose Oil.

These higher frequencies create an environment in which disease, bacteria, virus, fungus, cancer, and so on, cannot live. Throw in frequencies that work to destroy these organisms, and oh what power. Our cells respond to frequencies which is something we never really think about, but now knowing this information, we can absolutely utilize them for our benefit going forward.

A man by the name of Dr. Royal Raymond Rife discovered that the power of certain frequencies can help heal the body of degenerative diseases. These frequencies are directed towards the *bad* cells, and cause no harm to any other cell or part of the body.

Dr. Rife created what is known as the Rife Machine, an instrument that uses frequencies to kill or negate an organism, illness, or deficiency. Back in 1934, resonant frequencies cured sixteen terminal cancers within 70-90 days. He used frequency equipment where the people received two 3-minute sessions per week. Dr. Rife knew that everything vibrates at its own frequency. If you can discover the frequency of the disease-causing microorganism, you can destroy them with the same vibrational frequency.

Frequency healing which is also known as bioresonance, or vibrational healing, is a drug-free method with no side effects. This technique actually dates back thousands of years ago. It's an unaccessed goldmine of healing potential. In 1931, forty-four of the top doctors celebrated "The End of All Disease" but certain industries came in, ended this movement and pushed this science out of the picture.

They came up with their own science and methodology to *manage disease,* instead. The industry then took over getting rid of the evidence, information and research around frequency healing, as well as the Rife and frequency machines that were out there.

Lucky for us today, like anything good in the world, these methods have begun to return back to us and are slowly making themselves known again. We are presently understanding the quantum levels of our existence and bringing back all kinds of healing modalities, techniques, and devices that have been pushed to the side.

Nothing good can be held back forever. Today, there are several machines available on the market, as well as practitioners who are becoming well-versed in these methods, with an increasingly growing amount of information coming to the surface as well as testimonials.

At this moment, it's easy to access websites and videos around the power of the Rife machine, explaining how it works, how it's used, first hand stories of people who have completely changed their lives because of it, as well as actual frequency sound videos. I will list more info in the back for reference.

I read an article on Gaia.com about a study done in 1981 by a biologist named Helene Grimal and a composer/acupuncturist Fabian Maman, who studied the effects sound waves have on cells, mainly cancer cells. Through a microscope connected to a camera, they were able to record the effects that different acoustic instruments had on the cells.

The musical instruments when played, caused cancer cells to lose their integrity, eventually causing them to explode after the 14-minute mark. Frequencies affect the cancer *cell membranes* by disarming the cell, causing weakness, destruction and disintegration. Frequencies can cause destruction to specific cells while doing *no* harm to other cells. You can also target other malevolent organisms such as viruses, bacteria, and parasites.

We can adjust our state of wellbeing through the use of frequencies. We can use frequencies to detoxify our cells, and even to support and assist our DNA. We can uplift and raise our energy, balance our chakras, and create a more harmonized environment within our body.

Frequencies open us up to healing on a physical, mental, spiritual, and emotional level. When we raise our physical and energetic vibration, we enhance the flow and magnitude of our connection with God and our oneness with all things.

There is immense research being done around the healing benefits, powerful results, and outcomes these frequencies have. I'm a true believer that many of the healing modalities coming down the line in the near future are going to have do with frequencies. The best part is, once you have the equipment and knowledge, the effects are limitless.

Because everything has two sides, it's important to mention how some frequencies can also have negative, harmful effects on our bodies. We all know to stay away from microwaves when they're on and that it's been proven to be highly damaging to keep cell phones near our heads, or close to our body for that matter. Both of these objects have been proven to have negative effects on our biological tissues and cells, and cause damage and mutations to our DNA.

Some of these frequencies can influence our nervous system and cognitive performance. They do vary, as we are surrounded by frequencies everywhere, even the Earth has electromagnetic frequencies that it emits. This is to state, however, that some frequencies can cause real and serious harm to us, and that there needs to be more information put out there, as well as some bans on certain objects that do not belong near the human body.

Below I am listing the most well-known frequencies that have been studied and documented as to having profound effects on levels of all kinds. The knowledge dates back thousands of years, encompassing the wisdom of the ancients, our ancestors, and many healing practices throughout the ages. Some of the results for each of the frequencies listed below may seem a bit different, such as a frequency helping us to visualize our goals or restore our DNA, but again, this is a collective of information taken through and across all times and cultures. Choose what resonates, toss what doesn't.

There are tons of YouTube channels that have frequency music that I will also list, and all I can say is give it a try. I use frequency music almost every day. If I'm feeling anxious or down, if there's something in the world going on that's stressing me out, or I just want to create a more creative and motivating space while I'm writing or taking care of an important project, I play some.

They are so wonderful to listen to when we're studying, when we're going through a difficult time, or when we're feeling off. I promise you, frequencies can change your life and listening to the music created around it is without a doubt, transforming.

Once this becomes more widely known and eventually mainstream, there will be more options out there for us to use to enhance our wellbeing and bring on the healing that we so desperately need.

I believe in the next 10 years frequencies will be more commonly understood and widely accepted, as we move into the next era of healing. There are more health promoting modalities making their way into the picture that will indeed help us heal and transform our lives. Exciting times ahead of us!

(You can listen to each frequency by itself by listening on onlinetonegenerator.com)

174 HZ

- Helps you feel more grounded, connected to the Earth
- Calms you down
- Helps gain trust
- Removes physical, energetic, or karmic pain
- Natural anesthetic (pain reliever)
- Gifts your organs with a sense of security, safety, peace and love, inspiring them to function optimally

285 HZ

- Helps your cells remember what they should be doing & returns cells to their original form

- Sends your energy fields a message to restructure damaged organs and tissues, and helps them remember their optimal functioning
- Train your imagination
- Visualize your goals
- Revive your memory of great experiences

396 HZ

- Root Chakra
- Removal of fear and other negative feelings
- Clears, releases, and dissolves guilt and fear, and its origin
- Feel courage
- Remove obstacles to self-realization
- Helps ground and awaken you
- Returns you to your truth of what's for your highest and greatest good

417 HZ

- Sacral Chakra
- Leave traumas behind
- Removal of negative energy
- Dissolves emotional blockages
- Get ready for changes
- Look positively into the future
- Clears old and negative thought forms
- Helps you resonate with Oneness (God, Creator, Source Energy, the Divine)
- Clears feeling of alienation
- Encourages cells and DNA to function optimally
- Reenergizes
- Helps you use your full creative potential

528 HZ

- Solar Plexus Chakra
- *The Miracle Tone*
- Self-love, love yourself, trust in yourself
- Regenerate body and mind
- Returns your DNA to its original and perfect state- repairs DNA
- Increases amount of life force energy, prana, clarity of mind, higher awareness, spiritual awakening, and creativity
- Enhances deeper peace and joy
- Encourages dance and celebration
- Opens up to deeper spiritual experiences
- Live more authentically, return to true self

639 HZ

- Heart Chakra
- Love others
- Have more trust in others
- Strengthens relationships
- Enhances community and interpersonal relationships
- Heals relationship problems
- Encourages cells to communicate with their environment
- Tolerance and unconditional love
- Increases compassion and understanding
- Enhances communication with parallel worlds

741 HZ

- Throat Chakra
- Awakens your natural instincts
- Strengthens intuition
- Pure, stable connection to life
- Assists in changing the diet to foods that enliven and heal the body

- Detoxifies your cells
- Clears you from electromagnetic radiation
- Clears and heals infections- viral, bacterial, fungal

852 HZ

- Third-Eye Chakra
- Go with your gut
- Believe in a positive future
- Focus on inner strength and stability
- Awakens one to self-realization and empowerment
- Dissolves stagnant mental energy and indecision from over-thinking
- Clears blockages that hinder communication from one's higher self, spirit guides, & angels
- Clears distortion energy that confuses
- Heals and enhances the 3rd eye to open to psychic awareness

963 HZ

- Crown Chakra
- Activates and elevates
- Awakens you to your original perfect state
- Highest connection self: experiencing one's true, divine nature & higher self
- Enhances one's connection to the Divine, Course, God, the angels, and spiritual teachers
- Known as the frequency of God, the pure frequency tone

BINAURAL BEATS, WAVES, AND SOUND THERAPY

Binaural sound waves were discovered by Heinrich Wilhelm Dove in 1839. These sound waves can alter the state of our brainwaves. This is done by playing with two slightly different sound waves through each one of the ears. The *difference* in the sound wavelengths, alters the brainwaves (obviously best listened to through headphones).

What happens is that the brain finds the difference in the sound waves and sets itself into that frequency, putting the brain into an altered state. For example, if you use the frequencies of 110 Hz and 114 Hz, the body will create an internal frequency of 4 Hz which is on the Theta scale. Theta happens to be a state of deep relaxation, meditation, and creativity.

Through binaural waves, the body can achieve a state of lucid dreaming, relaxation, focus, better sleep, better recall, heightened states of creativity and positivity, even access to the unconscious mind when in the Delta state. Binaural beats can have a hypnotic, calming, and trance-like effect where we are more, deeply focused and have complete control over our thoughts. Binaural beats are great for grounding. They are incorporated with frequencies to create what's needed for the type of healing effect or conscious state we desire to be in.

***Please avoid these Binaural beats and soundwaves if you suffer from seizures, epilepsy, a serious mental health or psychological condition, and take those types of medications, if you're under the age of 18, are pregnant, <u>or while driving/operating machinery</u>.*

These are the states we can move into using binaural waves: <u>Delta:</u> 0.1-3 Hz Deep, restorative, dreamless sleep. <u>Theta:</u> 4-7 Hz Deep relaxation, meditation, mental imagery, intuition, memory. <u>Alpha:</u> 8-15 Hz Relaxed, lucid, calm, visualization, creativity. <u>Beta:</u> 16-30 Hz Awake, normal, alert, concentration, consciousness. <u>Gamma:</u> 31-100 Hz Insight, peak focus, expanded consciousness.

Another form of sound therapy which is so very powerful, is a sound bath. Sound baths are specific harmonic arrangements that can cause the body to become energized or induce it to entering a relaxed state of being. There are several different instruments used during sound baths, the most common are crystal or metal singing bowls and gongs. Sound baths create vibrational healing within the body and its energy fields. They can be an excellent way to treat physical ailments, as well as to balance the emotional and energetic states of the body.

In today's medical world, sound is used for diagnostics as well as in procedures, such as in breaking up gallbladder and kidney stones. Music is used in operating rooms to relieve pain with the benefit of having to use less anesthesia and medication. Cutting-edge research has shown the powerful impact sound can have on destroying diseases, just life we mentioned with frequencies.

Music is also used for relaxation, stress reduction, birthing assistance, for hearing and tone issues, learning disabilities, and to assist with the process of transitioning out of our body during meditation, or even when actual death is occurring. It's often used in medical offices, different types of business environments, treatment rooms, and varied therapy settings. Wherever one wants to create a tone or ambiance, this music can be utilized and created specifically for that particular purpose. Commonly used instruments used in sound therapy and with sound baths are:

- Crystal or bronze singing bowls
- Gongs
- Chanting, toning, and singing
- Chimes
- Tuning forks
- Digeridoo
- Water flowing
- Nature sounds
- Bells
- Shamanic drums
- Flute
- Harp
- Shakers, rain sticks

Here are some of the free resources and channels for Frequency and Meditation Music found on YouTube:

- Self-Healing Collective
- Jason Stephenson Life Expansion & Relax and Rejuvenate
- Good Vibes – Binaural Beats
- Idylic Melody
- Healing Your Soul

- PowerThoughts Meditation Club
- Meditative Mind
- ZenLifeRelax
- Lovemotives Meditation Music
- Spirit Tribe Awakening
- Relaxing Music

HOMEWORK:

1. What are you drawn to most about frequencies?
2. What part of sound healing do you feel most drawn to?
3. What would you want to use sound therapy to assist you in your life with?
4. Listen to some frequency music on YouTube. What did you notice happen to you? Physically, emotionally, or mentally?

ABUNDANCE & WEALTH MINDSET

'm sure most of us know that wealth and abundance don't necessarily have to pertain to money or attaining material items. We can have very few material objects in our possession, yet live an abundant life. If our basic needs are met and we feel good about ourselves, have our health, people we care about, and find we aren't constantly struggling with life, this can absolutely be acknowledged and felt as true wealth.

Everyone around this world needs money to survive. We have to pay for our food, water, electricity, housing, anything and everything to live the life we have wherever we are. Even if we own our home or land, we still need money on one level or another.

Without money in most of the countries around the world, people end up homeless and starving. There are of course people who live off of the land, and more heading that way, as well as that there are still tribal people in the world who actually live without money and material goods. Some don't even have a need to connect to the modernized, global society.

There are indeed ways to live without a need for money, it's not impossible altogether, though it's quite difficult unless you are someone who truly knows how to live this way, and that's very few of us.

In the dictionary, money means '*any circulating medium of exchange*'. There's no mention of coins or paper bills, instead speaks of money in terms of being a medium. Being a medium means to be '*an intervening agency or vehicle for transmitting or producing an effect.*' So basically, it's a vehicle used for exchange; to give something and get something in return. It's the catalyst that produces a new and different result.

It's like bartering and exchanging one thing for another. In today's day and age, we use money in the form of paper, coin, and plastic in exchange for the goods and all of the needs that we have. However, things are moving in a different direction as we speak, and much of what we use as money is now digitalized. Unfortunately, there's always a possibility that the grid could have interruptions and disconnection, so in my eyes, it's smart to keep other means of money in one's life, things that represent worth and value.

Seeing that we use money for just about *everything* in our lives; water, food, housing, clothing, electricity, health care, and everything in between, it's important to stay mindful about both our wealth and stay educated around it. There's more to wealth, and the mindset we hold around it is important, as it will reflect outward into our lives. How we take care of our wealth and finances is interchangeable with how we take care of ourselves.

Back in the day, precious metals like gold, silver, gemstones, and jewels were sought-after riches and considered very valuable. These along with other elements, different metals and crystals of the Earth have been used in the past, and are even utilized in our present-day as a barter or trade for goods and services. We even see that firearms, art, and old artifacts can be used as a form of payment and exchange.

Gold coins became a currency around 550 BC. The money around the world was once based on gold, but as things have changed, money and the exchange of goods and services transformed over time. Since 1971 our dollar here in the US was taken off the gold standard, and quite unfortunately so. However, gold and silver are still very valuable today.

Every person on the planet starts off creating their beliefs around money through their upbringing; their family and childhood circumstances, as well as from the beliefs and practices that we developed over the years of accumulating our *own* money.

Some of us grew up having little to no money, some just enough, and others had an abundance of it. The tone around money in the household we grew up in generally created the foundation and mindset that we have around money and wealth today; in how we see money, how we obtain it, how we treat it, how worthy we feel around it, and how we utilize it. We can grow up and keep the same concepts that we learned around money, or, we can decide to do something different for ourselves and work on changing it, and that can go either way.

Some of us grew up knowing nothing about money or finances because it was kept very quiet in our family. It's not always discussed, nor spoken of in the home. Maybe our home had everything it needed and there was no stress or discussion around money. Or, even if there was less, our parents made everything feel and seem okay, and we lived happily without the knowledge of having more than enough.

Or, the opposite occurred and we lived in a home where money was always stressed over. We constantly heard our parents verbalize their lack of having it, maybe even fighting about it, saying things like there was *"never enough... things were too expensive... times were hard... money doesn't grow on trees"* and so on. Money was a cause of stress and anger within the family. We took all of that in and it became a part of our perspective on money.

Whatever the experience was that we had and perhaps still now carry around with us, doesn't mean we are destined to end up being the same way or in the same position. Right now, is a great time to tune into all of that and see where are money concepts are rooted. Who's thinking and ideals around money have we adapted to?

As we know, children absorb so much that's going on around them, and they generally take on their family's beliefs and concepts around just about everything. The years of witnessing whatever it was that our family's concepts were, was what molded our mindset and carved out that neural pathway for us. We could have decided we were going to live a different way than them, or we fell in and got stuck underneath their patterning and mindset. We either learned to live in peace and abundance mode, or stress, survival, and lack mode.

Some people completely turn their life around, and I mean go from rags to riches. They purposefully transform their thinking, feeling, and belief system, first and foremost, to create a better outcome for their life and themselves. Something much more than what their family had. What they witnessed or went through, gave them the desire and determination to make change happen. They worked hard to move out of the struggle, hardship, negative, and limiting beliefs around money, by making different decisions. They worked on their mindset to ensure they didn't end up in the same place.

People can change their life regardless of their circumstances. We've seen it time and time again. People coming back from the darkest of places. We've all heard stories about people who grew up in poverty and totally turned their life around and did something good for themselves and others, ending up wealthy.

However it's gone for us, it's important that we get to work on tackling our old, imbedded beliefs and financial woes that are going on. Unless, of course, you are someone totally set in your wealth and financial aspect of your life, however, remember that wealth isn't just about money. If we have a lot of money but no friends, ill health, and difficulty with other aspects of our lives, things need some adjusting.

It's easy to identify with the beliefs we find ourselves saying most often. It's good place to start when we're looking at how things are going for us, if we struggle in our financial health. Writing down what we say, think, and believe about money can help us get to the root of where we stand in regards to money. We can then work from there and figure out a better way to think about or speak towards what it is we *do want*, over what we don't. We can change the limiting beliefs we've been holding onto, into more abundant, healthy ones.

Becoming aware of the concepts, mindset, and values we hold around money is always the first step. Then we can decide what it is that we really want, and deserve, which will bring us forward in the direction we want to go.

Our consciousness around money, our wealth mindset, and the energy we carry about money is embedded into our DNA, believe it or not. And it goes farther back than we realize. The famine, scarcity, survival situations, and crises that our ancestors may have gone through, is all written into our DNA. As we know, with each new generation our DNA is transformed, however, some of those feelings of unworthiness and scarcity may continue to linger on and carry through. That is, until someone in the family breaks the cycle. The one who figures out a way to overcome those limitations and build a wealthier mindset, is the one who breaks the pattern.

Money affects our feelings of security and worthiness. When we grow up without our basic needs met and a huge lack of financial stability within our family, we experience fear and struggle around not having enough. And it doesn't generally stop at money, it infuses into the other areas of our lives. Unfortunately, money can create a deep place of despair for many, especially in being unable to meet one's basic needs.

There are people who have everything they need, and then some. These people keep an abundance mindset and that feeling going continuously. They create a magnitude of positive and abundant thoughts around money and its circulation in their lives. It shines through in how they feel, act, and in what they receive. Some people who have an abundance of money choose to have very little of the material in their life, who give to others instead of giving to themselves. In my eyes, this is what it means to be rich.

Some people have all of the riches in the world and are the world's most selfish, miserable, and unfortunate people. We see this everyday as we log onto the TV and watch the wealthy people in the world deciding what's best for themselves, even making decisions for everyone else. They're never concerned about us having wealth and maintaining an abundant life, they're there to make sure they make more for themselves.

These people know only to keep it to themselves and it seems they can never have enough. They even harm or disregard others in order to obtain more. Money and wealth can change people and rip families apart. It can create huge imbalance and misfortune in other areas of life. As we all know, having all of the money and riches in the world doesn't make someone a happy or good person.

However, the right people who carry abundance in their life can make a huge difference in other people's lives, as well as to the world around them. Money has an enormous ability to transform people's lives and make a difference towards the betterment of others and the planet. If money was circulated evenly and used to create more goodness and beauty in the world, it would create a more peaceful planet for everyone.

It's good to think about what money could do for some of the countries and communities around the world who have so little. We definitely need a more equal distribution of wealth wouldn't you agree? There would be a better quality of life for all of the people around the world and I believe, less fear, strife, and conflict. If you look at who creates conflict, it's usually the ones who have a lot but want more for themselves.

Everyone no matter what country or culture we come from, deserve to live in a place of security and comfort, with an abundance of the basic needs in life.

For some people money is used as a replacement for love. These people might grow up having everything they want, with the unfortunate illusion that objects equal love, and never find out what it really means to be loved and cared for. With this disconnection, money then becomes a vessel to fill the void where love is lacking in their life. Mental health issues, drug and alcohol abuse, indulging in risky and negative behaviors, and suicide can actually sadly come into play. On both sides, not having enough money or the emptiness around it can create these unfortunate outcomes.

Spending money is known to boost dopamine in the body. When we make a purchase, our brain releases endorphins and dopamine, our pleasure and reward chemicals. Most people when excited about a purchase, get a boost when they buy something. This boost of dopamine gives us that high, elated, happy feeling, but eventually that rush of feel-good energy dies down.

This can act like a drug, causing us to make yet another purchase to get that feeling back again. Even the anticipation of spending money can bring in the feelings of pleasure and happiness for a brief moment. Of course, this is not the case for all who spend money, as it can be a super debilitating and stressful time and experience for some.

Those are stuck in and who have poverty thinking, fear, and worry around spending money, may even experience it physically. Their nervous system is largely affected. The fear and worry can create anxiety, depression, insomnia, and even ill health. Finding a healthy balance of giving and receiving money is not only vital to survive, it's also vital to our physical well-being.

There are poor people around the world with so little yet live a healthy life with a joy and peace that many of us could only imagine. They've learned that money and riches can bring unwanted effects into life, such as greed, conflict, desperation, and even violence. They do not see money in the same way as most of us do. They have everything they need with the basics of shelter, food, and water, and are humbly grateful for all that they have. They don't allow greed to corrupt themselves or their community.

We know money can drive people into some pretty dark places. Unfortunately, when a person holds a fear and scarcity mindset, it can cause them to put themselves and others in a negative or even worse, a horrible situation. We know money corrupts people causing them to steal, commit acts of violence, or lower themselves in order to obtain it. Desperation takes over, but considering the pressure we have to obtain and use money in these times we're living in, it sadly happens all too often.

Many of us have encountered some type of person, situation, or scenario like this at some point in our lives. Someone we knew, or maybe someone we didn't know, took something from us that greatly affected our lives. Some of us may have even fallen into a lower place ourselves at some point where we did something out of desperation or were at a very low point in our lives. Either way, this has been happening to human beings of all kinds for thousands of years.

The good news is that we don't have to stay in any one place regarding wealth, abundance, or finances for the rest of our lives. We can change things and move ourselves out of the place we're in if it's not serving us well. All we need is the desire and willingness to make some changes, which includes our mindset and the motivaton to take action.

Abundance and wealth can show up in our lives in so many ways. We are wealthy if we're in good health and our body is strong. We are wealthy if we have amazing friends and family in our life who love and care for us. We are wealthy if we have a roof over our heads, a warm bed, running water, and food to eat.

I believe as we change what our idea of wealth is defined as, we will find that the wealth in our life goes way beyond our previous expectations and thoughts around what it is. We will even find ourselves appreciating so much more about our lives, in all that we actually have, feeling more gratitude than ever before.

If we took a moment right now and felt truly thankful about where we're at in our life, and for all that we have, our present mental and emotional state would shift. Being grateful attracts more into our life to be grateful for. We might come to realize how wealthy and fulfilling our life already is, regardless of whether or not we have all of the material objects and money we might desire.

There's obviously a consciousness around wealth. We need to remember that everything is energy and that includes wealth and money. It's an exchange or transfer of one thing for another. If we think of money as energy, we realize that energy must flow freely in order to keep moving. There needs to be an ebb and flow to it, with a healthy balance of giving and receiving, however that looks. Whether you give of your time or your prayers, wealth can be exchanged in lots of different ways.

Money needs movement, but it also needs to be met with respect, integrity, and trust.

When we're stuck or fearful around wealth or money, we live in this constant cycle of fearful thoughts that we won't have enough. We feel like there might not be any more coming in, or we're going to be left without any. This thinking will stop its flow.

Instead of thinking about *spending* our money, it's better to think about *circulating* it. Spending means it's spent, gone from our lives. Circulating means, it's coming and going, into and out of our lives. There's a constant flow of energy and exchange, give and take.

Abundance comes with feeling and emotion. If we access the feelings that we would have if we *were* wealthy and had everything we could need and then some, we would find ourselves happy, satisfied, excited, and maybe even welling up with tears some of the time. It's good that we set the emotional tone for wealth and we can do this by purposefully putting ourselves into the joyful feeling of what it is to receive wealth, over dwelling in the fear-based, usual way of poverty, lack thinking, which had not gotten us anywhere good. Remember, the subconscious knows no different. It will find a way to get us that wealth that we're feeling so happy about and worthy of.

Worthiness is a big factor in this. I get that it's hard to feel the feelings of wealth and abundance when we aren't feeling worthy of receiving it. This is where some faking it comes in, which I will give power to, that it can go a long way for us. Worthiness is a big deal for those of us who don't feel abundance and wealth are possible. Especially in this case, it's more vital than ever to add more of these happy and abundance feelings into the mix, because it will set us up to understand better how to feel this foreign feeling, allowing our subconscious mind to get the jest of it. The more we think and feel it, the attraction to it will grow.

If we believe we are worthy and capable of attaining wealth, *and* we're willing to give energy in exchange for the wealth, as the basic law of science operates, like attracts like. This only works in our favor. When we add intention to it, like in having the desire to give to and help others with our wealth, we attract more of it.

First thing we really need to do before forging ahead, is to forgive ourselves for our past, as well as whatever present situation that we now find ourselves in. It's important to acknowledge that for one, each and every beautiful soul on this planet deserves wealth and abundance. And two, it's without a doubt possible for us to shift these areas of our life through our mindset and in creating new goals for ourselves. We can get into a better head space around wealth and ignite some changes.

We can call in the type of work, job, or career that we are better suited to or desire, and start motivating ourselves to turn our income and wealth around for the better. Mindset is usually the toughest part of it and letting go of the locked in thought patterns and feelings around wealth can be a tough one, but it's easily changeable. Just remember that stating something three times a day, for twenty-one days, will help anything stick.

Also, in order to gain wealth, we need to practice the gift of giving. There's an energy with giving that emits a higher vibration and feeling. It finds its way back to us in some way or form. That's why it's so important for us to watch what we put out into the world, is it what we want coming back to us? Everything seems to find its way back to us on one level or another.

There are so many ways we can give that don't cost a thing. Complements, kind words, being of service, an ear, a hug, helping out a friend, they don't cost us money, maybe just a little time and effort. A smile or hug has enormous benefit and reward for everyone involved. Even an outsider witnessing the smile or hug can be positively affected just in seeing it.

These free gifts can be given as abundantly as we so choose. Our heart is usually calling in these interactions, with the intention to give and receive good energy and vibes. We're all deserving of this abundance and wealth stuff, we just need to realize it isn't always about money. That which we put out comes back to us, and it can return to us in whatever form we happen to need. When we wish blessings and wealth for others in the world, it only moves us closer to achieving that of our own.

Offering our good deeds, kindness, and assistance to others, also helps us to transform our old thought patterns and concepts around wealth. Giving in this way helps us create a new version and reality of what we desire wealth to look like in our lives. How we want it to express itself, how we see ourselves receiving it, how we want to create it, how blessed we feel for it and by it, and how we use it to exchange energy. Wealth transforms lives for the better. We just need to decide what we want wealth to look like in our lives, and instill new values and standards for ourselves in how we treat it.

We can start with a journal or notebook if we want to identify the patterns and ideas we have around wealth and where we're at presently in this moment. Helps us to really look at where our wealth and abundance mindset are at. We can look back at when we were growing up and how we've grown because of it. From there, we can start breaking things down and change the concepts that are holding us back. Reworking to rewire our minds, and bodies, towards what we want to create for ourselves.

New ideas and thoughts around how we want to contribute to the world, will just come up for us. Recreating and transforming our money and wealth concepts will inspire us and bring more creative energy into our life. New ideas about how to create more money will show up. Our energy and mindset around wealth will begin to transform and our awareness around what wealth means will expand. In turn, we will find our desire to share more of it.

What would you do if you had more than enough wealth in your life? Would you want to do something to help out in the world?

If we had an abundance of wealth, we would have the ability to change circumstances for others who struggle and are in need, and there are endless ways to do that. It's also good for us to write down some of the people and circumstances that we feel most drawn to helping, see what comes up in that area for us. We can learn a lot about ourselves this way. It can show us more deeply what it is we truly care about, feel concern for, and who and what we love the most.

When it comes down to stating and claiming wealth and abundance to come into our lives, affirmations are once again, a great tool. They can help us to start reprogramming our subconscious, and our mindset and beliefs around wealth. Of course, the emotion and feeling along with it, will magnify it at a much greater level. Here are a few examples.

- I am abundant, rich, and wealthy.
- Money flows effortlessly and freely into my life.
- I always have enough.
- The Universe/God provides all the wealth I need and desire.
- I happily and gratefully receive wealth in all of its forms.
- New financial opportunities to come to me that bring wealth into my life.
- The abundance in my life is unlimited.

You can create your own affirmations or find ones that resonate with you. Again, there is tons around it online, there are beautiful books, and fabulous teachers out there. It's all so easy to find. Just remember to feel the bliss, joy, excitement, and gratitude behind them.

Let's face it, we all deserve the best in life, which includes wealth of all kinds. We've been misled for far too long believing that we're somewhat worthless or have to struggle with money, that there are only a few who get to be rich and wealthy. This couldn't be farther from the truth. There's truly more than enough for everyone on this planet. Don't limit yourself thinking and believing the limited thinkers who say there isn't enough. **There's more than enough**.

Imagine if we all had wealth and were contributing to the world on one level or another. What an abundance and windfall of goodness and wealth we could create together. Wealth doesn't just offer us a sense of security, it offers freedom, power, creativity, generosity, and a means to healing.

HOMEWORK:

1. What are your money concepts? Which ones work best for you and which ones do you feel need to go?
2. What does abundance mean to you? What areas of your life would you desire more abundance in? This can be finance, friends, experiences, and so on.
3. What new inspired actions sound like something you would begin to do to bring in more abundance?
4. How would you help the world if you had an unlimited abundance of money in your life? Dream big. What would you build or create? Who would you want to help the most?

CONNECTING TO NATURE

We have become so immersed in technology, working long hours, and dealing with the everyday stresses of life that we find very little time for resting, relaxing, or enjoying ourselves outside of the usual forms of entertainment. We don't even see the fact that we might be falling away from the things that are important to us.

One of the things many of us forget about, or leave for a more, rare occasion is connecting with and being out in nature. A lot of us take for granted the fact that it provides us with everything we need to exist, the oxygen we breathe, the food we eat, the water we drink, the medicine to heal ourselves with, and the shelter and clothing we need. And it's really not hard to do, we just need to step outside of our homes and we're instantly connected, even if we're in a city.

Spending time in nature is good for us on so many levels. The fresh air alone can uplift our physical and mental bodies. Nature brings with it a sense of peacefulness and calmness, that is so very needed in the stressful world that we live in today. It elevates our mood, nurtures our spirit, and it's often times the perfect medicine for whatever it is that we're dealing with.

Imagine a world where part of the medical care plan prescribed by our doctor was that we go outside and immerse ourselves in nature every day for at least 15-30 minutes. We can do this by taking a walk or just going outside and sitting in the grass, listening to the sounds of nature. However we choose to participate, we have endless choices and activities we can do on the daily to immerse ourselves in nature.

When we get ourselves outside, it benefits us in many ways. We are taking in the fresh oxygen that we need, receiving negative ions that uplift our moods, and we become easily energized by the beautiful scenery and visuals. Being outside soothes our soul, especially when we can listen to and watch water flowing or the waves crashing. So many aspects of being outside can be hugely beneficial to our overall health and wellbeing.

Nature generally brings with it feelings of bliss, relaxation, inspiration, motivation, creativity, and gratitude. It's honestly one of the most easily accessible spiritual experiences and connections to ourselves that we have. Nature acts as a direct link with spirit and God in tangible form. It helps to strengthen our connection in realizing the divine love that we have flowing deep inside of us.

Being out in nature exposes us to negative ions that are in the air. Negative ions help to regulate our mood by helping to increase our serotonin levels, which brings balance to our mental and emotional states. These ions can help us reset our mental mindset, as well as relieve symptoms of depression naturally, and even more so if we're exercising outdoors.

These ions also amplify the oxygen that gets into our cells and tissues, and stabilizes and strengthens our DNA. They assist our physical body by stimulating and boosting our immune system, our metabolism, as well as help to regulate our sleep patterns. These negative ions help increase the flow of oxygen to our brains, which brings an increase in our mental awareness and alertness. They further purify the air enhancing our absorption of oxygen.

Being outdoors and in nature, ultimately gives us the fresh and bountiful oxygen that our bodies need to survive. We have a symbiotic relationship with nature, one where the plants and trees give off the oxygen we use, and then take in and use the carbon dioxide that we breathe out.

This is an undeniable truth that cannot be ignored. We need nature in our lives to live, thrive, heal, and enjoy this beautiful life. Not to mention how absolutely powerful nature is in providing us with the food, water, medicine, and endless the resources we need to live, like we spoke about earlier.

There are many ways in which we can get ourselves immersed in and connected to nature, besides the obvious act of just going outside. We can increase the benefits of being out in nature by being barefoot and doing what is known as grounding, or earthing. This is when the body is in direct or indirect contact to the Earth's electrical charge.

Connecting directly to the Earth's electrical charge has so many benefits. The easiest and simplest way to do this is by literally standing bare foot on the ground and connecting to the earth through the soles of our feet, whether it be in the grass, dirt, sand, or even by standing on stone or concrete.

We can also use a walking stick, that is of course made of wood, as it will connect us to the earth and its electrical charge and vibration through the stick we hold in our hand. There are grounding systems available as well, created to bring the Earth's magnetic and electrical frequencies into our homes.

Our bodies have a powerful electrical charge of their own, and without it working properly, we can encounter heart issues, nervous systems problems, health issues and an overall decreased functioning of our entire system. There are scientific studies that prove that the effects of grounding are quite powerful for the human body.

Grounding, or earthing, has positive effects on inflammation, the immune response, wound healing, and the prevention and treatment of chronic inflammatory and autoimmune diseases. Studies concluded that grounding makes a measurable difference in the capacity and function of our immune system's cells, empowering the white blood cells and cytokines that assist our bodies with inflammatory issues. It is immensely helpful for injuries and muscle pain, as studies have shown the incredible impact grounding makes in reducing pain on great levels.

Grounding improves blood flow, decreases stress, improves energy levels, and assists us with a peaceful, restorative sleep. Another study proves that grounding has a beneficial impact on the *thickness of the blood* by helping to decrease red blood cell clumping. After studies were done on people who had cardiovascular disease and blood thickness issues, there was an undeniable change in the viscosity of the blood. The conclusion proved that grounding helped to reduce cardiovascular risk and cardiac events.

It also promotes a calmness that bring us back to being centered, especially if we are someone with an overactive mind or are dealing with a lot of stress. It's the easiest thing we can do for ourselves. Even for those who cannot get outside and put their feet in the grass, as I briefly mentioned, there are products to help us ground such as grounding mats, sleeping pads, and rods that we can use to connect ourselves to the earth from within our home. This is ideal for those who are unable to get outside or who have mobility issues, especially for the elderly who are stuck in their homes with ill health and slow healing wounds.

There is a free movie on YouTube called Grounding, that is worth the watch. The well-known author Deepak Chopra, shares the undeniable effects that come from grounding in this film as well as that it can be found in much of his writing, as well.

It's been said that the human's worst invention is the rubber-soled shoe. It breaks our connection with the Earth and inhibits the flow of electricity that we need from the Earth. Shoes with rubber soles began to be produced in the late 1800's and of course have been useful, so this is not to say stop wearing rubber soled shoes, as they've had great benefit for many reasons. However, it's just something none of us knew about that is quite interesting.

The suggested amount of grounding is twenty minutes, twice a day. Of course, we need to be mindful of where we are placing our bare feet. We don't want to stand in grass that's been treated with herbicides or pesticides, or with something that we don't want getting absorbed into our skin. Avoiding places with debris, animal feces, or possible hazards is a must. If you cannot be barefoot outdoors, as I mentioned there are the earthing mats, and they even have shoes and flip flops available that can be worn outdoors if barefoot is just not something you can or are willing to do.

We can incorporate meditative practices to our grounding, or to the time we spend in nature, especially while we have our feet connected to the Earth. It can enhance our connection to the energy of the Earth and its healing and grounding effects. Scott Jeffrey, the founder of CEOsage, mentions an easy meditative practice we can do while grounding.

Closing our eyes, we can quiet our mind and center ourselves into the energy of our heart. This energy can be seen as a warm, glowing light, which can be white, golden, green, pink, purple, or whatever comes to you. Envision that light coming from your heart and expanding outwards, filling your body. Then see in your mind the core of the

Earth as a fiery ball of light, imagining a beam of energy from your heart connecting to the Earth's core energy. Envision a similar beam of light coming from the Earth's core and connecting back to your heart forming a circular or oval shaped connection.

If we keep that vision going for 10 minutes, we will feel profound effects throughout our entire being. It's an amazing and life changing feeling and so magnificently healing.

Another way we can connect ourselves with the nature is simply just spending time observing it. Doing this can shift us out of being in a negative place. When we witness life in its most natural and perfect state, it automatically works to inspire us and rejuvenate our spirit, helping to reignite the connection that we have with ourselves and nature.

The amazing details and intricate designs of the plants and animals are other level, and truly awe-inspiring. Ever look at a flower and feel so amazed by just how perfect and beautiful it is? The sight of it alone can bring us immense joy and appreciation. Add to that, the aromas and smells that are present which can also shift our mood and energy exponentially.

The entire experience of immersing ourself in the observation of nature will quiet our mind and uplift our mood and energy. Many studies have been done proving the positive effects that nature has on those who suffer from mental health issues such as depression, anxiety, and bipolarism.

Getting into a body of water is other level. Being in a natural body of water has a way of moving us into a better state both mentally and physically. Science has proven that for example, swimming in the ocean, can help to decrease our risk of chronic illnesses and even improve the health of those with diabetes and heart disease. It helps to reduce joint pain, improves circulation, helps the muscles relax as well as gain strength, and has even been proven to have a positive impact on those suffering with illnesses such as cancer, cerebral palsy, and respiratory diseases.

Ocean waves generate negative ions which was just mentioned. Studies have shown that the beach in itself, is one of nature's number one cures for alleviating stress and *healing the brain*. People with brain injuries benefit from time by the ocean. Being in or by the ocean, also has a positive effect on our skin, and boosts and enhances our immune system, quite powerfully so.

Taking a stroll in the park or somewhere out in nature, improves our mood, lowers our stress levels, reduces blood pressure, boosts our attention span, reduces the risk of mental health and psychiatric disorders, and even is proven to increase our empathy and cooperation.

The truth is, we all have an innate desire to connect with nature. Studies have been done comparing the difference of someone being out in nature, to someone being in an urban, city environment. The person who was in nature with all the visuals and sounds around them had an improved mood and performed better on cognitive tests in comparison to those who were surrounded by little to no nature, concrete, car horns, and busy city sounds.

They even did this study where the subjects just listened to the sounds on headsets. Some listened to the ocean waves and birds chirping, while the others listened to the sounds of city life and it had the same result. Those who listened to nature did much better on all the tests, as well as had an improved outlook and mood.

This was even proven to be true when it came to *pictures and videos* of nature in comparison to pictures and videos of city, urban life. Taking in the colors, vibrant life, and the atmosphere of nature even visually, brought an elevation to the energetic state of the body lifting the mood and improving the strength and ease within the body.

Studies have also been done to show nature's effect on people in regards to how they treat others and life around them. This study was done with adults and children. The children, of course, responded the fastest and transformed almost entirely, after being out in nature.

Children are more responsive due to the fact that their bodies are in a more, pure state. They generally carry less mental and physical problems, and have a greater capacity and ability to letting things go. They are innately connected to nature because of their sensitivity and purity. Indeed, after the study was done, the children all responded by being more kind to one another, and were in more joyful and happy moods.

This just makes you realize how important it is for children to be outside in nature as much as possible. In today's day and age, children are trapped in buildings for 7-8 hours a day with maybe a small break to play outside. The sun is out yet they sit in chairs under fluorescent lighting. Technology has since taken over and has become a main focus for them, which sadly, has taken many children out of nature, creating a huge disconnection that is actually detrimental to their health and wellbeing.

Children need nature. They need to spend a lot of time outdoors to explore and take in the undeniable benefits to reset and ground their systems. With all that's been said about grounding and connecting to nature, it's obvious this is absolutely necessary for our children.

If you want to make it simple, just go outside and take a walk. Spend time observing the nature around you and find appreciation in the little things. Or, you can sit yourself down in the grass or up against a tree and do some breathwork, meditate, journal, read a book, or take a nap.

Being in nature is also a great way to spend and enjoy time with those that we love, including our pets! Speaking of pets, we can bring nature right into our home with our pets. Pets bring unconditional love, high vibrations, and healing benefits. We can also bring in many different kinds of plant life into our home. The plant life in our home produces more oxygen for us, brings beneficial grounding energy and positive ions into our home environment, as well as that they help to purify the air.

Some plant energy can bring in peacefulness, while others can bring in an active energy. Many plants are air purifiers that help to remove toxins out of the air, and some can even absorb radiation. There are toxins in so many parts of our homes from the carpets, to the paint, cabinetry, furniture, detergents, cleaners, plastics, rubber, insulation, and so on.

Plants can help to buffer and relieve us of some of these unseen burdens and toxins that get released into the air in our homes that absolutely, yet unknowingly affect our physical health. Plants have been studied for these properties by scientists and programs like NASA. Let's touch on a few common plants that can help protect us in our home.

- Rubber Tree not only gives off oxygen, it purifies by removing mold spores and bacteria from the air, as much as 60% of it, and that's because it needs to do this to protect its soil. It also removes formaldehyde from the air.

- Spider Plant removes 95% of the chemicals in the air including carbon monoxide, benzene, and formaldehyde.
- Snake Plants can grow in all types of lighting, easy to keep and they purify the air remarkably removing chemicals like formaldehyde and benzene.

Some others are the Palm family, the Peace Lily, the Ficus/Weeping Fig, the Fern family, Aloe Vera, English Ivy, Gerber Daisies, Chrysanthemums, as well as with many others.

We are continuing to discover the amazing abilities and effects plants have on us as the beautiful, living beings that they are. Science has found, and confirmed, that plants are indeed sentient beings, which means they are perceptive and conscious beings. They can perceive light, smell, touch, and water, as well are very sensitive to the energy we put out towards them.

Plants can sense us and even see us. They have receptors in their cells that are identical to the neurons that we have in our body, which enables them to learn, remember, and communicate. They translate information through electrical chemical signals, similar to how the signals and synapses work within the human body. The electrical signals of plants can even create sound and there are devices that can be used to hear this. And it sounds like beautiful music.

Plants are far more intelligent and sensitive than we realize, or give them credit for. We know that talking to our plants enhances their quality of life, growth, and how well they thrive. Surely, we haven't been taught enough about the intimate connection that we as humans have to plants, however the beautiful connections between plants and humans are being more deeply acknowledged and seen.

It's been found that genetically and biologically speaking, we as humans are closest to the mushroom family than any other plant or organism out there. There's a movie called Fantastic Fungi that speaks on the proven science around this discovery, and it's very fascinating to say the least.

Now let's talk about animals, whether it be our pets, or the animals in our backyard and out in nature. They are very healing, beautiful beings as many of us know. Anyone who owns a pet knows of the unconditional love, healing, and joy that they bring into our life. Animals are found to help lower blood pressure, decrease stress levels, even help heal a broken heart.

Pets can be life savers for a person's mental health, like in the case of having depression or anxiety. When we're playing with our pet, they can take our mind off the stresses and weight of the world that we're carrying, because they bring us into the present moment. A pet snuggling up to us or on us, is soothing, comforting, and provides emotional support and healing energy beyond what a human can. They can sense when we aren't well, when we're sad, sick, or anxious. It is said that a cat licking us can bring down stress and anxiety.

Pets can get us out of bed in the morning, motivate us, and make us feel like we have something or someone to live for. They can bring purpose to people who suffer with mental health problems, help those who are lonely, or who have suffered great loss in their life. They are our companions, our best friends, and will always be there for us when we need them. They are there to greet us when we arrive home from a long day and help us release the daily stress we're carrying with their unconditional love and presence.

According to scientific research, the frequency of a cat's purr can literally help mend a broken bone, as frequencies of 20 to 50 Hertz are helpful in healing bones and connective tissue. The vibration of a cat's purr ranges from 20-140 Hertz which can also help heal soft tissue injuries. As most of us know, cats have different vibes and personalities. Some are lap cats and constantly want to be around us, snuggled up against our body, and then there are others who want their space and hang out only when they feel like it. Cat owners speak of the unique love and joy, and mischief, that their cats bring into their lives. They are great companions, like dogs, especially for the elderly and those who live alone.

Dogs are also so incredibly healing, although they require more care and physical activeness than cats. They too, bring unconditional love to their owners and are as loyal as you've heard they are. They require exercise and walks which helps their owners to motivate, get outside, and be active. Like children, no matter how they are treated, they always return to the unconditional love they have for their owners.

Bees have also been acknowledged for their amazing healing energy and potential. Their buzzing and humming produce frequencies that range from about 150 to 250 Hertz, sometimes even up to 500 Hertz. The general bee frequency is 216 Hertz. Their humming stimulates various areas in our brain, as well as some of the glands of the Endocrine system including the Pituitary, Pineal, Hypothalamus, and Amygdala.

A pioneer of bee healing is a woman named Dr. Valerie Solheim otherwise known as the "Bee Lady". She created a recording of her bees during different seasons and activities. She used one of her recordings on a collapsing, struggling colony and it brought it back to life. These recordings have also been used for healing people with nervous system and physical ailments, with remarkable results.

Unfortunately, animals have gotten lost in the mix. Much of the time they've become seen as disposable and useful creatures. Of course, many of us see them as beautiful, intelligent beings, even regarding some as life companions and family, but that's not always the case. As we know animals are used for food, to serve us, and are even used to provide clothing and medicine for us.

There's been a loss of respect and compassion for them on so many levels, which is sad because they deserve our utmost love, respect, and compassion. We sometimes forget that they live on this planet too, and have every right to exist and thrive just as we do. They deserve to be regarded and respected for more than how they can serve us.

Of course, some of them can be seen as a threat, but in the end, humans have the ultimate power over them, as they can be killed quite easily, are hunted, sometimes sadly in the name of vanity and ego. We seem to forget that we, too are mammals. Humans work to be the dominators of the animal kingdom, however, animals also have emotions, intelligence, strength, and a purpose on this planet, even if we choose not to see it. There are endless injustices happening, and not as much concern as to what we can do to help them.

Every animal has its own unique power and abilities, along with special characteristics, features, habits, ways of living, eating, sleeping, and connecting to one another. Because they are so fascinating, it's hard to not feel in awe when you're around them. I know not everyone feels so passionate about animals but if you are, let's look at some of them and their beautiful story and spirit. To connect in and learn to understand them on a deeper level, only helps us on a larger scale, and believe it or not, it serves us to know and understand them.

Animals are all magical creatures in one way or another. Changing our perception about them can help heal a lot of things for us, as well as for them. Yes, humans are by far the most advanced species, but in my opinion, we need to let go of always feeling superior to them and believing their lives matter less. Animals have so much working against them these days, so it's good to remember just how delicate and vulnerable they are so we can look out for, and help them whenever and wherever possible.

I've mentioned this to some people who have the mentality that animals are here to serve us and as a source of food. The Bible even specifies that man will have dominion over every living thing, but in my eyes means that man with its power, should actually be responsible and take care of all animals and living beings, working to live in harmony with them. We are the protectors, and we should love and respect them, regardless of if we use them as part of dietary intake.

It's understood that animals have literally been sacrificed for thousands of years for our benefit, so where would we be without them? Today, we are empty, thoughtless, and just go on without thinking a single thought about the food that we're eating.

Back in the day, our ancestors actually gave thanks to the animal for the abundance of food that it provided, even speaking to the animal spirit in honor of what it was providing for them. This still exists a bit in the world today, but for sure man has become so disconnected and so detached, that we've created a huge disregard for them. We've lost the connection to and compassion that we once had for them.

We all come from blends of different cultures and races, so I'm sure our ancestors somewhere back in the day, revered and respected animals and the Earth. What better time than now, to reconnect back to what our ancestors once felt which was respecting the earth, its creatures, taking care of it, and only taking what we need. Besides providing us with food and labor through all these years, animals have also been incredible healers, messengers, and catalysts in our lives.

We spoke about their healing capacity already when it came to owning pets and the enormous gift that they are, especially in regards to lifting our spirits and helping us feel better when we're sick or depressed. Indigenous people and some religions believed that each kind of animal had different messages, meanings, and powers. The Native American people believed that every person was accompanied by nine animals that were their animal or spirit guides throughout their lifetime. These animal guides were there to offer power and wisdom, as well as healing medicine.

We've all heard of the myths and stories told through generations that seem other worldly. We hear about animal symbology in tons of cultures, so I thought it would be useful for some of us to touch on some of the old knowledge that is derived from these cultures and the wisdom of the ancients. Although this is not the usual, accepted, conformed knowledge that's out there at this time, and it may seem silly to many, let's remember that animals were once seen through a different lens that I personally believe is worth exploring and talking about. I find these aspects and animal medicine to be quite significant and powerful to know, regardless of whatever background or religious beliefs we hold. Animals deserve much more credit than they've been given. And when we realize their medicine, it will honestly change our lives.

THE EAGLE - Mastery. Fearlessness. Victory. Spiritual Knowledge. *You are on a spiritual journey; soar to new heights.*

THE OWL - Wisdom. Insight. Enlightenment. Intuitive Development. Transformation. Change. Mystery. Guardians of the Truth. *Open your inner vision and you will always see the truth.*

THE ELEPHANT - Greatness. The Peaceful Warrior. Power. Dignity. Harnessing. Wisdom. Strength. Loyalty. Leadership. *You are a natural born leader with love as your strength.*

THE DEER – Love. Gentleness. Innocence. Intuition. Grace. Peace. Beauty. Vigilance. Sensitivity. Kindness. *Your gentleness and love bring light to the world.*

THE DRAGONFLY – Transformation. Change. Illumination. New Perspective. Diving Deeper into Emotion. Joy. Lightness of Being. Honoring Inner Truths. *I courageously change and transform for the better.*

THE DOLPHIN - Play. Life Force Energy. Playfulness. Freedom. Harmony. Cooperation. Protection. Peace and Harmony. Self-Love. *My freedom is in the joy and play that I seek every day.*

THE BEAR – Power. Personal Strength. Courageousness. Protection. Dream Time. Self-Healing. Sovereignty. Confidence. Leadership. Standing Against Adversity. Going within. *Strength and love guide my power.*

HOMEWORK:

1. How can you add more nature into your life?
2. What parts of nature most excite you? What parts calm you?
3. What parts of connecting to nature resonate? What parts of nature do you see as healing and beneficial for you personally?

GRATITUDE

Gratitude is the best medicine. It's a powerful emotion. When we feel grateful, we're in a state of appreciation, one that sometimes hits us so deeply it may even bring us to tears. Naturally, we feel good, humbled, and full of positive vibes. The feeling of being grateful brings with it, more reasons to be grateful.

It even moves us into a place where we're drawn to do things for others. When we feel honored and elated by all that we're grateful for, we want to bear the kindness and goodness onto others. We want to run out there and find a way to pay it forward.

Being grateful has so many benefits. For one, our vibration and mood are uplifted. We feel more heart-filled, love energy than we might normally feel, generally speaking. We enter into a state of bliss with the realization that life is indeed, good to us regardless of the hardships and struggles we may have.

Although, I had always felt and expressed my gratitude throughout my life on one level or another, I didn't realize how powerful it was. The first time I truly understood the power behind gratitude was when I first watched the movie *The Secret*. The film amplified how gratitude was such a powerful emotion and creator. With gratitude comes the ability to attract more of what we want into our life. We can essentially enhance our lives by just feeling and being grateful for the everyday things, no matter how small they may seem.

The emotion behind our gratitude is everything. When we feel grateful and experience those heart-filled, joyful emotions, we open ourselves up to receive even more of the gifts and beauty that life has to offer us. Of course, we can just speak the words of gratitude, and although they do have an effect, it's the feeling we have behind saying it that carries all of the gold.

Even if things aren't exactly perfect in our world, and we would prefer our life to be different, the act of being grateful will actually draw more of what we want towards us. When we're grateful even if just for the little things we have, we resonate with a higher vibration and energy, as gratitude is very high vibrationally.

What we put out there will find its way back to us, giving us more reasons to be grateful. Appreciation pulls things in and towards us. As stated perfectly by Dr. John Demartini, *"Whatever we think about and thank about, we bring about."*

When something wonderful or exciting happens to us, or for us, we automatically feel grateful. It's usually an emotion that hits us without even having to try, although if we're in a heavy, negative place, this can sometimes be hard to move into, feel, or acknowledge. Negative energy can have a way of cancelling out the gratitude feeling by bringing in more fear or worry. But eventually, the more we work on expressing our gratitude, the less negativity will present itself, and the more accustomed we become to the feeling of being grateful.

Let's gain some insight into what gratitude can actually do for us beyond making us feel more elated and good about our life. Gratitude quite literally has scientifically proven, positive effects on our *physical* bodies, it doesn't just affect our mental and emotional bodies.

Dr. Joe Dispenza brings this to light. If we spent just *four* days straight feeling and expressing our gratitude, it literally strengthens and boosts our immune system by fifty percent. In just four days! He figured out this immune response by doing an experiment and study with one hundred and seventeen people. He asked that they stop feeling negative or worrisome emotions, two to three times a day, for ten to fifteen minutes at a time and to replace those emotions with feelings and expressions of gratitude. The study showed that every single person's immune system was strengthened by fifty percent in this short period of time.

Speaking gratitude and the positive vibration that it puts forth, helps our immune system release immunoglobulin A, which is our body's primary defense against bacteria, viruses, and other organisms.

The pain and inflammation the people in the group were experiencing began to dissipate or disappear altogether. Food allergies, immune conditions, even cancer began to transmute and leave the body, thus proving how powerful the thoughts and positive emotions of gratitude have on making us well and work towards our healing.

Gratitude literally acts as a protectant and a strengthener that enhances our immune system. On the opposing side of things, fear and anger will act to defeat our immune system, making us more susceptible to illness and less able to defend ourselves from foreign invaders. We literally weaken our body and immunity with fear, and even weaken ourselves muscularly, as fear is even proven to weaken the heart muscle. Gratitude, however, makes the heart muscle stronger, and we really don't need science to realize this.

Let's face it, gratitude makes all parts of us stronger. It works to free us, strengthen us, and blesses our life on every level. Our body is impressed upon by how we're feeling. It doesn't know if something has happened in real life or not, so it responds to the feelings that we have, and whatever it is that we're focused on.

Just by expressing and feeling gratitude, we can create a *favorable condition* where things in our life have the room to transform for the better, including our physical body and our health. Whether it be through boosting our immune system or in helping us to create a more positive environment and room for good things to happen in our lives, the resonance of being grateful has an undeniable, powerful, and positive impact on us.

When we experience the effects, seeing and feeling the difference in how we feel about and receive life, we will without a doubt, absolutely continue to keep expressing our gratitude as often as we can think to, and more freely so.

World renown author and speaker, Tony Robbins, spoke about gratitude in a beautiful way. He said that when we feel and express our gratitude, we see life as the unbelievable gift that it is. Gratitude indeed invokes positive emotions that have an effect on how we see the world. These positive emotions go out into the day ahead of us and towards our future experiences. Experiences we would be so happy to have and welcome into our lives.

It's easy to get caught up in what's wrong in our lives or in the world, and understandably so, as it's nearly impossible to fully avoid when life presents us with challenges, struggles, sadness, and loss. Keeping ourselves trapped in those feelings is however, going to keep us in a lowered state, unable to receive the good or look at other perspectives and sides to life.

It's absolutely important to feel all of our feelings and emotions, but also very important to do our best not to get stuck in them or be held down by them. Honoring our feelings, good or bad, is necessary, even when they're uncomfortable. However, we can always find it in ourselves to work our way out of being stuck in fear or anger, and back into reasons to be grateful, even in some of the worst-case scenarios.

If we're not used to feeling grateful about things, when we first start out, it might feel foreign or difficult to drudge up from inside of us. We may even feel like we have to force ourselves to find a reason to be grateful. At some point after putting the continuous effort into it, we'll find that it becomes something we like to spend time doing, especially as we realize that it makes us feel good.

We may even return to feeling our sadness or upset, but as long as we keep pushing ourselves to find things to be grateful for, the simplest of things even, it will move us into the energy of goodness. It might even change the outcomes of our not-so-great situation or circumstance on some level or in some way.

The more grateful we become, the better life will feel, no matter what it is that we have going on. Things may still be a mess or be going wrong on some level, but the way we handle it will change.

Gratitude has truly changed my life and my expression of it has increased enormously over the past year alone. No matter what bump I hit in the road, I find myself more at peace. I find that I get less angry, I speak less negatively, and get less overwhelmed or stressed out about things. I even say thank you at the things that brought a lesson or reflective moment, even when they weren't the most wonderful occurrence. Being grateful is a gift that helps us to move through and overcome some of the tougher times and challenges in life.

Gratitude is a gift that we give to our nervous system, as it works to soothe and calm our energy. When we get into the practice of doing it more frequently, we will find our nerves more calm, more balanced, and find more ease in even the most stressful of times. It nurtures our nervous system by giving it support and time to rest and feel at ease.

Being grateful also helps to dissolve fear. It has a beautiful way of healing our mental and emotional well-being, relieving depression and anxiety, even if it's just for a moment. It can have long-term, superior effects in helping to decrease depressive states and setbacks that happen. It's even being used in the mental health industry to help move people out of feelings of hopelessness, or with those who have the desire to harm themselves, proving to be an absolute game changer.

Focusing on the good in the world serves us and others, as the feeling and energy around it reverberates and goes out into the world. It reflects off of us to the people who surround us. Not only do we release our own negative energy that we're holding onto, but as gratitude expands, it nurtures the energy around us, carrying with it the ability to help others. It sends out the grateful energy that we're feeling, into the world in front of us. This may sound silly or even somewhat fictional, but the truth is, when you study energetics and quantum physics around the impact that our emotions, thoughts, and words have, you will realize just how powerfully true it is.

On a soul level, we are all innately tuned into the frequency of gratitude. It's a part of who we are, even a part of our DNA, because it's how our ancestors aligned themselves with the beauty and goodness of life. No matter how life went for them, this was a practice that came with all religions, cultures, and the ancient teachings of the past. No matter where we've come from or what's happened in our lives, this is true for each and every one of us, no matter what traumas we may have been through.

There are people out there who have been through some of the worst experiences one could imagine, who've completely turned their life around. They found strength in the art of forgiveness and gratitude changing the course of how they saw, handled, and felt about everything going on around and in front of them. They found reasons to be grateful in even the smallest of things, and put in the work to make changes for themselves. The outcome was powerful.

There's truly so much to be grateful for, and the more we give thanks for the things in our life, the more reasons life gives us to be grateful.

It's really that simple. The act of gratitude is such an easy practice and worth every effort. As we practice gratitude more often, we'll find ourselves saying thank you for just about everything we have in our life. For the shower we're taking, for our car as we get into it, for the computer we're working on, the bed we're lying in, for the food we're about to eat, the person we're spending time with, for the song that we're listening to… whatever it is we're looking at, experiencing, or observing in the moment. All of the simple things in our life become reasons to be grateful. Life truly does begin to feel more like an honor and blessing to us. We move into appreciating everything on a much deeper level and we even find that our love and concern for the world around us grows because of it.

When the power of gratitude starts flowing through our life, we experience positive changes. Unexpected goodness makes its way into our life. It's truly a universal law that exists, what we put out there, comes back to us. When we're in a state of gratitude, we emit a higher, more profound vibration and frequency which attracts more high vibrational things to come into our lives.

The author and narrator in the movie *The Secret* spoke about how we can incorporate gratitude so simply into our day. One of the most perfect times for it is when we first wake up in the morning, before our feet even hit the floor. This is a great time to spend a few minutes to say thank you and feel grateful about whatever it is in our lives that we feel thankful for, and for what we appreciate in our lives. It's easy to feel thankful for the new day ahead of us, right down to the pillow we're resting our head on. It's easy enough to wake up in the morning and simply say, *"Thank You"*, without having to attach it to a certain thing or situation.

We can also focus on what we're grateful for before bedtime, which is another powerful and easy moment we can use to put out some goodness and feelings of thankfulness. It sets us up for a more peaceful, restful sleep and can help us to carry that energy in through the night, right into the next morning and day ahead.

Sometimes just being grateful in our heart for life itself, or for another day before us, is enough. Regardless of the challenges we're facing and the issues we encounter in our lives, gratitude will help shift our reality on unseen levels. When we pour good feelings into our day, we've now opened ourself up to the *receiving* mode. It takes all of about 3 minutes on either end, in the morning or at night, and the return comes back ten-fold.

Starting our day on a note of positive, loving, grateful emotion, sets us up. We experience a deeper feeling of satisfaction, safety, and a loving connection to ourselves and our environment. We also find ourselves feeling blissed out about something as simple as seeing the sun in the sky or hearing the birds chirping. After a while, the reasons to be grateful become so much easier to find and so much more empowering to us. Things that make our heart happy begin showing up for us more often.

The act of gratitude helps us to attract more good into our life. It also creates the space for us to become more giving in return. We'll find the desire within ourselves to help others and do more for the world, when we feel good about ourselves and about life. Gratitude opens us up to the natural flow of giving and receiving, and works to break down the barriers that are preventing us from experiencing life to its fullest.

When we move out of the feelings of not having enough or being without, we realize that we no longer need to project feelings of lack and distrust. We can give without feeling like we're going to lose something or go without, because the reward is much greater than our fear of missing out. We become more open to give of our time, words, kindness, and assistance.

We become more patient, present, and thoughtful throughout our days. We lose the need to constantly consume and attain more, because the desire to have more is no longer as important to us. We also lose the need to be as negative as we once were, because gratitude literally shifts around so many aspects of who we are, how we see the world, and how we are in the world.

Gratitude offers us the space to be a better human. It brings more light and love into our lives, enabling us to put more love and goodness out into the world. And that's just what the world needs right about now.

HOMEWORK:

1. What are 10 things you are grateful for in this moment?
2. What practice sounds easiest to you. How can you set yourself up to practice gratitude daily?
3. Do you see deeper meaning in being grateful? If so, what does it mean to you now, knowing it's more than just stating a few simple words.
4. If you felt grateful each and every day, what do you think might open up or come into your life?

GiViNG BACK

I found several short, online video clips of a man who helps out the homeless in his neighborhood. He goes and buys them food, brings them sleeping bags and other gear, gives them nights in motels, haircuts, money, you name it. He befriends them; even helping some of them try and get their lives back on track by providing a month's worth of housing, along with everything they need for the month. He even helps them to get job interviews.

Obviously, this man has more than enough money to be able to do this, and he also has a ginormous heart. It's beautiful to see the exchange happen and just how much of a difference it makes in those people's lives. You can see their facial expressions, their tears, and overall feelings of gratitude. It really touches a deeper part of you, and all that it took was someone to care enough to do what they could, even if just for a moment.

Imagine if all of the people in the world who had more than enough, gave to others so freely?

This gentleman also spends his time raising money for some of them. He organizes a fundraiser online and even helps to sell some of their artwork. He makes things happen; giving others the opportunity to contribute to these beautiful people as well, helping them get back on their feet, or just to get them some food and a warm bed to sleep in. This opens up a beautiful space of love and compassion, letting them know that they matter, and that people do care.

He selflessly spends hours of his week being completely in service to others who are less fortunate than him. In doing this, he not only adds to their lives, but he puts this powerful energy of love and giving out into the Universe which vibrates and resonates in more ways than we can see.

He's contributing to humanity in a bigger way than in just giving some money and food to people. The good he puts out there reverberates out into the world.

Doing things for others that they wouldn't otherwise expect, opens up the space for them to see their value and their worth. Some of these people might have ended up in these places because they never felt special or learned to love themselves. They might have grown up around people and in situations that were heavy, negative, and unsupportive. They may have never learned what it was to succeed or feel like they were worth enough to even do so. Doing something kind for no reason other than to show someone you care, goes a long way. We all deserve to feel appreciated, loved, and worthy, and equally so.

It's even in how he speaks with them, his sincerity and kindness just channel through. You can feel that he is there without judgement and is genuinely concerned for their wellbeing. This is an example of the beauty of one human being reaching out to inspire the beauty in another, extending love and kindness without expecting something in return.

Any one of us could be this guy on some level or another. He's just one example of how we can have such an enormously positive impact on other people's lives through our kindness and action. He could've chosen to treat his money like some of the other wealthier people who are out there, keeping and spending it all on himself and whatever he desired. Instead, he understands the power that money has, in that it can bring positive and loving change to the world, even if it's just in doing a few things for a handful of people out there. The power is behind his intention and his actions. He understands the energy of money and how powerful it can be when used to help others.

Even if we only have a few extra dollars or some spare change, there's a lot those few extra dollars can do for someone else. But it doesn't always have to be in monetary form. We can give of our time, love, and service to others. It doesn't have to cost us any physical money, to give.

Imagine what the world would be like, or feel like, if we all gave more to one another? Lending a hand, an ear, a tool, a ride, whatever it is, our time, concern, kindness, compassion, and assistance goes a long way.

We would probably have a more blissful, peaceful existence in this world. We surely would not have the depth of poverty, homelessness, and despair that we have today. There are so many ways that we can help people, even the smallest of gestures and acts of kindness can move mountains for some people out there who are really struggling. A smile is the easiest thing we can do, and it can have a big impact uplifting and brightening someone's entire day.

Our time, prayers, random acts of kindness, and loving, encouraging words all create an impact and can make a huge difference in people's lives. They might even save someone's life one day. They're not hard to do, and as free as it gets. There's no reason why any of us should refrain from giving to others when we all have the capacity to give on one level or another.

If we only spent our money on what it is that we truly needed, and I mean the basics of housing, water, food, clothing, and a few essentials we might desire, we'd likely all be much more monetarily wealthy. However, it's gone differently and we've gotten to a place where we purchase and consume much more than we need, gathering stuff which leads to clutter and really only throws off the natural flow of abundance. When things go too much in one direction or another, there's always an imbalance created and we don't realize just how much this affects our own life.

Thankfully, there will always be wealthy people like this gentleman who will always strive to give of his time and money to other's who are in need. He is an example of someone who is truly grateful for all that he has in life and who understands what abundance really means.

When we give, our body releases endorphins, or our *feel-good* hormones. Giving makes us feel good on a chemical, physical level, literally increasing the flow and feeling of bliss. I think this is why, once we start giving to others in whatever ways we can, it creates a momentum for us that we end up wanting to continue doing it. Giving *feels* good.

Some people have a mindset of lack where even giving of their time or even a smile feels like too much. They're so caught up in their own life and everything happening to them that they just can't see how they could possibly give of themselves in any way.

Perhaps, something inside of them is too afraid to let go, even if it is just five minutes of their time. This is a form of protection and self-preservation. Somewhere in life they learned this either through someone else or because of a situation that they had in our lives. This is a form of lack, feeling as though they're never going to have enough for themselves. Generally, they don't feel they are worth as much as they are, but once they tackle those self-limiting beliefs and move them out of the way, they'll will be able to open themselves up to giving more which will open the door for them to receive, as well.

What they need to understand is the energy of giving and the value behind it. Giving to others on even the smallest of levels, will *always* attract and bring with it great benefit, both to the giver and receiver. The energy of giving attracts more into our lives, and even attracts our ability to give more. It's a circulation of energy.

If our consciousness was built on poverty or scarcity, we do have some work to do. Again, it's just like rewiring our mindset and rewriting the language, as rewiring applies to all aspects of our life including giving. Although, it may be the complete and total opposite of what we presently think, do, and know, when we work on rebuilding our mindset around giving and receiving, so much changes for the better.

There are always those people who would give us the shirt right off their back, and we always notice those people. They humble us and really put things into perspective. It makes us think a bit more deeply. How when they have may have next to nothing could they feel so free to give of their only or most important possession? Well, this is what it's all about. Life is not just about attaining and owning things, it's also about how we contribute to the world. It's finding the beautiful balance between giving and receiving.

The world needs us to get back into this balance now more than ever. There are so many people in need, so many suffering in the worst of ways right now and there really is so much each and every one of us can do, that will serve others and help create the change that we need. And we can do it in our own way…

There are endless situations and people that are in need of our help. It could be our next-door neighbor who just needs some company and a human to talk to every once in a while. There could be someone we know who needs assistance getting to and from their doctor's appointment, or people who just lost everything in a fire who need all they help they can get to rebuild their lives. Doing things to help others is not that difficult to figure out, and we're all capable in one way or another.

Acts of service and giving to others is naturally a part of who we are, and as we know, children are the best examples of this. They start off in life as such open and loving little beings. They are some of the most, sincere, giving beautiful people on the planet.

Children are born with a purity and a natural capacity to love and give to others. It's in their blueprint, which means, it's in our blueprint. Still. It would serve us well to learn a little bit more from children, as an example of how to be in the world. Perhaps we can even reconnect back into those hibernating parts of ourselves, because no matter the years of conditioning that we've had from our parents, elders, society, or our life experiences, we can bring this beautiful, innate part of us back around.

The consciousness of giving is reawakening in people. More of us are finding ourselves with the desire to serve and give to others, especially because times are so fragile for so many people in this very moment. We can make a huge impact that brings more ease and love into being.

There's a pouring in of love as we all wake up to what's happening in the world. It's as though our hearts are activating without any effort on our behalf. We are naturally coming back into who we are; the loving, giving, beautiful souls that we've always been. Giving to others doesn't have to look like anyone else's way of giving, we just need to do what feels right and good to us, and whatever it is that comes from within. We each have a unique and special way of giving.

We can make someone's day with a smile or a hello, offer a complement, or our help. We can even just say a prayer for people or for situations to resolve. Prayer and intention have a powerful impact and are so very easy to give.

When we focus on and put intention and energy into what we *do* want, over what we don't, it sends that vibration out, sending love, healing, and protection towards what it is, or who it is that we're thinking about. Giving is ultimately energy, so spending our energy on intending for the resolve and healing of a situation, will indeed help in ways unseen.

We no longer need to block the flow of this beautiful energy.

We all deserve to be a part of the energy of giving and receiving which brings in some of the most amazing, profound, and loving experiences. When we realize that each and every one of us truly have an endless supply of love and energy to give, it hits home. The love in our heart can never run out, as it's infinite at its source. The more love we give, the more love that returns to us. Our heart actually gets so full up, you can't even explain the feeling in words. All I can say is there is truly nothing greater.

Open up your heart, allow the surge of love that is just waiting for your permission, to flow. Giving won't feel like a chore, task, or burden, it will feel so deeply rewarding and better than we could've ever imagined it would. Our whole body will feel it, too. And soon we'll find that we want to give to so many more people on so many new levels. The ways and resources to be able to do so, will show up. We will attract more to us that will help us give on a larger scale than we had imagined ever being able to do. All because we have the deep love and desire to help.

One last thing to remember, is that it's just as important to make sure we give to ourselves, and that we act kindly and lovingly to ourselves, first and foremost. It's of utmost important, my beautiful friends.

Giving to ourselves is just as vital, because we don't want to feel like we've just given and given leaving nothing for ourselves. The genuine care and concern for ourselves has to be number one, because without us doing well and receiving what it is that we need, we can't do much for others. It's important that giving never feels like it's draining or emptying us on any level, nor causing discomfort in our life.

Abundance comes our way when we give ourselves the permission to give freely, lovingly, and unconditionally. When we want nothing more than for other people to be relieved of their suffering, goodness has a way of flowing back towards us. Life works that way, you know, and so wonderfully so. Along the giving journey we will find new ways to help and give to others. It's a win-win situation for everyone.

I know that so many of us out in the world genuinely care about people. We naturally feel love and sympathy for the lives of others, especially for those who struggle. So, remember that our thoughts and prayers for other's well-being makes a big difference, never discount or underestimate the power of this. Our intentions indeed always have an impact.

We can also give back to the Earth, the animals, and the environment. It can be as simple as feeding the birds outside or getting food for the animals at our local shelter or sanctuary. We can pick up garbage when we take a walk on the beach, we can volunteer at the nearest homeless shelter or food kitchen, whatever it is, we can always find a way to help a cause of some kind.

Of course, we can give money to one of the many organizations working to help save people and animals. We might even find ourselves inspired and end up starting our own foundation, organization, or line of work towards something that we're passionate about. You never know what will open up for you.

And lastly, no matter how small our contribution is, it still has a profound effect. What we put out there does so much more than we can see. Intention and love are more powerful than we give credit to.

My advice is to keep the energetic flow of giving, going. Keep filling up that basket with good deeds and intentions. Giving helps our capacity to love more deeply, to grow, and it only changes us for the better.

HOMEWORK:

1. Let's begin with you. How do you give to yourself? In what ways are you compassionate, loving, and caring towards yourself? It's important to fill our own bucket up so that it's easier to give to others.

2. In what ways do you give to others in this moment? Think of the little things, too.

3. Do you notice your ego creeping in telling you things like you don't have the money or time to give? Do feelings of lack or stinginess come up? Observe this without judgement. Write down your struggles or barriers to giving more.

4. Write down a few people, groups, or causes that you feel drawn to help. Next write several ways you could possibly help each one. Be creative. Now get out there and do it!

KARMA & LiFE LESSONS

This isn't necessarily a concept we are all raised with, some even think that it's nonsense or just a superstitious belief. But, if you think about the phrase '*What goes around, comes around*', it makes total sense; like common sense. We've even all experienced it on one level or another.

Karma, if you don't know what it is, is a fundamental law that seems to originate and is rooted in Indian philosophies and religions, relating to the consequences of one's actions, words, or deeds. Basically, what you do, say, or create in the world will somehow return to you and bring some type of experience or consequence, whether it be a good or bad, back to you. It all depends on what you put out there. Karma encourages people to seek and live a higher moral life to avoid the negative from coming back into their lives.

Here in the West, we see karma as a fate of some kind. The concept and my consciousness around this, didn't hit me until I was into my late twenties. I never really thought about consequences too much before that. However, at this age, I began to notice that a lot of what I was experiencing in my life, was reflective of what I had done or chosen prior. And it wasn't all good. It became obvious that my past actions were catching up to me.

Also, along with these realizations came some serious life lessons. Life lessons that were not for the weak. Life lessons generally aren't that easy, as we all have lived and learned. But it shows us that, we can get through some of the more challenging times because we're built with the innate ability to do so.

The truth of the matter, was that I had made some choices that weren't in the best interest of myself or others, especially in my teen years. When I started to realize that things were returning back to me, it was clear as day. I knew like I knew, like I knew. It was as though my past was now flashing before my eyes, showing me what I had done previously, and exactly why I was in the predicament that I was in. I couldn't avoid it, and it surely didn't feel good, but I wouldn't have traded it for anything in the world. It forced me to wake up, face my shadows and negative aspects, and it changed my perspective on how I lived life. I walked forward much more conscious of what I said and did, and it's always a work in progress, as it is for any of us.

The truth is, it took me repeatedly doing things over and over again before I realized how my choices were actually affecting my life. Things today show up almost immediately, it's as though our karma is speeding up, wasting no time whatsoever. Once we realize all of this stuff, things seem to amp up. Our good choices and their effects come in way more quickly and frequently, and we create less room for regret or negativity to take hold. Our perception around our choices changes dramatically.

We can all learn how this goes by taking a look at some of the things that have happened in our life, the good and the bad. Perhaps we lost something or something was stolen from us. Perhaps we took something we weren't supposed to or that wasn't ours. The little things we do can build up, and sometimes come back to us in an even bigger way.

I now make my choices more thoughtfully and lovingly, living more truthfully and honestly with myself. I do this of course, for me, but also for others. And it's not *just* because I don't want the negative stuff to come back around to me, but more so because being more conscious around my decisions adds more to my life and it feels better in the long run.

It makes you want to do better in life, make more honorable decisions and do less of the stuff that complicates things or hurts people. As none of us are perfect, we still need to work these aspects of our reality on a daily basis. In truth, we all want to do things that *add* to life or *helps others*, not things that bring in chaos or harm to them or ourselves.

Once we start tuning into how we are creating karma or consequences and feedback in our life, we start making better decisions. We even have some truly eye-opening moments. This universal law of what goes around comes around, in my opinion, it's a law that no one escapes. Not even the world's most terrible, wrong doing folks. Things will eventually catch up to them and come back their way, even if we can't see it initially. Their consequences cannot be held off forever.

Whether or not you believe in karma, I think the idea around it, is a good gauge to live by. Knowing that what we put out there will eventually come back to us, makes a lot of sense. It makes us want to think more closely about the things we do or say before making a decision. We think more closely about what the outcome of our words and actions might be. If we put out love, kindness, and service to others, it will return to us tenfold. If we put out anger, hate, or selfishness, that too will return to us.

If not seen on a spiritual or universal level, then we can think of it on the scientific level where like attracts like. For every action there is an equal and opposite reaction, which is Newtons Law. Everything has an outcome or a reaction.

Deep down, we all have a big heart that just wants the best in life, for both ourselves and others. This outlook, concept, or tool, however you want to see it, is here as an opportunity to help us make better choices and be a better person all around. Life can be more fulfilling because of it. It even helps us honor our life more.

We've all seen the evidence in how something can manifest or take place because we focus on, or speak of something so much. I've seen myself and other people repeat something over and over again, and that thing actually finding its way into culmination. I see it like wishful thinking, of sorts. But did we really want it? We focus so intently on the details of what we *don't* want that almost every time, we get that which we didn't want.

For myself personally, I knew it was vital to reprogram my usual thinking and ways of being in the negative, in order to stop calling the wrong things into my life. For example, when we're always talking about getting sick, it's like, do we really want that?

I've always disliked greatly when people stated something awful like, *"I'm going to have a heart attack… or a stroke"*. I've always thought to myself, *no! Stop with that thought!* I never liked hearing people even joke about things like that. Why set something awful into motion that we don't want? I know, people don't always give power to this, but I'm not sure why they don't. Words are proven to make a difference in things, so unless you really want a heart attack, why say it.

We all do this in some form or another in just about every area of our lives, from our money talk, health dialogue, even with our life events and our everyday goings on. Redirecting our language from the negative to the positive will definitely help shift the outcome. We can change what we say and change our thoughts by replacing them with something we *do* want. Instead of *"I'm always sick"*, we can replace it with, *"my body is healthy and strong."* In the money department, saying things like *"I can't afford it!"* or, *"I don't have enough."* is focusing endlessly on the negative side of our circumstance, which is never what we want to continue. Instead, it makes sense to say, *"I always have enough. I am always provided for."*

Why continue to attract what it is that we don't want. Some people just can't see it this way. They're stuck in a negative cycle or victim mode. They don't believe that they are part of, nor a reason as to why things are happening to them. They're usually stuck in denial, and hold a lack of accountability. Most of us get plenty of signs to help wake us up to things, but some people choose to ignore them, finding it easier to blame something or someone else instead.

In the end, we reap what we sow. We all do. It's time for us to decide what we really want to receive and how we want to continue moving on in our life. At a core level, most of us want positive, good things to come our way. Whether it be good health, love, to have all that we could ever need and want, a peaceful life, peace for others, all of it, we can speak to it and act in a way that reflects wanting those things to happen.

There's no better time than now to take a look at how we're doing in this part of things. To be able to figure out what no longer serves us and how we truly want to exist as a person in the world. To me, it feels easy enough to live by the golden rule to *"Do unto others as you would have them do unto you".* The term karma is an all-encompassing law of the Universe, and excludes no one. What goes around comes around. Let's go live our lives with this is in heart and mind, so we can create a better life for ourselves and others.

LESSONS

Our lessons in this life begin upon conception. We pick up and absorb information, emotion, and energy from within the womb. We learn about trust, how safe our environment is, what it's like (or not like) to be properly cared for, nourished, and loved, all while in the womb. How our mother takes care of herself creates a base for our experience.

When we finally make our way out into the world, we're either in a loving, supportive situation or we may end up in a rougher, more difficult situation. Either one brings in lessons and experiences with it, and our life expectations are formed around that. We learn what life looks like and feels like through our first and earliest experiences.

If our needs are met, we learn that we trust in life and feel secure knowing what it is to be cared for. Our nervous systems are kept calm and balanced and life stays somewhat steady for the most part. If we are neglected or abused, and our needs are *not* met, we will likely learn something along the lines of the world being unsafe, that life is a struggle, and we may end up feeling utterly unworthy, stuck in survival mode. Our nervous system is activated and stressed out.

Our life will be guided by what we learned early on as it is programmed into us, into our subconscious whether we realize it or not. We learn to function from this place, either feeling like we're on survival mode or in a relaxed, peaceful state. Everything that comes our way afterwards, we receive based on our early experiences and handle however we do, because of them.

Either way, whatever we came into the world with, we are more powerful than we realize. The truth is, we are powerful beyond measure regardless of our circumstances. Even those of us who went from one struggle and bad situation to another, we've proven time and time again that we can get through almost anything life throws at us.

And from these lessons, we've grown and changed so much. It's just important that we remember after learning from these lessons that we work on what we want going forward. It's important to start truly looking at what we want our lives to look like in the future and learn how to rebuild ourselves to be someone that is strong and loved regardless of our past.

I understand that not everyone survives their hardships and the truth is, people don't deserve all of the things that happen to them, especially when we're small and helpless little ones. My heart goes out to children and people who are needlessly harmed or mistreated.

There are many of us who *have* made it through some of the most difficult of times, and even though there's likely still work to do, we can ultimately use these experiences to make changes in our lives. Hard as it may be, we want to ensure that we don't have to keep experiencing these hardships the same because of programming and the poor experiences of the past. We can actually accomplish some pretty amazing things because of it.

We can choose not to allow the abuse or trauma that we experienced in the past to rule our entire life and continuously drag us down and hold us back. Instead, we can use it as the fuel we need to help rebuild ourselves, however that may look for us. Though, it does take a lot from us.

We need to work through the issue and the pain around things first, and this isn't necessarily very easy. However, we'll get nowhere if we still hold onto the fear, sadness, and anger behind everything. Of course, this takes time, so it's important that we are patient with ourselves, but as we work through those emotions and birth out the pains of the past, with determination, support, and the belief that we have what it takes to move forward, we can move beyond these limitations. We can turn that which was unhealthy and ugly into something more beautiful and into something we deserve.

Abuse and hard lessons are very challenging to overcome. Many of us learn to dissociate from and push the events or memories away, but in the end, things have a way of showing back up if we don't deal with them. The emotional and mental effects essentially change how we view the world, as well as how we respond to it. We may heal from what someone did, even forgive them, but there could still be a residual effect that interferes with some area or aspect of our lives.

Unfortunately, there are a lot of people who've abused others, who don't always feel remorse. They might never apologize, nor ask for forgiveness. They might be immune to learning the lesson and continue on the same path of harming others. This is unfortunate on many levels. We don't get the apology nor the closure we might feel that we need.

However, from this we might find that the lesson we learn is that we only ever have ourselves, especially when no one is there to listen to us or come to our aid.

The first lesson we can take away from a terrible situation of abuse is that we need to build more loving compassion for ourselves and create some boundaries. We can tune in and talk to ourselves, giving ourselves the recognition that we are still a beautiful, amazing human being regardless of what's someone else has imposed upon us.

Our strength, no matter how hard someone tries to disable and crush it, is always pushing through, even if at times it feels like we've lost it. We never really do. If we hone in on our inner strength, we'll realize that it helps us to hear when the alarm bells are going off- sensing when people around us are untrustworthy and capable of causing us harm. When we recognize the strength that we have, it can give us that extra push of energy to get ourselves out of a situation or away from a scenario or person. It helps us to identify much more easily, people and circumstances that we need to move away from and how to say *no* when we feel so strongly about it. Tuning in to our strength gives us power and in this we will learn how to set new boundaries for ourselves.

We actually gain power, unknowingly, from some of the harder events of the past that seemed to have harmed and hurt us the most. Lisa Nichols, a best-selling author and speaker refers to as the '*Get up*'. It's not about the *what or who* caused us fall down, nor how hard we fell, it's all about the **getting back up** and how we handle things after, or because of the fall.

We can either sit there and wallow in the pain and misery of how or why this happened to us or, we can create a new state of being for ourselves. It can bring in the motivation to do things and see things in a different light. We can look at how the experience and pain we felt brought us into even greater strength than we had noticed in ourselves before. This speaks to just about everything we've been through, right down to our health challenges.

We can decide and declare that we are clearing our slate and starting over in whatever way we choose. In a more wise and compassionate way, we can *use* the energy of the fall to create something greater for ourselves. We can take these events and experiences, learn from them, and create something new and more powerful for ourselves; being the cause of something good to come into our life.

Some of our lessons create the feeling that we can never trust people again. How many of you, as I know I've been there, have felt like you would never be able to trust people again because of how badly someone hurt or betrayed you? Many of us have experienced being hurt by someone more times than we can count. We stay in this place of self-preservation to protect ourselves from things happening to us again, and maybe because of *just one* person who betrayed us.

In this, we close ourselves off and even temporarily lose the ability to connect with people altogether. We end up missing out on all of the good people and the good in the world that *does* exist. The lesson we got from this was how to cut ourselves off.

The hard lessons we learn create our armor, which can absolutely be a good thing on some levels, but we don't want that armor to stop us from experiencing life and all the joy that comes with it.

I believe that, all that we've been through, especially the more difficult of times, is meant to wake us up. To ourselves, to our power, and to help open our eyes to how we exist in the world. These events help push us to greater levels, and help us find our voice, our strength, and our truth. They show up in our lives to help us to access our incredible depth and the wisdom we have within us.

This deeper connection that we end up having with ourselves in light of these lessons, strengthens our instincts and intuition so that we know when to move away from people and situations that insult or negatively impact our health and wellbeing. As our inner connection builds, we become more aware of some of the things that we need to work on clearing out of our life. It gives us better vision to be able to see that we have more power inside of us than we ever realized.

I get that a lot of it's easier said than done, but I'll tell you this much, once we overcome our worst past event or experience, and take our power back, the shift that occurs, is beyond words that can be expressed. It's like going from level one directly up to level ten. The benefits from getting through and out of difficult, painful experiences, and seeing the lessons on the other side of it, are endless.

Our confidence in who we are, increases. It becomes easier for us to speak our truth, as well as speaking up for ourselves and others, much more powerfully. We can finally see that we're our own boss and the creator of what comes into our life next. We get to decide who and what we will, and will not allow into our lives.

We also find a place where we begin caring more deeply about ourselves. A new place of peace within. We have more empathy for ourselves and others, and we find it easier to give more support and good vibes to ourselves and others, just like we deserve to. It's way more worthwhile to be in this state than it is sitting around stuck in victim mode, feeling helpless, or endlessly wallowing in the pain and hurt from the past.

Seeing everything as a lesson only serves us. It helps us to be more aligned with what we desire and want in our life, and to move forward in the best way. We always have the unseen forces to help us get through our lessons, if you believe in God, Source, our Creator, the Divine, guides, angels, or passed away loved ones and ancestors. They are absolutely there to support us and love us especially when we're struggling.

It's useful to look back at different times in our life and try to look at them from an alternate perspective. Do they still have a big impact on us and if they do, how so? Do we sit in fear, worried about that same thing happening again? Are we still stuck in that painful place, still feeling it as though it just happened? Are we feeling like a victim? Where does being in this place affect us in our life? Are we stuck in negative patterns or thought processes because of it? How is it serving us?

Being stuck in this place around any type of issue or problem keeps us trapped. It stops the flow of more of the good things that we need and deserve to have coming into our life. We prevent good people, wonderful experiences, and abundance from coming in. Actually, we may indeed have an abundance of something coming into our life, but is it something that benefits us or something we want? Being stuck and in fear attracts and brings more of the same in along with it. We then find more reasons to stay stuck, in fear, in pain, or as a victim. The Universe will give us more of what we project outwardly.

When we fight against something that has happened to us, we actually keep ourselves strongly connected to it, and is that what we really want? It also makes us use our energy on it rendering us drained and tired, unable to enjoy and do the things that we love. We continue to dance with the memory of something that happened thirty years ago, and for what? What we're not realizing is that we're keeping ourselves chained down to something. Something that causes us pain.

I know it's not easy to deal with some of the things of our past because what happened was just down right horrible. But, to give it the energy to actually continue feeling it still, so enormously so, isn't very fair to us. We need to access it, look at it, and remove it from our conscious and subconscious minds, as best as we can. At least to clear the emotions we have around it.

When we access a painful memory or event of the past, it's important to know that the past event or situation can no longer hurt us, unless we're presently still in something, which is a whole different story. But if it's in our past, we need to, and deserve to, move ourselves out of it so it no longer steals our energy and our joy.

We don't have to relive so much of what happened, we just need to see ourselves in the situation, with eyes of compassion. We can send healing and release to ourselves so we can realize that we're going to be okay. Hec, we already got through it, now we just need to end the chapter. We can create an ending where we end up as the champion with an even stronger soul, who healed themselves and won in the end.

We can even see the scenario in a totally different way, change the movie and how it goes. We can make up new details and occurrences that create a better story and outcome. Kind of like pretending you can travel through time and change things. I know it sounds crazy but the imagination and mind can do some pretty amazing things we wouldn't otherwise expect. There have been studies done around this and the synapses in the brain reconfigure themselves towards that new story, creating it to be as though that was the story that actually took place. A new memory replacing the old.

Any which way we choose, it's important for us to have our own back. To do things to help ourselves heal, move forward, and free ourselves from the chains of the past. Learning the lessons within all of our experiences, always enhances our power. This is how people who have been through some of the worst even things in their lives can move mountains out there in the world. They heal themselves and find their power to be able to help others heal from things that are similar and to find their own power. Sometimes the worst things that happen to us are actually meant to break us open to see the beautiful and unlimited power that we have inside of us, where we would not otherwise have seen it.

Healing through our experiences and learning the lessons from them, brings with it great power. No one can actually take our power away from us in the end, but there is something to reclaiming it that is a beautiful gift.

I feel for everyone who's been through rough, unfortunate, nightmare-like experiences in their life, but if you're here right now reading this, you've already overcome more than half of the battle. Now it's just time to reclaim yourself, your power, and the much deserved, amazing, and good-feeling life that you deserve.

If we see that our lessons can teach us so much more about ourselves, with it will come the discovery of some of our hidden, most amazing gifts and potential. Never underestimate the power of a lesson. It's time we start using them to our advantage.

HOMEWORK:

1. What life lessons have you had that have made you grown?
2. Have you ever noticed something coming back around to you (karma)?
3. How can you take your 2 most difficult lessons in life and use them for your growth and transformation?

LETTiNG GO & FORGiVENESS

When you forgive, you heal, and when you let go, you grow.

We all know there are times that letting go of things isn't easy. Just talking about learning lessons was an eye opener about letting go of the past to learn from them. Letting go of certain events, memories, and experiences can certainly be a challenge, however, we know that some of it is so very necessary.

There's an enormous benefit to letting go of things that we hold onto that no longer serve us. The things that we no longer need or cause disruption in our lives and they aren't just past events or traumas, there's tons of other stuff that we hold onto that isn't healthy for us to keep.

Letting go can look like a lot of things. We can let go of objects, people, ideas, beliefs, events, feelings, situations, habits, whatever we can think of, most everything can be let go of to one degree or another. Whatever it is, if we feel its presence in our lives in one way or another, can be let go.

Certainly, not everything in our lives needs to be let go, nor should it be. However, if something is causing significant discomfort and strife for us, wavering into and out of our lives, it may serve us and be necessary to release it. Sometimes we hold onto something so tightly, that we don't realize just how much of a hold it has on us or how it's affecting our world.

There are many meaningful items and memories of the past that are good to keep around and hang onto. Things that are sentimental to us, that bring us happiness, and still add to our life. Things that elevate us are usually the things that are worth keeping and holding onto. This includes beliefs that we have, people, cherished items we keep, as well as values that we know help us and guide us in a positive direction through life.

Sometimes, not everything that we've held onto, such as our beliefs and values, are as beneficial for us as they once were. Many of us hold onto religious or cultural beliefs because they were ingrained into us. However, as we get older, some may no longer resonate with the path we're choosing to take and no longer fit into the world we are creating for ourselves.

As an example, I was raised Roman Catholic and felt strongly about letting go of some of their thought processes, particularly their shame and guilt mentality, so I could follow a more loving and heart-centered path in my life. I took the things from within it that resonated with me, and left what didn't.

Some of us carry with us a lot of heavy, negative stuff or we keep things that are a total drain in our life, without even realizing it. We hold onto things for a variety of reasons however, this heavy, cumbersome stuff can really take a toll on us. We generally aren't even fully aware of this being the case, as we don't necessarily associate thought processes or a few objects that we have lying around, to be the cause of any heaviness in our life. Some of these things can literally drain and stress us out endlessly, yet we have no clue as to why we might be feeling that way.

Things, situations, and people can keep us feeling down, stuck, or unable to get ahead. We're often unaware that certain things are unhealthy for us and can drain our energy. Objects, people, obligations, jobs, or even a past experience can all cause shifts in our energy and emotions.

Not only does holding onto these negative things drain us, they spill out into other areas of our life, including our health. We don't realize just how much our health can be affected by the things, situations, or even people that we hold onto. These can also hold us back from our growth and movement forward, or can cause a lot of chaos and discomfort in our life. One argument or experience that we have and hold onto, can rule our entire way of life without our awareness.

We might not see it or recognize it now, but as we get older and wiser, things start to show themselves much more obviously. We come to realize that a lot of the stuff that we've been holding onto wasn't necessarily a good idea to keep around, nor is it working towards our benefit to be holding onto.

The things we hold onto can often times cause a vague, uneasy feeling, or worse case, cause issues to erupt in our lives. We go from one bump in the road to the next, feeling like it must be us, that it's our fault something is happening, or sometimes, that life is unfair. The truth of it is that, yes, part of it *is* us, but not because we're a magnet for these things that are happening, and certainly not because we want it, but because we've held onto something so tightly without even being aware. Things that can indirectly affect our life on so many levels.

We might realize that something that we've been holding onto has a negative effect on us and doesn't feel good to have around, but we hold on for dear life because of one reason or another. This can be stuff, a grudge, a person, or just something that happened to us. A lot of us have a fear of releasing something or someone thinking it serves us to keep it, maybe even feeling bad if we let go of things, not knowing that its actually causing us more harm than good.

Maybe somewhere along the way, we were led to believe that we can't let it go, or that we needed it in our lives for one reason or another. We may keep it as a reminder of the wrongdoing or broken promise that we experienced, so it can never happen again. We might hold onto things out of guilt or fear of the consequences that we believe will come if we do, so we keep holding on.

Many of us learn to live with the heaviness, anxiety, or depression that goes along with keeping these things around, again being unaware of the fact that we are adding more stress to our lives. We don't realize the extra weight that we carry because of it.

The thing is, as humans, we've almost been taught to be attached to things. We have a difficult time letting go, in general. We've learned to attach ourselves to different ideas, experiences, thought processes, material items, beliefs, and of course, people. We end up forming an emotional bond with whatever it is we feel attached to. Unfortunately, this bond doesn't always feed us on a positive level, as it can create feelings of insecurity or fear, and grow into a very, unhealthy dependency.

Most of us have held onto at least one object or item that holds special meaning to us. We cherish an heirloom, something special that was given to us, or an item that holds sentimental value because it reminds us of someone, or a time in our life that brings us good feelings. It can definitely be something that nourishes and comforts us, adding to our lives. This is a positive expression of holding onto something.

It's pretty common to feel as though it's hard to let go of things, however, some people hold onto just about anything and everything. They don't just keep one or two special things, they keep *all the things*. Whether it be old clothing, a piece of mail, an event, a feeling, an experience, or some type of material object, they feel the need to hold onto all of it.

Something about getting rid of stuff feels scary and uneasy for them. There are usually reasons attached to why they feel that way. Generally, it's based on fear, maybe something might have happened in the past, it could be a way that they learned, or a combination of things that occurred in their life.

Sometimes we hold onto something because we paid for it and we don't want to have *wasted* our money. We see getting rid of things as throwing our money away, or that if we do get rid of something, we'll regret it and never be able to get back the value that we put into it.

We've all held onto things because they still work or we think we might need them later on, and we consider them valuable. We keep things because we believe that it might be worth more money later on, which may or may not be true. If it's something that can hold value, or is a rare item that could be worth a lot a few decades down the line, then this is understandable.

As this can be true for some things, there are people out there who believe this in just about everything they own. Surely, there's a collectible or two in the mix that might be worth holding onto, but chances are that some, or a lot of what they're holding onto, may never end up worth much, nor looked at again. There are tons of people who have storage units full of stuff they no longer need or use, just sitting there collecting dust.

Keeping things that are useful, is by all means still a good idea. We're not going to get rid of the only hammer or cooking pot that we have, or our favorite childhood book from forty years ago. But, it's about all the other stuff. The knick-knacks, the endless mug collection, the old, ragged stuffed animals in a bag in the attic, all of the old mail from the last forty years, the empty boxes for every purchase we made, the baggies we saved from every bag of bread we ever bought, the old, broken things that will never be used again. It's that stuff. That stuff is what clogs up and congests so many people's lives, even causing mental and physical issues, and they're totally unaware of it.

The kind of stuff that's likely no longer useful that just hangs out taking up energy and space, can often times can overcrowd the actual space that we live in. This is where the intrusion of *stuff* begins. When we are overwhelmed with so much stuff, and let's face it, people even keep garbage laying around, it creates a heavy, stagnant, stuck energy that affects them, with each and every passing day that goes by.

This is very much where things need to be addressed. The people doing this don't realize just how much this collection of stuff has on creating negativity and burden in their life. They don't see just how deeply it interferes with their life on so many levels, and it can absolutely have a negative impact on them, even on their health.

Energetically, an overwhelm of stuff can make our life more difficult. Being dead set on not letting go of certain things (or everything) can create stress that we're completely unaware of. We may find ourselves sick more often, depressed, mentally unstable, unhappy, and unable to cope with some of the situations that life brings our way.

Granted stuff isn't always necessarily the sole cause of all that's happening in our lives, as obviously there are many reasons for things. However, the accumulation of stuff can absolutely cause an energetic drain, mental stress, and a huge imbalance in our lives. The amount of stuff we have can impose a lot of stress on us, without our conscious awareness of it doing so. Being surrounded by loads of stuff gets in the way of living a clean, healthy existence. The accumulation can weigh us down.

It usually gets to a point that we're so overwhelmed by all of the stuff, that we begin to dissociate from it and disconnect from the reality surrounding it. We begin ignoring things and render ourselves *okay* with how things are, when in truth we're not actually comfortable with it. This undoubtedly affects our mental and emotional state, as well as our nervous system, immune system, and overall state of physical health.

I've had a patient, or ten (when working in home health and hospice) tell me that the clutter and overwhelm had a way of comforting them. Some people prefer to have stuff around them so they don't feel so alone, and this is sometimes seen after the loss of a loved one or partner. The clutter feels almost serves as a safety net and comfort for them.

Although this is quite unhealthy, it's not hard to understand the reasoning and emotional need behind it. Some people grew up with clutter and know nothing but that. Others who grew up without much and lived in a survival state, may have a hard time letting go of things because they feel they were finally able to obtain and own things that they never had before, so as adults they don't want to let them go.

With others, clutter and a collection of stuff can exist because they actually don't care about themselves, their home, their life, and often times suffer from mental health issues such as depression or dissociation, which causes them to ignore it. They may not know how to take care of themselves, keep a home, or maintain a balanced, healthy, stable life for themselves.

In turn, these people learn to exist with an overwhelmed energy, both physically and energetically, sometimes even keeping literal garbage laying around. We've all heard of people who hoard, we might even know someone, and there's even a TV show about it. There are some very extreme cases, although it's becoming more common these days than we realize. Serious clutter that also contains garbage, becomes toxic and is undoubtedly harmful to the person physically, mentally, and emotionally. They remain unaware and disconnected, which is utterly heart-breaking for any human being.

One can hope that they may have an epiphany or something that happens that shows them the light, somewhat granting them permission to move out of being in that space, but most often times, that does not happen. They might have grown up in a home that was dirty and unkempt and are just so used to it, but even if we grew up with this mess, there comes a time when we need to honor ourselves and decide what's good for us and what isn't. Again, this is not easy for people who've lived fifty plus years this way. People in this sort of position need help and assistance to work their way out of it.

And I get that it's not that easy for everyone. It's a hard, long road ahead for a lot of people who live like this. These people who are in dire straits absolutely need some form of help, including mental and emotional healing work so that they can overcome the reason behind why they've allowed this into their lives. If it's left up to them, chances are, not much is going to change. They likely lack the personal strength, or perhaps the awareness *of* their strength, and their ability to do it without assistance.

When over-crowding and uncleanliness gets out of hand, it's not uncommon for depression or anxiety to kick in, as well as a host of physical health problems, if it hasn't already been an issue. When this is happening to someone, their sense of self becomes harder to acknowledge. They lose themselves in the overwhelming clutter and have a difficult time processing the reality around them. Mentally, there is a great suffering occurring.

People who have tons of stuff sitting around in their life might have some form of poverty consciousness happening. They might feel scared of going without. Having broken items or garbage around, is better than having nothing at all. Poverty thinking is most likely created early on, through and during our upbringing, (or it can happen at a later time in our life, as well).

How our parents or guardians took care of money and material items they owned, the statements they made around money or having enough, the value they held around money or material objects, and their overall mindset that they projected outward, all affects us as we move through our life.

We may even have had everything we could have ever needed, but suddenly lost it all due to some type of circumstance or situation. This loss would absolutely change a person. It would likely throw us into fear and scarcity mode, creating a new, fear-based, negative consciousness around money or having enough.

Although, it's easier said than done, this needs to be shifted soon after it happens so as to not to forge a new pathway with this mentality in mind. I know it's unrealistic as things don't happen as perfectly as we would wish, receiving help and support early on would save us from a future of deep depression and the inability to survive on our own.

Holding onto clutter, especially in our homes, is greatly detrimental to our physical health, and emotional and mental stability. I've known a lot of people who have suffered from keeping things; they have clutter everywhere and seem to experience many difficulties in their life. It's as though something is always going wrong, they're always unhappy, and their home literally feels like an energy drain hole.

Having too much clutter causes unnecessary turmoil in our life even creating issues in our personal relationships. The people who hold onto the clutter often complain about how much of a struggle their life is, when maybe all they need to do is let some things go.

This brings us to another area of letting go that needs attention. The stories we hold onto. Those old stories that we live by as though they're still happening in the present. The ones that shape how we see life and our existence and that affect how we think, feel, act, or live our life.

We've all held onto different stories and situations, good and bad, holding on out of joy, pain, or fear. The unhealthier stories we hold onto are usually around some type of pain we encountered from an event, trauma, loss, or because of something someone did to us. Sometimes it's even something we did to ourselves. We find ourselves constantly repeating this story to the people we meet, even to ourselves, telling it over and over again, and using it as a reason for our behavior or way of being in the world. We might even hold onto a mistake that *we* made to ensure we never make the same mistake again, or even as a form of self-punishment.

We can play a story over and over again, as if it just happened yesterday, keeping it alive and present. Sometimes, we even make it a daily habitual thing we use in one form or another, believing it to be to our advantage. Our mind gets stuck in a loop and it overwhelms a lot of our thoughts and feelings. We might use it as a form of protection, or we can use it to gain something, as some of our stories may bring us some sort of attention.

We might feel we deserve the attention or sympathy, or maybe we just desire other people's energy and concern. We use it to what we believe is to our benefit, but of course, that's not always the case, sometimes it attracts the not so good to us.

Sometimes we hold onto stories in order to have an excuse to stay locked in victim mode. Unfortunately, some people seem to love living in victim mode, they believe it serves them. They use their painful stories to grab the attention that they seek sometimes getting others to help them because of it.

They realize that when others feel bad for them, they get more of what they want, and the more they talk about it, the more attention that comes their way. Their focus sits on how sad or terrible it was for them and they try to ease things for themselves through external means. Unfortunately, this doesn't always end up well for them, especially when they use a situation or past hurt to their benefit.

Soon enough, the people around them grow tired of it and they not only lose people in their life, their story no longer serves them. They then go out looking for a new story to work for them, as I'm sure we've all known people like this.

We can become obsessive to a point. Obsessed with holding onto something we view as helpful or that renders us some form of satisfaction, but unfortunately, it's not always a healthy thing as we've been saying. Holding onto something like a painful story or situation can end up leading to mental health issues and illnesses.

It's understandable that sometimes when something or someone *has* ruined a part of our life, that we may have a hard time moving passed it and letting it go, but undoubtedly, we need to move on, get the lesson, and do some very necessary healing around it.

There's never room to make light of anyone's traumatic or life-altering events, nor their experiences or present state of being because of them. We cannot force someone to get over something and let it go of it, just like that.

I'm sure we can all relate. I've definitely been there, stuck in victim mode, depressed, blaming someone for ruining my life with what they did, allowing it to affect my life for a long time, and never for the better. I get that there are some serious life ruining events that feel like something we can never fully recover from. Especially in the instance of losing our innocence in one form or another as a child, or if we encounter a terrible loss that cannot be understood.

How do we then let go of such things? Especially when there is nothing we can do about it, and it affects every aspect of our existence. Sometimes it's so hard to let go of such a loss or difficult betrayal. In these types of circumstances, especially when things happen to us as children, we generally bury those memories deep down, or we forever live feeling like a victim, unsafe, and unable to trust people.

A lot of times these memories are buried so deeply into our subconscious, that we don't even realize that we're functioning from that place or how strongly it's affecting our lives. We just exist believing that it's who we are and how we live. Fear always lingering in the background.

It's extremely important for us to move into an awareness and the feeling that we *want* to make a change, even if we feel like it's near impossible to do so, and that there's no way we can do it alone. Without that agreement, there can be little to no progress made, nor the ability to receive the help we need.

However, when we decide that we're tired of living that way, usually an overwhelm of emotion comes up. It might be all of the sad issues and depressing situations that we've been avoiding. We will likely need a lot of help getting through those emotional issues.

We may experience a strong feeling of relief, which can help us to start moving out of the unhealthy place that we're in. The decision and acknowledgement that we need help and our desire to be free from the heaviness will make it easier to work through. It gives us the permission that we need in order to move ahead. We end up feeling lighter, less burdened, and finally have the room to let go.

Hands down, we can get help from others to process through things, clear things we no longer need, out, so getting a therapist or coach to help us get through releasing and letting go of things can be such a blessing for us. Ultimately, we don't want to be stuck with something and carry it around like it's the weight of the world on our shoulders for the rest of our lives.

When need to find a surrender moment in there somewhere, so we can create a calmer environment for our nervous system and our mental health. One where we to come to realize that it's not healthy to hold onto this thing that's been weighing down on us, anymore. So, we can let go more freely and openly.

I know from experience, that it does take time to get through letting go of something that's been difficult to release, so patience with ourselves is so important. The desire of wanting to be free will alone be the spark that we need to push us forward. The emotions behind it give us the extra energy we need in order to help release it from our life.

Yes, letting go of some type of traumatic experience is no walk in the park, however, it doesn't have to stay so painful.

The long-term effects of holding onto things keeps us held back, and greatly robs us of many parts of ourselves. It interferes with our vision of the beautiful life that we want and deserve. It messes with our perception and how we respond to things that aren't even related to the situation. It's an entanglement that latches on to other areas and aspects of our life.

We can make the decision to move on and find our way to let go of something at any point in time. At whatever moment we so choose, we can decide that we're done holding onto this thing. It's quite empowering to declare that we no longer will allow this situation or stuff to keep a hold on us. Doing this creates a new neural pathway in our brain, helping to realign our thinking and perception towards what we *actually* want, instead.

Our brain will then move onto that pathway more often, no longer connecting itself to the more limited, fear-based one we've been having. The old neural pathway will no longer be used. We can do this with all of the events and the reasons why we hold onto things. Things will indeed be so much easier to release.

Our whole life can change through declaration especially accompanied by confidence in that which we declare. If we're done with feeling pain over something someone did, we can declare this. *"I will no longer allow this to affect my life. I am healed and this event no longer has a hold on me. My life is blessed and I walk forward with a new sense of freedom and in love with my life."*

Our vision gets clearer as we start deciding what it is that we want our life to look like. We can even see our gifts and passions more clearly. So much shows up for us when we decide to release and let go of things that no longer serve us.

All we have to do is stand firm in our decision to let go of the object, event, or story and declare our freedom from it. It gets easier to do this over time with just about everything that comes up.

We'll soon find that stuff we didn't even know was there, shows up to be released. Once we set things in motion, we might find that we needed to process much more than we thought and we realize, better out than in.

Because all of the little things together can take up big energy in our lives.

Sometimes we might feel like we're going backwards, emotions flare up, things aren't looking as bright as we thought, but it's all just a part of the journey. We just need to keep forging ahead because the benefit outweighs those momentary setbacks. Things will absolutely change and shift in our life, for the better.

We'll naturally stop allowing things to accumulate in our lives, whether it be objects, stories, experiences, or negative people that we do not need. We gain a new sense of strength and find ourselves naturally evolving into a more powerful and peaceful human being. We find and connect back into our truth, who we really are, and into the amazing strength that we've always had within.

Letting go opens us up to a much happier, peaceful existence. We aren't here to hold onto things and limit ourselves and our potential. We're here to be the best version of ourselves. Ultimately, nothing should stop us from living our best life. Nothing.

Remember that holding onto something like a grudge, only ever hurts us. We're the ones continuously experiencing the pain and negative emotions, keeping us in an alarmed state of being.

We can start by shedding some layers of our life and donate a few boxes worth of stuff to our local shelter or thrift store. Things don't have to be thrown away altogether, someone else may find good use for our things and feel so grateful to have them. We are adding to the benefit of others by releasing and letting things go.

Getting rid of boxes worth of stuff creates room for the new; new items, new blessings, or whatever else wants to come in. People don't realize the blockage and cutting off of abundance that happens from holding onto stuff. It can literally act as a barricade to our being able to receive the things that need to come into our life. When we release something, there's a new opening and opportunity to receive. Circulating our stuff and letting go of the excess, only opens us up for the arrival of new blessings and things to come our way.

I'd rather breathe easy, feel at peace, let go, and know that I'll always be okay, than to live in constant stress mode. Seeing life through this new lens helps us to gain perspective and insight into creating a better future for ourselves. Letting go opens up new doorways that would have otherwise stayed shut. It invites in new experiences and opportunities. It brings freedom into our lives.

FORGIVENESS

In order to let go, we need forgiveness, and forgiveness is a gift that we give to ourselves.

However, forgiveness does not always prove to be easy, nor does it even at certain points, seem realistic or possible. Especially, when we are deeply hurt by something or someone, it's not so easy to do, at least not in the beginning.

Sometimes it takes years for us to even consider it, let alone work on doing it. Though, as we begin to ease ourselves into considering and doing it more often, we realize the beautiful wisdom and healing within it. Our willingness grows.

It's easy to start with the little things, like forgiving the guy who cut us off on the road or the person at the cashier who's holding up the line. Although these can even be somewhat of a challenge, they are in truth, the smaller things to work through. It's an easy way to start if we're someone who has difficulty forgiving. It also gives us insight at just how well we do with it.

Of course, the biggest thing to remember is that forgiveness is never allowing or excusing the bad behavior of others. It's never saying that something was ok that obviously was *not*. However, what forgiveness does do, is it frees us from the huge burden that we carry, the one we've taken on because of someone else's actions.

We've all likely done a thing or two in our lives that required someone's forgiveness, as none of us are perfect. As we get older, we understand more clearly that there is an effect or consequence to every one of our actions, be it good or bad. We learn from our mistakes and (hopefully) move forward making better choices.

We understand that what we do and say affects others. As we learn some pretty hard lessons through our life, we do our best to learn from them and choose more kind and loving actions. We understand things on a deeper level, and we certainly don't want to attract unnecessary karma or situations down the line.

Forgiveness allows us to free ourselves from being trapped in continuous cycles of stressful, unhealthy emotions. When we're stuck in one of these cycles, we tend to blame our emotions and troubles on another person or situation. In this, we give our power away. We give it over to something that frankly, doesn't deserve our attention or energy.

In the end, we're the ones who suffer when we hold onto a grudge, not the other person. Keeping a hold of something we refuse to forgive only makes it more difficult to deal with as time goes on. When we hold onto something that's from way in the past, we don't realize just how heavily it's been affecting and draining us for all those years.

Forgiveness is something that we do for ourselves. We realize that we are only hurting ourselves because of what it is we refuse to forgive, let go of, and move on from. When we forgive, we give ourselves permission to no longer hold onto the pain and feelings of the past. We learn that we can break free from the chains, and no longer need to be bound by them again.

Within forgiveness, we are honoring ourselves. We're allowing the room for more good things to come into our life and for new, wonderful things to happen. The gift is in the releasing of the heavy weight, the anger, hurt, or sadness we've been carrying around, allowing a space for so much more to open up to us.

The red flags, signals, and warning signs that come, as they usually do, are much easier to see and catch. We build more trust in ourselves through forgiveness. We find that it's gets easier to stop allowing people and situations to come into our life that in the end, will need our forgiveness.

We have more clarity, confidence, and assurance in ourselves to make better choices whether it be in situations and circumstances, or in the people that we let into our lives. Forgiveness strengthens our mind, emotions, and our senses. We are stronger in our vision and our insight.

Of course, life around us is not always in our control, so there's still room for things or people to insult or harm us. However, our heightened awareness can cause us to respond more quickly and in our favor. We can get out of a situation with more speed and ease.

Having a connection with God, our Creator, the Divine, our ancestors, passed away loved ones is powerful, if you believe in them. We can always ask for their support. Often times forgiveness can feel too difficult to get through on our own. This can be our first line of support especially because it's available to us so instantaneously.

Working with a therapist, is familiar route that people will take to process and talk about forgiving and letting go of something, or for some of us, confiding in a loved one or friend is the most helpful. Talking to others about things, helps us to work through more of what happened, work out our emotions that are trapped behind it, and to see all of the setbacks we've had because of it.

We can also figure out different ways to release, detach, and forgive, as well as create some plans and goals for ourselves once things clear out. There are always people in the world who can be there to assist us on one level or another. We can work to close that chapter so another one can begin.

Forgiveness, of course, comes with a bit of work on our part. We do have to make our way through whatever it is that's binding us in order to get to the other side of it. We need to figure out where our emotions are and set ourselves up for where we *want* to be. We can proactively use affirmations, visualizations, prayer, meditation, and other methods to help us realign ourselves and move into a new perspective.

Moving on requires that the event or situation has been completed, and no longer affects us. This means it no longer stirs up the emotions and even better, we don't think about it anymore. If something still affects us, it's still got a bit of a hold on us so chances are, we need to work on some other level of forgiveness. Sometimes we actually have to forgive *ourselves* in these situations.

A lot of us have issues forgiving ourselves for things. I know this one all too well. When there is nothing we can do to change what we may have caused or done, it's hard to ever forgive ourselves fully. We know we cannot change what happened, what we did, or how everything went down because of it, but we'll never live a free, healthy, peaceful existence if we're holding onto something that we did in the past. It can actually show up as a health issue or disease process if we hold onto it long enough.

We're never excusing what we did or what was done, we're just no longer allowing things of the past to swallow up our energy, mental health, or entire life. We honestly learn so much through all of these experiences and though forgiveness, we grow immensely.

We can realize the impact everything caused, feel the all of the emotions, and change ourselves because of it. It's okay to forgive and move on. There's no way to become the more beautiful, powerful version of ourselves that we need to if we're busy holding onto the pain of the past.

We are not our past. We do not have to allow it to control our every moment and future ahead of us. We are not what someone else did and we certainly don't have to allow our lives to be controlled by it. If we choose to hold onto the feelings of disappointment, guilt, shame, anger, and distrust, and allow our past troubles, pains, and traumas to control our life what good does that do for us, or anyone else for that matter?

Moving on and into a better version of ourselves will help us to attract more good in our lives. Once we see how good it feels to let go, forgive, and move on, we start experiencing less that requires our forgiveness.

It's only ever good to get through and release the stuff of the past. Move it out, forgive it and let it go. It's no longer serving us, we learned our lesson, now it's time to move on.

The reward in doing this, is beautiful.

We can learn how to allow things to come to the surface so they can be looked at, forgiven, and healed. We just need to be patient with ourselves and know that some things need and take more time than others. Forgiveness doesn't happen overnight.

Working through things can be done simply by using prayers or meditation, or we can even work on it while doing chores or exercising. We can intend to help move through forgiveness even while we're asleep as our subconscious mind does a lot of work while we're sleeping. You'll be surprised at just how much we can resolve in our allowance. Little by little, things will begin to transform, and we will begin to notice the profound affect forgiving has on all aspects of our life.

Everything happens in the perfect time, space, and sequence. As soon as we give ourselves permission to process, let go of, and forgive all the stuff we've been holding onto, we'll feel a freedom like we've never felt before.

HOMEWORK:

1. What are some things that you absolutely have a difficult time letting go of? What objects or material items? Is your life overcrowded with *stuff* on some level?

2. What events, circumstances, or stories do you continue to talk about and hang onto. Ones that are continuously causing you to relive those times. What part of you feels like you need to keep them? What is it doing to serve you?

3. What do you desire to let go of? What do you want to finally forgive and end in your life?

4. How do you want to feel in comparison to how you feel presently keeping a hold of these events, things, or people in your life?

5. How do you think your life change for the better if you let go of and forgave some events and people in your life? How can you begin to create the space for yourself to do this?

FiNDiNG yOUR BALANCE

Sometimes we fall out of sync. Things are going on in our life and we forget to spend time taking care of all the areas of our life that we need to. We might have lost sight of a couple of them, even downright neglecting some.

Deep down we know that we would benefit from changing a thing or two in our life to give more room to the areas that we know we're neglecting, but we just keep doing the same thing, and those areas and things are left unchecked.

Life gets overwhelming sometimes and not everything is *as important* as the others. We might even give more of our energy and time to other people, more so than we give to ourselves, so we might find ourselves forgetting about different parts of our lives that need our attention.

Truthfully, deep down, we want to create a better balance in our lives, we don't want to be neglecting anything. We can actually feel the results of the neglect, and some of it doesn't feel good. It might even pain us and we might be reminded of it all day, every day. But we're so overwhelmed that's it's difficult to find our way back around to get things back in order and cared for.

I'm sure we all know that instead of us waiting for things to fall apart and keep crumbling, it's better to get on top of things sooner than later, if we can. We've usually had the same ones falling to the wayside, for the most part. Usually having the same struggles in those areas for a long time, or maybe not, and they're new for us. Whatever the case, we just can't seem to get a hold of things well enough to add to, or change the things we need to.

There are reasons behind why we struggle more in one area, than we do in another. We learned about all the different areas of life through our upbringing, our schooling, and whatever social, cultural, religious situations we found ourselves in. Much of what we learn from others molds our perspective, the way we do things, and how we handle things throughout our life.

As we get older, we definitely learn to change and alter how we think and behave around all of these areas through watching what other people do that we might also like to do for ourselves. As we get older we gain new insight and perspective on certain things, which can help us on many levels, but we might still ignore certain parts and areas altogether.

When we allow one or two areas in our life to become neglected, we'll notice that it affects many other areas of our life. There can be some unwanted and negative effects that occur because of our neglecting things, that we otherwise didn't really want. For example, we might allow our attention to self-care and our health to fall to the side. Suddenly, we find ourselves feeling discomfort in some part of our body, a health issue arises, and suddenly we find ourselves hitting a wall. We end up in a very challenging place, now faced with the reality that we need to spend *even more* time taking care of things. Now we need to put more energy and work into healing our body and getting our health back into a good place, so our career and the time we spend with our friends begins to take a hit.

The walls we hit in any of the areas of our life are just telling us that they need more of our time, attention, and assistance. That we're out of balance. If our health is having an issue, it might turn out that we're being the least conscious in that area, hence the problems. We may be inflicting more harm on ourselves in an area, like if our finances are weak, it might be because we always we sit around and dwell on the lack of money, and the fear of never having enough. Or we're busy using our money more than we spend time making it.

Perhaps the time and energy we *do* spend on some these areas is are negative and unhealthy ways. We might truly need to change the way we're spending our time, thinking, and energy on these areas, and could really use some help in shifting things around. We might need to change our perspective and what we believe is best for these areas of our life.

The truth is, deep down we are capable and strong enough, no matter who we are, to be able to take care of all of these areas well enough and maintain a good balance. When some of them are out of balance we find ourselves *unable to take care of everything,* which renders us feeling incapable and doubtful of ourselves, creating nothing but more stress on ourselves.

Being out balance can cause our mind to scatter, because the imbalances are busy pulling our attention in all kinds of directions. We struggle with negative self-talk about how much we're failing at maintaining one area which consumes even more of our energy, causing us to neglect other aspects of our life that might have otherwise been doing well.

It becomes a vicious cycle, back and forth as the imbalance is yet again, pulling other areas out of whack. We're too busy dealing with negative, limiting thoughts and putting out fires to deal with maintaining the good things that are going on.

If only there was a tool or reminder that could help us to keep our attention on all of the areas of our life so we can work on them equally. Having a tool can help us look at all of the areas of our life and make the adjustments that we need to, and help us pay attention, checking in on things before they fall off track.

In my early twenties, while in my holistic, nutritional schooling, I was shown a diagram that was designed to help a person do this exact thing. A diagram that helps you look at your life, all of its aspects, and how well balanced everything is. This diagram gave good insight into each area of my life personally, and just how well I was doing.

It was a pie chart called the 'Wheel of Life', from the book *Business Mastery,* by Cherie Sohnen-Moe. Throughout the last twenty-five years, I've seen it being used in many places by coaches, teachers, in workshops, and classes. It's become a popular way to give perspective on all of the areas of our life; where we're thriving and where we're lacking.

Needless to say, I was inspired by it, but I was also in shock at how out of balance things were for me. It was totally eye-opening. I saw how much I was neglecting different areas of my life and where most of my attention was going. Needless to say, it helped me figure out where I needed to add my energy, and I was soon on my way to working on things. I tried to bring the balance back to every category by spending a little extra time on the ones that I neglected the most.

The categories aren't all fixable with physical, material means, as you might imagine. There is quite a bit of mental and emotional work that goes into working on these categories. Why we neglect our health may be more than food deep. So, it's important to take our time and be gentle with ourselves while working on things.

No matter what, we need to commit ourself to ourself. As long as we work on things gradually, taking the baby steps that are needed, we can keep working on things and make progress no matter what. Eventually we'll find that the balance has returned to us and our life becomes much easier to maintain.

The pie chart contains 8 sections: Relationships, Home Environment, Spirituality, Social Life, Joy, Health, Career, Creativity, Finances, and Education.

Let's take education as an example. If we are someone who does the 9-5 and come home to the TV (which we have all been there at some point) then likely, we aren't giving any of our energy over to learning something new (unless we watch educational content). And I mean something *we want* to learn about, not just what we get at our job. It's easier to learn things these days, because we don't necessarily have to go to school to learn about something. We can get a book on it, listen to information online, watch a video, do some of our own research, even take a class online or in person. There are so many avenues available for us to use and access to strengthen that area.

Basically, we can create new goals for ourselves in each of the areas and set ourselves up for more empowering outcomes. It helps to try and incorporate as much goodness, lightness and fun into things as we can, while we work though helping ourselves spend more time and attention on the things that we need to.

This chart is a great way to take note of where we're at, as it gives us a wholistic overview of things. It can highlight the areas we're totally overlooking and neglecting, opening up our awareness so that we can create the energy behind whatever it is, that we need to do. We can see and really take a look at what needs our immediate attention, as well as how well we're actually doing in certain areas of our life. It's a great tool that helps us acknowledge where we're at. We can give ourselves some kudos for that which we *are* doing well in our world. It's so important that we are kind to ourselves even on the areas that we've been neglecting so that we can stay positive about making the changes that we need to.

We'll soon find ourselves doing extra things in each of the areas, dedicating more attention and spending additional time contemplating the reasons why things may be out of balance. This only helps us to take on and manage the parts of our life that need us the most.

You can absolutely adjust the pie chart categories to resonate with you more, even creating your own. The example below, is just an adjustment of the original.

You might notice that each piece of the pie has a few categories within it, so if you wanted to, you could even divide the pie chart into more sections. The ones that go together can often times be worked on as a whole, but this is totally up to you. You get to design and formulate it in whatever way works for you.

I'll use the 'Wealth, Abundance, Finance' pie piece as an example. On the original chart, which was in fact more, simple, it just stated '*Finances*' on that slice. Back when I used this simpler version, I was surely in a different head space at twenty-three, perhaps a bit clueless even. Having the category say '*finances*' was enough to help me to look at where I was with my money and how it was circulating in my life. Basically, my income, bills, and spending habits.

However now, twenty plus years later, things aren't quite as simple, or I don't see things in the same way altogether. Although income, bills, and money circulating are still a major part of this category, my ideas around money and finance began to translate into wealth, abundance, and the movement of energy.

How I see my wealth, my feelings around wealth and wealthy people, my relationship with money, the abundance in my life, and what that all means, has transformed over the years. In my eyes, abundance is a state of having more than enough, so it's good to look at what we are getting an abundance of, and where we're going without.

Also, we can make a hefty salary, but if we have an unhealthy relationship around money, we might spend it all foolishly, gamble it away, and lose it all too quickly. It's important to know the thoughts and ideas that we carry around each area and work on realigning them as per what we actually want in our life. We need to start speaking into practice that which we want to see.

We can certainly use some affirmations when things aren't as great as we want them to be. As an example, on the finances or money category, we can say something like "Money loves me. I am a money magnet. Money circulates through my life. I always have enough money. I am abundant. I always have all that I need." This is part of how we can work on the area, incorporating whatever resonates with us as we work on things.

We may certainly have to change a few things. Letting go of the past is always helpful so we can release any old concepts or patterns that no longer serve us. We can reconfigure our mindset and transform our belief system around whatever category we're focused on and what it means to us. Release, reset, and realign. Or, we can keep everything the same and stay stuck struggling to find a way to help ourself.

Gratitude comes in handy with all of this as well. Being grateful for the health that we *do* have, the money that we *do* have, or whatever it is we do have is just as important as focusing on the lack of things. Stating what we're grateful for, in even the weaker areas and categories we have, has an empowering effect and boosts those areas towards getting stronger.

When using this chart, we mark a dot on the pie piece according to how strong or weak we are in that area. Either we're saying, yes, we spend a good amount of time and energy on that area of our life and it's thriving, or, we're saying, nah, we even forgot it existed until now, and we barely ever look at it.

For the areas that we give more time and energy to, we mark our dot closer to the outside of the circle (more expansive). For those areas that we neglect, where we are much weaker with our time and attention, the closer in towards the center of the circle the dot will go.

So, now's it's time to grab a pencil and start thinking about how you're doing in each area of your life. After you figure all of that out, you can start making some plans and goals for each of the areas that need more of your loving attention.

It's important to try and find a way to enjoy doing it, and not to beat yourself up for what you've been neglecting to do. We all have room for improvement, we all have our ups and downs. Just be easy on yourself and remember the goal here- to work towards living your best life.

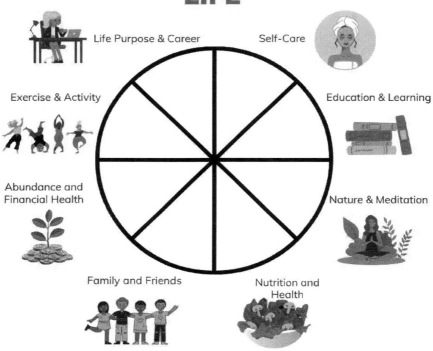

The Pie Chart of **LIFE**

FALLiNG iN LOVE WiTH yOURSELF

magine yourself, so happy with and enamored by who you are. Captivated by what a beautiful soul you are. You're in love with the vibe that you put out into the world, and absolutely adore who you've become. You are honorable and loving. You appreciate in yourself just how much you take care of the world and the people around you. You are at home with yourself, in love with this person that is you! You admire the deepest parts of yourself, how bright you shine and how you love yourself in the face of darkness.

You're proud of yourself for the many challenges and problems you've overcome, and just how strong you were throughout the trials and tribulations of your life. Your innate, beautiful, and unique energy adds so much to the world, and nothing can take that away from you.

Imagine we all saw ourselves this way.

Well, there's never been a better time to do this.

No more waiting around for perfect to happen, for things to be fixed, or a certain way. No more waiting for the perfect body, the forgiveness of everything, or the perfect job.

The time has never been better than right now.

Every single person on the planet *is* *this*. A perfect, magical, beautiful being who belongs on this planet and deserves a wonderful, fulfilling life. We were fooled somewhere along the way, falling into some sort of broken wisdom that caused us to lose sight of our beauty and magnificence. Somewhere in there, we were led to believe in a lesser version of ourselves, and it went on for what feels like, thousands of years.

To be here right now at this particular time in history is next level goodness. We're at a time and place that is so transformative, and things are evolving at such vast, exponential levels. People are expanding and opening themselves up to a lot more wisdom, their *own* wisdom, and are busy making mountains move because of it.

It's time we stop seeing ourselves as small, as we have a much greater potential than we ever imagined.

We've been getting caught up in the negativity that's happening all around us, and we've been spending too much time focusing our energy on what's wrong in the world. This only leaves us depleted, feeling like there's nothing we can do, which only takes power away from us. In fact, we have the power to do something, and it starts with us realizing the truth about who we actually are.

A divine, special, beautiful majestic being.

We are indeed *very* powerful, and we can create and bring about great change if we wanted to. If we spent even half of the energy that we spend on feeling down about what's wrong in the world, we could accomplish way more than we ever thought we could. We could change the course of things and not only help ourselves, but help so many others.

The truth is, it's up to us to get our own minds and thoughts right. To realize the truth about of our greatness and power. These things need and deserve our attention, so it's time to take off the mask we've been wearing, and let go of the false beliefs that we've learned to live with.

The ones that were created and built through who we *thought* we were or needed to be. With this, we can then create the space necessary to provide ourselves with the much-needed love and compassion that we deserve, along with the energy to be the best version of ourselves.

Deep down we all have such beautiful, amazing gifts to use, as well as true hearts of gold. We just need to work on seeing that and connecting to it again.

When we finally give ourselves permission to step into our greatness and be the best version of ourselves, we can more clearly see these amazing, unique gifts that we have inside of us.

Over time, it gets easier to recognize all of this in ourselves and to be able to stand strong in who we are and what we believe in. In this, we can take better care of ourselves on every level and actually live a life we love.

We can finally let down our walls knowing that we are perfectly safe, which allows more love in. We can let go of all that no longer serves us and needs to be released. We no longer have to include things that insult us or that don't agree with our soul.

The deep love that we develop for ourselves opens us up the expansive potential that enables us to create more of what we want in life, and to be able to heal ourselves on every level. In the end, recognizing all of this helps us to give more of ourselves to the world. And the world needs us so very much.

We no longer need to put on a show or pretend to be someone else.

As we truly get to know and love ourself, the journey is unlike anything else, with so much to be realized. We're like a shining star that burns bright for all those who need it. It is said that we're made up of stardust, afterall. Our bright light is needed in the world. This divine light is a part of who we are, and it's in each and every single one of us, meant to shine bright.

We've finally returned from being in a place of forgetting who we are, to seeing just how utterly powerful and magnificent we are. I know this may sound so esoteric and out there, but it's a truth that we haven't been hearing enough.

I know it's hard to see ourselves this way altogether, because we're not used to thinking this way. Maybe it doesn't sound like a reality that we can even think to step into, considering the planet that we live on right now and all that's happening, when other people are suffering so greatly. But, this is why it's *so* important to do this and feel this way, at this time.

Seeing ourselves as this divine, beautiful, powerful being has been needed for a very long time. We can all feel a shift happening, whether we can explain or not. We feel as though things are somehow speeding up, time is just flying by, all sorts of extremes seem to be happening on so many sides of things.

Many of us have already decided to stop playing small. We've begun to realize so much of our greatness and that we shouldn't dim our light anymore. We've come to realize the power and potential that we hold and have decided that we're going to start living our life differently because of it. One with passion and purpose. We've chosen to move back into the true essence of who we are, where we can accomplish the amazing things that we're meant to do.

When we do this for ourselves it not only opens us up to our greatest potential, it reflects upon and helps others to shine *their* light and understand *their* greatness, as well. People feel more comfortable and able to step into themselves and see the loving, creative, amazing soul that they are. Like a beautiful ripple, we affect one another. *'In lakesh'*... *'the light in me honors the light in you'*.

We can transform ourselves every day. We don't have to have the perfect job, the perfect body, the perfect situation, or perfect relationship in order to feel like we're *this beautiful, powerful, amazing person* that exists in the world. We're already perfect.

Take a look at the beautiful, wonderful soul that's already inside of you. Look beyond all of the *stuff* (the past, decisions, mistakes, emotions, experiences, etc.). That stuff is not who we are. Our circumstances and experiences do not make us who we are even if they've strongly affected how we act, think, and create in the world. In truth, they have nothing to do with *who we really are.*

We can stop feeling that we need to accomplish or succeed at something in order to be good enough. We're at a point in time that doesn't work anymore. We accomplish so much more when we live from a place of loving, accepting, and believing in ourselves. Seeing our glory and how truly amazing we are, puts us into a more empowered state.

Self-love and acceptance may seem foreign, it might even sound silly at first, but it's one of the best places we can focus some of our time on. Delving into these parts of us is one of the most rewarding things we can do for ourselves.

As adults, we have the power to change how we live, and decide from what part of ourselves that we want to be living from. Do we want to live endlessly through our old stories, fears, and the same old beliefs and limitations? Or do we want to rewrite our story, change our beliefs, and carve a new path or two, so we can live a more empowered and loving life?

No matter our circumstances or past experiences, we deserve the best. To be our best selves. It's time that we start appreciating ourselves, as well as forgiving ourselves.

The old thinking and limitations will begin to fade away as we realize what a perfect and beautiful human being we are. As we always have been. The decisions we make going forward will begin to reflect this and we'll find ourselves more guided by the love than ever.

It's also the time to be *grateful* for ourselves; everything that we are, all that we do, and for all that we've gotten through all of these years. I know, it's not been an easy road, but upon reconnecting with ourselves, the journey lightens and more beauty presents itself. It's time to learn to trust ourselves on the deepest level.

We are here to remember the truths that lie within us, that we are already perfect and loveable. Even better, we are all connected to each other and all a part of the greatest love that's out there. When we realize how amazingly perfect, full of love, and awesome we are, life will shift in the most profound, beautiful, and powerful ways imaginable.

HOMEWORK:

1. What emotions do you feel, when you think about loving yourself? Or about how perfect and beautiful you are? What comes up for you around this.
2. What are your general thoughts about yourself? How do you see yourself?
3. How would you like to see yourself? Write down the wonderful qualities about you and the ones you want to work on. Who are you beneath the surface of things?
4. How can you love and support yourself more right now in seeing how perfect and amazing you are in this now moment?

AFTERWORD

Now that we know how amazingly, beautiful and powerful we are, and that we can actually transform our health and create a better life for ourselves, it's time to align ourselves with our undeniable power. The power we have within that can create change and transformation in our life.

We have the power to truly change our lives. The power to find out what's most important to us, what we love, and who we want to be in the world.

It's time to stop limiting ourselves and believing in our smallness, instead realize and trust in our greatness. We have so much more to experience and give to the world, more than we ever thought was possible.

We once gave our power away, and what a shame that we lost touch with this part of ourselves. But now that we know, we are more informed, aware, and connected than ever, and doing what's right, comes easy. We know what is or isn't in our best interest, and have begun to really listen to and follow our heart.

We are here on this planet to realize our greatness so we can assist the quality of life on this planet. We have the power to do amazing things. As we work on ourselves by making positive changes, changing our thinking, forgiving others, letting go, eating healthier, and helping our bodies to heal, life rewards us in ways we hadn't ever imagined that it would.

No matter who we are, where we come from, or what the past held, we all have the freedom and power to change our lives. As we grow and learn how to be in our power, we can be an example for others who need and deserve to access *their* own power. Through this, we can change what no longer works in the world and create new pathways for the future generations to come.

We're all born as the same tiny human, with a glorious, bright light within. Creative geniuses, ready to explore and help create an impact in the world. No matter what's happened to us in the past, no one can take this away from us.

Every step we take towards improving our lives, with our relationships, careers, finances, mindset, and our health, creates momentum towards becoming the best versions of ourselves and more powerful than we ever knew possible. Our power has yet to even be felt, as we've been living at such a small percentage of what we actually could.

Taking care of ourselves and the planet around us is being in our power. Doing what we love and living with passion, is being in our power. Make sure to express your power in everything you do; with every move you make, every thought you have, and with every word you speak.

We are meant to live, thrive, and be in love with this life… and we deserve nothing less.

Now go out there and be the most powerful version of yourself. The world is waiting!

REFERENCE LOVE

THE NURSE TOOLKIT

Most people have a few band-aids on hand, maybe a bit of gauze and some ointment. It's pretty safe to say that people should have some basic medical supplies on hand, a little tool box of sorts to keep all of your stuff in. We can use a container, a tool box, some Tupperware, or even a sturdy shoe box.

It can take a little while to accumulate and purchase all of the things we may want to have on hand, as some medical supplies can be more costly. So not to stress. We can always work our way to build it up over time. Having this *tool box* on hand is definitely a stress reliever and good to have on hand.

I thought I'd share items that I've found helpful over the years, especially after doing home care and hospice nursing for so long. However, this *does not mean* you have to get them, or purchase anything for that matter. This is just a guideline of sorts, should you want to create or enhance your medical kit.

I always say, better to have a few items than none at all. Some of it we can even find at the dollar store. As a nurse, I've grown fond of certain brands over the years, so I may mention them, but get what you can afford. Beautifully enough, all of them can be purchased on-line.

I'm all for putting the power back into our hands. We should all have the basic skills around how to care for our bodies, that includes caring for cuts, wounds, and other injuries. I'll be creating videos down the line on taking care of simple and common injuries.

I want nothing more than for people to be empowered and know how to take care of their basic needs *with confidence.*

Of course, this is **_never a replacement_** for seeking medical care. Always go to the hospital or emergency room when you've injured yourself in a big enough way. If your gut tells you that it's bad, go! Get the help you need.

If it's not critical or urgent, then to know the basics and what we can use in the case of an emergency, is only ever a good thing.

It's important as well, to make sure that our self-talk during a health issue or crisis, is as positive as we can make it. It's great if we can have a bit of confidence in ourselves, even when we have no idea what we're doing.

Calm is *always* better than frantic. If you are someone who gets nervous when it comes to dealing with medical things, step back, take 3 deep breaths, then come back in and try again.

We're not always going to know everything and that's okay. We weren't taught that much of this in school, but it's also never too late to learn a thing or two.

Most of all, give yourself a break, things aren't always easy. Especially when emotions are running high. Throw in a statement like, "*I can do this*". I promise it helps immensely, especially when you say it over and over again. Do it every time that self-doubt creeps in. In time, you'll get to know and trust yourself more with the process.

Do some research and watch some videos, there is a lot of information out there from many wonderful doctors and nurses explaining first aid and at home medical care.

These tools are for when you need to take care of yourself or your family, if medical help isn't available right away. Please, do not take on situations all by yourself, especially if it's not just a small physical event, <u>seek medical attention</u>.

- **Coban**

Who doesn't love this stuff! Coban was originally made for horses and animals. It has so many uses. It holds gauze and bandages in place, it can be wrapped around almost any part of the body, and used in different ways as a means of support. It's a great means when tape cannot be used, as it does not contain adhesive (good for hairy areas).

Coban can create compression, which is good for edema and

swelling, but can also <u>cut off circulation and cause more problems</u> if stretched too much and wrapped too tightly. My go-to brand is 3M.

- **Gauze (pieces, rolls, non-stick)**

Also known as a sponge. Gauze is necessary for cleansing, protecting, and helping wounds to heal. They keep medicine applied, as well as they help to absorb drainage. They protect wounds from dirt, debris, or interference so that the wound can heal with very little interruption. Gauze comes in various sizes; you can buy sterile gauze and they come in separate packs or you can buy bulk in big stacks.

There are gauze *rolls* that are good for wrapping and holding dressings in place. They're soft and easy on the skin. Dry gauze can end up sticking to a wound, causing further trauma to it, so there is non-stick gauze called Telfa. Non-stick gauze is excellent for burns, skin tears, and wounds that are delicate.

- **Bandages/Band-aids**

It's good to have several sizes of bandages on hand. Some are sold in variety packs with different sizes. The fabric ones have good stretch ability. There are sensitive band aids for people who cannot handle adhesives and break out in rashes. They also sell ones that are latex-free. Band-aids can tear off skin, especially on the elderly and those with fragile skin.

- **Ace Wrap and Braces**

Ace wraps are very handy to have around. They protect and keep dressings and bandages in place, and are especially good to wrap around an arm or a leg. They can be wrapped around part of the body and used as a brace lending support to something such as a weakened joint (i.e. the knee, wrist, or ankle). Many are self-closing with Velcro, although they still sell the ones with clips. They sell variety packs that come with a few different sizes which is ideal, and it's pretty cheap.

Braces are different from ace wraps, as they are formed, fitted, and designed for whatever area they are made for, like the knee, elbow, wrist, or ankle. They're great for a weak joint, or when we need support while doing an activity.

** When you have a sprain or injury, the best thing to do is to rest the affected area, ice it, elevate it, and when up, wear a supportive device. Go see a doctor for more serious injuries. It's *never* smart to push one.

There are sleeve braces that are made of soft, elastic material that can be pulled over the area. There are also adjustable ones with Velcro straps, as well as the ones we get from our doctor, especially related to surgery. Always make sure to have the correct size, because wearing a brace that's too small or too big can cause more injury than good.

There are also back braces that are great for those with weaker abdominal muscles or back injuries, when heavy lifting and bending is required. They help to prevent further injury. There are also abdominal binders which are wonderfully supportive to the abdomen, especially in the case of a hernia or after abdominal surgery.

- **Hydrogen peroxide**

Hydrogen peroxide is a powerful cleanser and oxygenator that is popularly used to disinfect cuts and wounds. The standard version that is used for this is 3%, however there are other percentages available such as 6% and 12 %, labeled as food grade.

Hydrogen peroxide is an amazing alternative to bleach. It can be used as a disinfectant because it kills germs and fungus. It's a great treatment for plants that have fungus gnats. You can do your laundry with the higher percentage version, as it gets stains and odors out of things. You can even use it as a face wash or rinse, of course, *diluted*. It helps to exfoliate the skin, can assist with the rebalancing of overly oily skin, disinfects to decrease bacteria, combating skin infections and break-outs.

- **Rubbing alcohol**

Rubbing alcohol kills bacteria, viruses, and fungus. Rubbing alcohol can be used as a disinfectant. It's never good to pour into a wound, it's better to be applied with a cotton ball, gauze, or QTip. It can clean and disinfect hygiene and personal items and tools. It can remove adhesives and sticky substances (at a concentration of 70% or higher) helpful if bandages or tape have left a residue on the skin.

Rubbing alcohol has been found to be helpful with post-surgery nausea by smelling an alcohol swab. Often used by people with medical devices or to prep the skin before injections. Widely available and easy to find. Always good to have a bottle or two on hand. The common percentage available is 50%, up to stronger concentrations of 70% or 91%. The higher versions are the best at removing sticky residues from surfaces.

- **Saline – Sodium Chloride 0.9%**

This is the liquid solution of sodium chloride (salt) and water. There are saline solutions made for many purposes; wounds, the sinuses, the eyes, the mouth, and some for internal use. It's largely used medically for wound care, during procedures and surgeries, and to hydrate a person through an IV (it gives the body the salt it needs to maintain fluid balance and blood pressure, rehydration, amongst other things).

Saline is used to cleanse and flush different parts of the body, and is the most used solution in hospital settings. It's good to have a saline wound rinse and a saline eye flush on hand. When you have a wound, if the area is delicate, saline is most gentle on the tissue. Good to flush the eyes with when something gets in them whether it be chemical, debris, or in the case of general irritation.

- **Wound ointment**

Ointments are used to protect wounds, cuts, and burns. An ointment serves as a protectant keeping bacteria from interfering. Some ointments kill these unwanted organisms and are used to assist with the healing process. The most well-known over-the-counter versions are the antibiotic ointments, namely bacitracin, neomycin, or polymycin. These ointments kill a broad range of bacteria and are sometimes effective against staph and strep of the skin. However, they are petroleum based and contain parabens which are man-made chemical preservatives.

If you would like a more natural ointment without petroleum and chemicals, there are several.

There are two other popular types of ointments that are used widely in the medical world, are 100% safe, effective against bacteria and other organisms, as well as assist with wound healing. One that is gaining momentum is, manuka honey ointment. Manuka honey helps to heal open cuts and wounds, as well as heal injured tissue after wound closure. Manuka honey has been used for centuries, if not thousands of years, because of its strong anti-microbial properties, killing bacteria, as well as that it is proven to heal wounds faster. It is great for burns, even severe ones, as it maintains a moist environment to speed up healing. It is gaining popularity in the medical industry. When people were using triple antibiotic ointments with no results, they applied the honey ointment and healing began to occur. All depends on the situation and individual.

Another commonly used ointment is colloidal silver. It comes in a cream or a gel ointment. Silver is another highly effective antimicrobial product that kills bacteria, fungus, and viruses, including candida and ringworm. Silver is also well known in the medical community, used for burn treatments and wound healing. A common cream used in the medical industry is silver sulfadiazine cream. It is used for healing *bedsores,* as well as wounds that will not heal. There are silver ion infused gauze products used by surgeons for post-surgical incisions to ensure healing and protection. However, the gel is not to be used on a closed surgical incision, at home, unless specified by your doctor. Silver gel can be used on your dog or cat, for skin issues and infections. There are products specifically made for them, they can even take the tincture, which is available as well for internal consumption.

- **Burn ointment**

There are several over-the-counter products for burns. We just mentioned silver and manuka honey being helpful for burns. Depending on how bad the burn is will depend on what you need to apply or should do. For severe burns that burn through several layers, seek medical attention *right away.*

Aloe vera is great for surface burns like sun burns. Most of the ointments for burns that you buy at the drugstore contain silver. Some of them also contain pain relieving ingredients such as lidocaine or arnica. There are over-the-counter manuka honey products specifically made for burn healing. Then there are hydrogel pads and patches, that contain anti-microbial and cooling properties while keeping the area moist and protected during the healing process. When covering a burn, be sure to use non-stick gauze because you don't want to dry out the wound or have anything stick to it.

- **Pain cream, gel, or ointment**

Most pain-relieving products on the market are numbing agents that take away pain and create loss of sensation. Most over-the-counter products contain some form of lidocaine. You can buy a tube of lidocaine gel at 4-5% which can be applied to the skin. It's very effective, but not good for issues such as chronic or severe pain. It can however, relieve acute pain from an injury, hemorrhoidal pain, and is safe for burns and bruises.

There is a well-known herb called Arnica, that is used for its pain-relieving properties. It comes in gel, cream, or ointment form and can be used on the skin for muscle aches and pain, bruises, as well as that it can also be found in several wound ointments. Arnica comes in an edible pellet form known as a homeopathic remedy, that can be taken as directed to assist with muscle pain and soreness.

CBD ointment made from hemp or marijuana is amazingly effective. It can actually be a temporary pain reliever for chronic or cancerous pain. CBD can be taken in capsule or liquid form, and is even available as a gummy or chocolate.

CBD is quite because it has so many healing properties. As for its use in pain relief, it reduces inflammation and works with pain receptors in the brain. My absolute go-to is Robin's Nest Naturals CBD balm, which helped my mother with her back pain during her struggle with cancer. It's great for muscle injuries, strains, sprains, and works for both acute and chronic pain.

Of course, there's no exact formula that works for everyone. You will find the best one for you through trial and error. Pain expresses itself differently in each person. And if you live in a place that marijuana THC products are available, balms and lotions that contain THC, have well-known and powerful pain-relieving properties.

- **Tegaderm**

This is a clear, transparent adhesive dressing used to keep gauze or other dressings in place. It is great for skin tears that occur on very fragile skin, usually with the elderly. It is best known for its use as the clear covering over an IV, if you've ever had one. If sealed well, it can serve as a barrier to water, but not if submerged and sometimes works while taking a shower (not 100% though).

They are very thin which can make them a bit precarious to work with because once it sticks to itself, you're moving onto to the next one, so always be mindful of that when working with them. They come in a variety of sizes and some even come with gauze already embedded within them which is wonderful, especially for people with bed sores or wounds. The best brand and original one is 3M. Easily found online and in stores.

- **Silicone adhesive foam wound dressing**

This wonderful soft, flexible dressing is a God send for bed sores and bedbound people, as well as active ones. Flexible, great adhesive and does not harm fragile skin. It has an absorptive padded gauze area that absorbs moderate drainage. Can be used as padding for protruding bones and vertebrae. They come in many shapes and sizes, ones especially for the sacral/buttock area which come in a heart-type shape which is amazing for people with difficulty healing their bottoms from pressure sores.

- **Tape**

Medical tape is a must. Having a few options on hand is great, but at least one kind is sufficient. It's a wonderful tool to help keep gauze in place, and of course, for securing just about anything to the body. There are several kinds of tape made of different materials and are mostly latex free. Paper tape: easiest on the skin, great for fragile skin. Cloth tape: some are made with a nylon fabric, strong, easy to tear, very sticky. Soft cloth tape: known as Medfix or Hypafix which is a flexible, soft-woven fabric that is wonderful for holding dressings in place and good for moderate drainage. It is safe for fragile skin and has some stretch to it. Transpore or Micropore tape: made by 3M, a somewhat clear tape that's easy to handle and tear, often used as a surgical tape.

- **Scissors**

A pair of scissors that are strictly used for medical purposes is necessary to have in your kit. There are many kinds available, easy to buy at the pharmacy and online- which is generally less expensive, just type in a search for medical scissors. You can use alcohol to clean them after each use.

- **Tweezers**

Having a pair of tweezers is another essential, with the obvious use of pulling out a splinter or bits of debris off a wound, and just overall helpful to have around. A slanted tip pair is wonderful to have, but any will do. Keep these tweezers strictly in, and for your medical kit, and clean with rubbing alcohol after each use. Available in the beauty section at any store.

- **Cotton Swabs**

Otherwise known as Q-tips. Easy to obtain, any brand will do. These are very versatile, used to clean small areas, apply ointment, and when saturated with saline, can help remove something from the eye. There are some with *long* wooden 6-inch sticks that are great on many levels, a longer stick creates ease of use in harder to reach areas, just *don't* use them in your ear. Q-tips are the main brand but you can find cotton swabs almost anywhere, and medical ones are usually found online.

- **Over the counter medications**

These are your typical medications that can be found in almost every person's home. Having them on hand can serve a variety of ailments and come in handy upon an emergency. Lots of precautions on any pharmaceutical medication, even if over-the-counter, so please check with your doctor on taking these as they do interact with other medications. There is information all over the place online, highly recommend doing some reading.

Benadryl (aka Diphenhydramine)

USES: Allergic reactions, seasonal allergies, rashes, itching, sneezing, runny nose, motion sickness, can be used to induce sleep. Used for poison ivy, poison oak, insect bites, sunburn, to relieve itching and pain. It's an anti-histamine, sedative-hypnotic, and anti-pruritic (skin).

PRECAUTIONS: Can cause drowsiness, do not operate machinery or drive while taking this. Can cause dizziness. Can cause the *opposite* reaction in some- instead of drowsiness they can cause hyperactivity. This drug has an interaction with alcohol; some have blacked out from the mix of the two- DO NOT DRINK ALCOHOL with this medication. Not for *children 2 and under,* and **always** use with caution with children. Also use with caution while breastfeeding, as it will get absorbed by the child, as does any medication taken while breastfeeding. Our immune system attacks an allergen by releasing histamine, which is what causes allergic reactions and responses. This drug suppresses the histamine response.

Tylenol (aka Acetaminophen)

USES: Fever-reducer. *Minor* pain reliever.

PRECAUTIONS: Liver toxicity if taken in large amounts; Do not take if you have liver issues or disease. NEVER take more than 3,000 mg per day (this number was recently reduced from 4,000 mg per day)- it *will* cause liver damage. An overdose can cause death; there are tons of reported deaths each year from Tylenol overdose.

Aspirin

USES: Pain reliever. Reduces fever. Thins the blood. Decreases swelling.

PRECAUTIONS: Thins blood, <u>do not use if you have a bleeding disorder</u> or <u>are already taking blood thinners</u>. Seek advice from your doctor. NEVER give it to a child with fever, flu symptoms, or chicken pox, as it can cause **fatal** consequences.

** Very good to take on the onset of a heart attack or stroke that is occurring, or has just occurred.

Ibuprofen (Non-steroidal anti-inflammatory)

USES: Decreases swelling and inflammation. Pain reliever. It reduces the hormones that cause inflammation and pain in the body.

PRECAUTIONS: Thins the blood. Can damage stomach lining and intestines, causing intestinal bleeding (which can be fatal) and ulcers. Can *increase risk* of heart attack or stroke. DO NOT give to a child under 6 months old. *Hard on the kidneys* so do not take if you have any type of kidney disease.

- **Immune strengtheners**

I believe it's essential to have immunity boosters in your tool kit. Many of these were mentioned earlier. You can get formulas with several of these immune boosters *combined*, so it's easy to just have one bottle for your toolkit. These are some of the main ones to have when you're feeling under the weather: Echinacea, Goldenseal, Elderberry, Zinc, Vitamin C, Vitamin D, Quercetin, L-Glutamine, mushrooms like Chaga, Reishi, Lion's Mane, Cordyceps, Turkey Tail, Shitake. These come in in powder, capsule, or gummy form and are easy to find.

- **Digestive assistance**

Ginger tea, Peppermint tea, Chamomile tea, papaya enzymes, activated charcoal, digestive enzymes, and pro-biotics can all be helpful to have on hand, although just having one or two is great. Ginger encourages digestion, stimulates blood flow, and relieves nausea. Peppermint is soothing, cooling to the stomach, good for upset stomach, bloating, and gas. Chamomile has soothing and anti-inflammatory properties, good for upset stomach, diarrhea, gas, relief from irritable bowel and Crohn's. Papaya seeds contain enzymes that assist with food breakdown, improve digestion, reduce inflammation, and even recently have been scientifically proven to combat infection. Papaya enzymes are also good for bloating, constipation, and gas. Activated charcoal is a wonderful detoxifier, as it is a pulling and absorbing agent. It helps remove toxins by binding to drugs and poisons in the tissues of the body and helps to remove them from the body. Good for heavy metal removal. Assists with bloating and gas. Important that you have decent bowel movement when using charcoal, sometimes bowel herbs are good to take such as GI Renew. Digestive enzymes are available to take before meals to assist with digestion. Probiotics are becoming more widely known and are recognized for helping to reestablish the good bacterial balance in our digestive system. People think of yogurt as one of the top sources, however, yogurt is dairy and is often loaded with sugar. A better version of the dairy probiotics is Kefir. There are various probiotic drinks, powders, and capsules. Kombucha, sauerkraut, kimchi, tempeh, and miso are all a good source of probiotics. Good capsule formulas are not always cheap, but having them on hand for stomach issues is a good idea, *especially after a dose of antibiotics,* or for those on chronic medications. Best kept in the fridge as heat can cause the live bacteria to die.

- **Ice Pack**

Any ice pack is great, even ice cubes in a zip lock baggie if it's all you have on hand. Gel filled ice packs are easy to use and can be molded around an area. You can make an at home gel ice pack by combining 1 part rubbing alcohol, 3 parts water in a well-sealed plastic bag and freeze it. Always cover ice packs with cloth when applying to the skin. There are fabric covered ice packs formed in many shapes and sizes available to purchase. Cold is a number one go to for <u>swelling</u>. It is wonderful and essential for an acute injury to the skin or muscles, great to prevent or lessen bruising, good for strains, and excellent for pain relief. Cold reduces blood flow to the affected area. Blood flows to injured areas and tissue, which is what causes swelling and pain.

- **Reheatable warm pack, hot water bottle, heating pad**

Reheatable warm packs are sold everywhere. They even come as snuggly stuffed animals. There are some that come in a specific shape for a certain area like the neck or shoulder area. They heat up in your microwave, though please heat with *caution*, and set a safe time on your microwave in case you should forget about it, as they can cause a fire. Safe timing is one-and-a-half or two minutes, and then you can work your way up for more heat.

A hot water bottle is an iconic classic that has been around for centuries, if not thousands of years. It's a rubber bottle that gets filled with hot water to use however and wherever it is needed. Great applied to the abdomen for belly discomfort or menstrual cramping. There's also something very soothing about the water element. Needs refilling to keep hot, but is a great tool for healing, soothing, comforting. A hot water bottle can also be bought with attachments and can be used as an enema. A heating pad is wonderfully convenient, though needs to be plugged in. They are lightweight and great when one feels cold for heating oneself up. Heat is great for cramping (*also Magnesium is great for cramping* as well as for heart function), muscle aches, and pain. Heat brings blood to the area.

- **Emergency antibiotics**

There is an emergency antibiotic kit available through a company known as Jase Medical. This kit is not meant to be used casually or in replacement of medical care. It comes with 4 different antibiotics *for emergency use* and there are instructions with it. Use ONLY IN case of a disaster or survival event, which may we never have! Do not purchase or take if you are sensitive or allergic to ANY ANTIBIOTICS. Jase Medical also has a program to have up to one year of your regular medications on hand, check them out to find out how. There are also other companies coming out doing this as well, another one being Duration Health.

- **Towels, rags, garbage bags**

Always have spare, clean towels on hand for personal or medical use. Rags come in handy for any cleaning, old towels are great for that, can be cut up for whatever need comes. Garbage bags go without saying- to discard of trash especially waste that contains bodily fluids or waste. They are also great to use as an ice bag or even a sling.

- **Iodine Tablets**

The last one I will mention that might be a good option to have on hand is Iodine, or Potassium Iodide tablets. It's a great means of protection for your thyroid in the case of radiation poisoning (for short term management). If in the case of this type of emergency, public health and emergency officials are supposed to notify us however, I'm not sure how we would hear them if such an event occurred as I would not expect our electronics and TVs to be working. Hopefully we never have a need for them, but they are available online.

It's also a good idea to have a few extra months of your regular medications on hand, if in case of an emergency. Jase Medical, mentioned a moment ago, can provide these, but there are other ways to get at least 6 extra months, worth of your meds. As a nurse I know, expiration dates can always be pushed when in desperate times. Your doctor will usually allow several months of medications in advance, though of course, not the controlled substances or narcotics. Your general disease management pills should be allowable.

A FEW FOOD FACTS

"THE DIRTY DOZEN" – foods that are the <u>most</u> contaminated with pesticides and chemicals:

1. Strawberries
2. Spinach
3. Kale, Collard, Mustard Greens
4. Nectarines
5. Apples
6. Grapes
7. Bell & Hot Peppers
8. Cherries
9. Peaches
10. Pears
11. Celery
12. Tomatoes

"THE CLEAN 15" – foods that are the <u>least</u> contaminated:

1. Avocados
2. Sweet Corn
3. Pineapples
4. Onions
5. Papayas
6. Frozen Sweet Peas
7. Asparagus
8. Honeydew Melon
9. Kiwi

10. Cabbage
11. Mushrooms
12. Cantaloupe Melon
13. Mangoes
14. Watermelons
15. Sweet Potatoes

(Both lists from the EWG- Environmental Working Group)

Food Products that available in the US that are *banned* in other countries:
(collective data from online resources)

1. Citric Acid- a common food preservative once derived from citrus fruits, now made from Aspergillus Niger (**BLACK MOLD**). Found in most foods, candies, and body care products. There is *naturally derived* citric acid made from sugar cane or cassava available, it can be found @ Mountain Rose Herbs.
2. Partially Hydrogenated Oil- This is a trans-fat, the worst kind of fat you can consume. Banned in a million other countries. Fried and processed foods are the biggest source of these fats.
3. Rice Krispies, Frosted Flakes Lucky Charms, and other sugary, GMO cereals. At this point, all popular brands contain GMOs. Now stated on the box as Bioengineered ingredients.
4. Skittles and M&Ms- banned in Europe and other countries, due to GMOs, red dyes and other chemicals found in then. Highly promoted for children in the US.
5. rBGH or rBST hormones in milk and dairy products- used in the US
6. Pop Tarts- contain artificial dyes and propylene glycol
7. Bread products made in the US- they are made with azodicarbonamide which is a whitener and *dough conditioner*, and potassium bromate used to strengthen and help dough rise. Both are found in packaged baked goods, cereals, breads, frozen dinners and boxed pasta dinners. Azodicarbonamide causes respiratory and other health issues, in Singapore you can get

fined $450,000 and go to jail for up to 15 years if it is found to be used. This chemical is found and used in making yoga mats and soles of sneakers. Potassium bromide causes cancer, kidney damage, and nervous system damage.

8. Gatorade- contains food dyes, flavorings, loads of sugar
9. Chlorine washed chicken
10. Coffee Mate- contains hydrogenated soybean and cottonseed oils. Contains corn syrup solids and also contains a compound that contains aluminum which might be why you can ignite it and it catches on fire.
11. Instant Mashed potatoes- contains hydrogenated soybean and cottonseed oils. Contains corn syrup solids. Some contain up to 4 preservatives, including citric acid.
12. US Pork- almost all US pork contains ractopamine, a drug injected to increase lean muscle growth
13. US Chicken- chicken are sometimes fed with arsenic which makes the meat appear pinker and fresher. They have been genetically modified to grow bigger in the breast region, as well as that hormones are given. During processing, chicken is injected with salt and chemicals to add size and juiciness. Chicken is also washed in chlorine. We already spoke about processing our chicken in China... so many questions with that.
14. US Beef- contains ractopamine a drug injected to increase lean muscle growth, amongst other hormones and drugs.
15. US Corn- genetically modified, heavily tainted with Atrazine. Atrazine is an herbicide that's been known to cause birth defects, reproductive issues and tumors, skin problems, and muscle weakness and degeneration.
16. US Soy- genetically modified, heavily tainted with Atrazine.
17. Food colorings- RED 40, YELLOW 5 & 6 in particular. All are very harmful to nervous system, are cancer-causing, toxic, disrupt functioning of the immune system.
18. GMOs- Genetically Modified Foods. Now also called Bioengineered Food. Linked to cancer, autism, nervous system problems, allergies. Modified with virus proteins and all kinds of other stuff. Banned in other countries but the FDA here in

the US say they're safe and *carefully studied*, so not to worry. But I would.

19. Sugar Cane crops from the USA. The US uses <u>Atrazine</u> on nearby weeds and grasses that ends up in sugar. Atrazine is an herbicide that's been known to cause birth defects, reproductive issues and tumors, skin problems, and muscle weakness and degeneration. It is found in 90% of US sugar cane products. It also leaks into the water supply and harms wildlife.

20. Fat Free Snacks made with Olestra, which is a chemical that causes the body to be unable to absorb nutrients.

21. Chewing gum which contains BHA. BHA is also found in cereals, snack foods, nut mixes, butter, meat, and dehydrated potatoes. BHA is linked to cancer according to all studies except here in the US. Also found to impair blood clotting when consumes in high doses and promotes tumor growth.

22. Farm-raised salmon or fish. They are fed synthetic chemicals that make them bright pink to add color, known as <u>astaxanthin</u>, which causes loss of eyesight. Antibiotics and other drugs are also given to these fish that aren't safe for human consumption.

23. High Fructose Corn Syrup- A more processed corn syrup that is not processed by the body. Ingestion causes insulin resistance, obesity, and Type 2 Diabetes. It increases appetite, causes inflammation, and raises cholesterol. It is also leads to non-alcoholic fatty liver disease. Completely banned in the UK and Europe.

24. Artificial blueberry in fruit bars. The color is derived from petroleum, linked to nerve cell damage, brain cancer, and hyperactivity.

25. US apples- chemicals are used to keep the fruit fresh and the color vibrant -DPA is a *pesticide applied to apples **after** they're harvested* and is linked to various cancers. Also have wax and Appeal, a new coating produced by Bill Gates. That alone, says enough.

26. US Potato chips- contain BHT preservative (look for this as it's on many processed and packaged food products) -stated by the FDA as "generally safe" however, studies show it causes cancer.

27. Palm Oil- found in peanut butter spreads, chocolate, cookies, bread, and ice cream. Studies show link to cardiovascular disease, as well as devastating to the rainforest. Banned in Europe and other countries mostly because of deforestation.
28. Artificial sweeteners: Aspartame, Acesulfame K, Saccharin, Sucralose. Damaging to GI system, immune system, and are a neuro-toxin (damage to the nervous system).
29. Processed meats preserved with Sodium Nitrate- Linked to cancer. Europe banned it.
30. Trans Fats- used to cheaply create long shelf life. They raise your LDLs (bad cholesterol levels), increase your risk of strokes and heart issues. Found in microwavable popcorn, crackers, cookies, fast food, frozen pizzas, coffee creamer.
31. Hershey's- there's nothing chocolate about this "chocolate". It contains edible plastics otherwise known as polymers, as well that heavy metals recently found.

** Some products may look exactly the same and be from the same company, but the ingredients are different in the US versions.

RESOURCES

BOOKS

The Body/Disease:

1. Body Into Balance by: Maria Groves
2. Become Younger by: Dr. N.W. Walker
3. The Detox Miracle Sourcebook by: Dr. Robert Morse, N.D.
4. Heal Your Body by: Louise L. Hay (also Heal Your Body A-Z)
5. Healing Beyond Pills and Potions by: Steve Bierman, M.D.
6. Body Electric: Electromagnetism and the Foundation of Life by: Robert Becker
7. The Complete Guide to Natural Healing by: Tom Monte
8. The Wisdom Codes by: Gregg Braden
9. A New Health Era by: Dr. William Howards
10. The Wisdom of Your Cells0 How Your Beliefs Control Your Biology by: Bruce H. Lipton PhD
11. The Live Food Factor by: Susan Schenck
12. The 80/10/10 Diet by: Dr. Douglas N. Graham
13. The Encyclopedia of Ailments and Diseases by: Jacques Martel
14. Self-Heal By Design by: Barbara O'Neill (ebook)
15. God Helps Those Who Help Themselves by: Hanna Kroeger
16. The Truth About Contagion by: Thomas S. Cowan
17. The Healing Power of Sound- Recovery from Life-Threatening Illnesses Using Sound, Voice, and Music by: Mitchell L. Gaynor, M.D.
18. The Psychic Roots of Disease by: Björn Eybl
19. Alkalize or Die by: Dr. Theodore A. Baroody

20. Vitality Supreme by: Bernarr Macfadden
21. Life Force by: Tony Robbins
22. When The Body Says No by: Gabor Maté

The Mind/Transformation/Spirituality:

1. You Can Heal Your Life by: Louise L. Hay
2. Becoming Supernatural: How Common People are Doing the Uncommon by: Dr. Joe Dispenza
3. Bringers of the Dawn by: Barbara Marcinak
4. Breaking the Habit of Being Yourself by: Dr. Joe Dispenza
5. Change Your Paradigm, Change Your Life by: Bob Proctor
6. Think and Grow Rich by: Napoleon Hill
7. The Tiger's Fang by: Paul Twitchell
8. The Breakthrough Experience: The Revolutionary New Approach to Personal Transformation by: Dr. John Demartini
9. All For Love by: Matt Kahn
10. The Gratitude Effect by: Dr. John Demartini
11. Say It Out Loud by: Vasavi Kumar
12. Waking Up in 5D by: Maureen J. St. Germain
13. The Peaceful Warrior by: Dan Millman
14. Healing with Light Frequencies by: Jerry Sargeant
15. Everything You Ever Need by: Charlotte Freeman
16. The Alchemist by: Paulo Coehlo
17. The Body Keeps the Score: Brain, Mind, and Body in Healing the Trauma by: Bessel Van Der Kolk
18. Ikigai: The Japanese Secret to a Long and Happy Life by: Hector Garcia & Francesc Miralles
19. Journey to Peace and Healing by: Dawn Michelle Jackson
20. Wise Up: Women, Inclusion and Self-Empowerment by: Dr. Myra K. Hubbard

Food:

1. Whole Foods Companion by: Dianne Onstad
2. The New Whole Foods Encyclopedia by: Rebecca Wood

3. The Mucusless Diet Healing System by: Professor Arnold Ehret
4. Don't Throw It, Grow It by: Deborah Peterson & Millicent Selsam
5. The Acid Alkaline Food Guide by: Dr. Susan Brown
6. Conscious Eating by: Gabriel Cousens

Herbs:

1. The Little Herb Encyclopedia by: Jack Ritchason, N.D.
2. Herbal Medicine For Beginners by: Katja Swift
3. Rosemary Gladstar's Medicinal Herbs by: Rosemary Gladstar
4. The Lost Book of Herbal Remedies by: Claude Davis and Nicole Apelian
5. A Modern Herbal- Volume I & II by: Mrs. M. Grieve
6. Dr. Sebi Encyclopedia of Herbs by: Emily Wilson
7. Breverton's Complete Herbal by: Terry Breverton
8. Evolutionary Herbalism by: Sajah Popham
9. Medical Herbalism by: David Hoffman
10. Herbal Antibiotics by: Stephen Harrod Buhner

Detoxification, Cleansing:

1. The Detox Miracle Sourcebook by: Dr. Robert Morse, N.D.
2. The Grape Cure by: Johanna Brandt
3. The Complete Guide to Fasting by: Dr. Jason Fung & Jimmy Moore
4. The Liver and Gallbladder Miracle Cleanse by: Andreas Moritz
5. Your Liver… Your Lifeline by: Jack Tips, PhD
6. The Complete Master Cleanse by: Tom Woloshyn
7. Juicing, Fasting, and Detoxing for Life by: Cherie Calbom
8. A Consumer's Dictionary of Food Additives by: Ruth Winter
9. A Consumer's Dictionary of Cosmetic Ingredients by: Ruth Winter

Cancer:

1. Chris Beat Cancer: A Comprehensive Plan for Healing Naturally by: Chris Wark
2. Understand Cancer Series by: Dr. Otto Warburg
3. How To Starve Cancer by: Jane McLelland
4. World Without Cancer by: G. Edward Griffin
5. Crazy, Sexy Cancer Tips by: Kris Carr
6. The Cancer Industry by: Mark Sloan
7. Cancer Secrets by: Dr. Jonathan Stegall

Alternative Therapies:

1. The Healing Secrets of the Ages by: Catherine Ponder
2. Radical Healing by: Rudolph Ballantine
3. Acupuncture Points Handbook by: Deborah Bleecker, L.Ac
4. Good-Bye Germ Theory by: Dr. William Trebing
5. Ayurveda: The Science of Self-Healing by: Dr V. Lad

Mushrooms:

1. The Fungal Pharmacy by: Robert Rogers
2. Christopher Hobb's Medicinal Mushrooms by: Christopher Hobbs L.Ac
3. Mushroom Cultivation for Beginners by: Carole Smith

Sungazing:

1. The Healing Sun by: Richard Hobday, PhD
2. The Mysteries of the Light by: Tom Rees
3. Sun Gazing by: Bob Finklea
4. Sun Gaze for Success by: Jerome Shaw

EDUCATION:

Spiritual Development, Alternative Healing, Ancient Origins:

1. GAIA – www.gaia.com – This streaming channel/service is chock full of amazing documentaries and information. You can get a free trial for 30 days to check it out. So worthwhile.
2. Dr. Joe Dispenza – www.drjoedispenza.com – Doctor of Chiropractic, Neuroscience, Quantum epigenetics, mind-body medicine, brain-heart coherence, Dr. Joe Dispenza is an author, researcher, teacher and has written many books, as well as has guided meditations and programs that are very powerful.
3. Gregg Braden – www.greggbraden.com – Author, Scientist, Visionary who speaks about many topics such as ancient civilization, DNA, quantum physics, healing, globalization, and new thought wisdom.
4. Dr. Robert Morse, ND – www.drmorses.com or www.drmorsesdetoxcenters.com – Dr. Robert Morse N.D. is a master teacher and naturopath who sees the intricate connections and simplicity of the body and its healing, as well as how powerful our spiritual lives are and their interconnectedness.

Herbs:

1. Mountain Rose Herbs @ Mountain Rose Herbs on YouTube – www.mountainroseherbs.com – Education of herbs, herbal formulas, and making products.
2. Healer with Dr. Justin Sulak – www.healer.com – Education around Cannabis, CBD, hemp, the endocannabinoid system.
3. Clover Leaf Farms Herbs – www.cloverleaffarmsherbs.com – Herbs A-Z listing information on herbs and foods. History, cautions, actions, uses, and biology along with other information.
4. The Herbal Academy – www.theherbalacademy.com – Great online school with amazing programs from beginner to advanced, if you want to get in some personal educating or

start helping others. They also have workshops and intensives, even a kid's online nature camp!

Mushrooms:

1. Paul Stamets – www.paulstamets.com – Mycologist and scientist with amazing resources and information on his website.
2. Fungi Perfecti – www.fungi.com – Learning resources on growing mushrooms as well as the ability to purchase all kinds of mushroom products and growing supplies.
3. North Spore – www.northspore.com – Learn anything and everything you want about mushrooms, growing them and the science behind everything mushroom including making tinctures and medicine.

Reiki:

1. Medical Reiki – www.medicalreikiworks.org – Dr. Sheldon Feldman was a cardiac surgeon who witnessed what alternative healing did for his sister, and embarked on his journey to bring complementary healing methods into the medical system, mainly Reiki which is now being used at renown medical centers around the country.

Frequencies:

1. Rife Frequency – www.spooky2.com – education as well as on YouTube @ Spooky2 Rife
2. Dr. Joe Dispenza & Gregg Braden both offer valuable information of frequencies – www.drjoedispenza.com & www.greggbraden.com
3. Neural Sync – www.neuralsync.org

Cancer:

1. Chris Beat Cancer – www.chrisbeatcancer.com -Chris Wark healed himself from cancer (after having stage 4 and surgery for his colon cancer) his course "Square One" is everything you

could need or want in terms of the what, hows, and whys of cancer and how to rid the body of it.

2. Dr. Robert Morse, ND – www.drmorseherbalheathclub.com or www.drmorsesdetoxcenters.com
3. Cure Your Own Cancer – www.cureyourowncancer.org

PRODUCTS:

Herbs:

1. Mountain Rose Herbs – www.mountainroseherbs.com – Bulk herbs, spices, essential oils, teas, skin care products, natural supplements, elixirs, and capsules, natural product ingredients, pet products, kitchen and product making tools, books, education.
2. Dr. Morse's Cellular Botanicals – www.drmorses.com (or can be easily found at www.pureformulas.com) – Amazing botanical herbal formulas specifically targeted at certain organs and systems, strong, powerful, potent, and easily assimilated by the body. Come in tincture and capsule form. Dr. Morse's Green Powders are by far, my favorite!!
3. Pure Formulas – www.pureformulas.com – This is an amazing source for all the best of supplements, herbs, glandulars, vitamins and minerals. They always ship for free, you build up points which takes money off, and you get things super quickly! Highly recommend.

Mushrooms:

1. North Spore – www.northspore.com – Buy mushroom grow kits, growth chambers, cultures, supplies, culinary items, and books. They even have a cool monthly grow kit subscription.

CBD Hemp Based Products:

1. Robin's Nest Naturals - www.robinsnestnaturals.com – CBD tinctures, gummies, pain relieving ointment, and Pet CBD

products as well as their new Delta 9 gummies. Use code FIRST15 for 15% off your first order.
2. ThoughtCloud – www.thoughtcloud.net – CBD tinctures, vape cartridges, pre-rolls, gummies, capsules balms, face wash bar, Pet products, and even sell distillate and CBD isolate powder that you can make your own products with.
3. Secret Nature CBD – www.secretnaturecbd.com – High quality CBD flower, pre-rolls, Live resin softgels, hemp flower drops, vape cartridges, gummies, capsules, and Delta 9 gummies.

Suppository Molds:

1. Cure Your Own Cancer Store - www.cyoc.store - Suppository Molds and other wonderful products are available as well as information on healing.
2. Amazon – There are many kinds of suppository molds now available, many are silicone kits for about $25-30. There are vaginal applicators if you should need them also available.

Enema Kits & Coffee for Enemas:

1. Mikacare – www.amazon.com – Mikacare is my favorite enema kit available online although you can find many and choose whichever is to your liking and within your budget.
2. S.A. Wilsons – www.sawilsons.com – High integrity company that produces gold roast coffee specifically roasted for enema purposes. They also have an estate blend for drinking. All beans are mold free, organic, pure, and clean.

Water Purification and Filtration Systems:

1. Water Distillation – www.megahomedistiller.com – Wonderful distiller, easy-to-use at home. Removes fluoride, lead, arsenic, viruses, and other contaminants from the water. There are other brands to purchase as well.
2. Berkey Water Filters – www.berkeywaterfilters.com – Highest quality filters out there that remove approximately 203 chemicals

and toxins from the water, including the *forever chemicals* that do not come out from the municipal water treatment plants in your area. They can also remove fluoride if you get the fluoride filter. Also removes bacteria, viruses, and all sorts of parasites, eggs, cysts, and larvae. The new news is that recently, the FDA banned the use of Nanosilver in their water filters, which removes **viruses** from the water. The filtration system is a free standing, gravity filtration system that does not require anything but space on your counter. Their website has some resources and information on it. Amazing company.

3. Multipure – www.multipure.com – These water filters do an amazing job like the Berkey filters do, also removing viruses and all of the *forever chemicals,* as well as hundreds of other contaminants. The have filtration systems for the counter top, as well as systems for the entire house. Tons of information on their website.

4. Kangen Water System - www.kangen.com or www.enagic.com – This water system filters the water as well as can change the acid or alkalinity of the water. Acidic water can be used for washing fruits and vegetables as well as for washing our face, whereas the alkaline water can be used for drinking, to incorporate more alkalinity into the body. However, it does not alkalize the body just by drinking it, one must work on alkalizing with their diet and other means.

Frequency Instruments:

1. Spooky 2 – www.spooky2.com – They have several versions of a rife. Machine for purchase

Irish Sea Moss/Zeolite/Shilajit:

1. Irish Sea Moss: You can buy dried sea moss many places, Amazon is my go to for easy access. I buy the Happy Fox Sea Moss and then make my own gel with it. You can buy premade sea moss and some come with flavors, which is great for kids.

2. Zeolite: My go to brand is Touchstone Essentials – www.thegoodinside.com – the second one I love is ROOT – www.therootbrands.com/product/clean-slate/ Zeolites are a class of mineral formed by the chemical reaction of volcanic ash with seawater. Detoxify heavy metals and toxins from the body, as well as the effects of EMF.
3. Shilajit:
   a. Lotus Blooming Herbs – www.lotusbloomingherbs.com
   b. Cymbiotika – www.cymbiotika.com
   c. Pure Himalayan Shilajit – www.purehimalayanshilajit.com
   d. CHOQ – www.choq.com

Castor Oil Packs:

1. Amazon – They have a variety of castor oil pack wraps, even ones for the neck/thyroid.

Grounding Products:

1. Earthing – www.earthing.com – They have a variety of products for in home use.
2. Earthing With Shoes – www.earthingwithshoes.com

Faraday Bags:

1. Go Dark Faraday Bags – www.godarkbags.com – Great bags for shielding EMP, cell phone tracking, and EMFs.

Ozone generator:

1. Ozone generator - www.ozonegenerator.com_– Great ozone generator kits. They also have a wonderful steam sauna cabinet

CENTERS FOR HEALING:

1. Dr. Morse's Detox Centers – www.drmorsesdetoxcenters. com – Dr. Robert Morse's clinic. You can have either online or in-person health and detoxification visits and care. Food and herbal protocols are created on individual basis, with loving guidance and healing practices around helping the body to heal naturally.

2. Fountain Life Centers – www.fountainlife.com – Preventative Health Care and Wellness Centers located in Naples, FL, Westchester, NY, and Dallas, TX. This is the absolute newest and most magnificent and most advanced diagnostic centers with new, profound tools that can detect every aspect of illness including cancer in the body through new technology and systems. New healing technologies and therapeutics to create a vibrant, health-filled life.

PRACTITIONERS:

Meditation, Emotional Empowerment:

1. Ruth Kemp - www.ruthkemp.co - Spiritual Mentor, Ascension Coach, and Teacher who can help to guide you through the powerful experience of returning to your core essence and wisdom. Through her programs, meditations, and spiritual teachings, Ruth will help elevate you into a more powerful and connected version of who you are on the path of ascension.

2. Kristen Braid - www.soulinspired.ca - Visionary, Creator, Teacher and Guide through her gift of compassion she leads other towards greater experiences of love, health and harmony. She takes her clients on a healing journey of self-discovery, health restoration, and finding their spark so they can live in their truth.

3. Dawn Jackson – www.dawnmichelejackson.com - As a Certified Grief Recovery Specialist®, Retreat Facilitator, Wellness Coach, Author and Nurse, Dawn assists individuals who desire to

heal their hearts and transform their lives. Her mission is to help others find their inner light and move from surviving to thriving.

Reiki:

1. 3 OMS - www.3oms.com – Laura Ahern, an advanced Reiki Master level 3 practitioner, healer, and teacher locally in Florida, does one-on-one healing sessions, performs long-distance healing, and excellent spiritual counsel. She also has group programs available.
2. Anchored Soul – www.anchoredsoulri.com – Alana Almonte, a Reiki Master level 3 practitioner, healer, teacher, and artist located locally in Rhode Island for Reiki sessions, trainings, and art workshops.

MOVIES:

1. The Lost Century
2. Frequencies
3. Inception
4. The Connection – Movie about meditation
5. Conversations With God
6. What The Health
7. The Earthing Movie: The Remarkable Science of Grounding
8. The Sound of Creation
9. Fast Food Nation
10. Food Inc.
11. Fat, Sick, and Nearly Dead
12. Forks Over Knives
13. What The Bleep Do We Know
14. They Live
15. The Secret
16. I Am
17. Peaceful Warrior
18. Inner World, Outer World

19. Burzynski: The Cancer Cure Cover-up
20. The Meat Lobby
21. It's A Wonderful Life
22. Life Is Beautiful
23. Cowspiracy
24. Fantastic Fungi

Lots of documentaries can be found on www.documentaryheaven.com

Made in United States
Troutdale, OR
03/18/2025

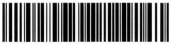

29872184R00231